INTRODUCTION TO PUBLIC HEALTH 5E

INTRODUCTION TO PUBLIC HEALTH 5E

Mary Louise Fleming PhD, MA, BEd, Dip Teach

Public Health Consultant and Non-executive Board Director,
Adjunct Professor, School of Public Health and Social Work
at Queensland University of Technology,
Brisbane, Queensland

Louise Baldwin PhD, MHSc (HProm), BEd (Sec)

Public Health Academic and Researcher,
Fellow Higher Education Authority, School of Public Health and
Social Work Faculty of Health; Design Lab, Creative Industries,
Education and Social Justice Faculty and
Australian Centre for Philanthropy and Nonprofit Studies,
Faculty of Business and Law
at Queensland University of Technology,
Fellow Higher Education Authority, Brisbane, Queensland,
Australia

ELSEVIER

ELSEVIER

Elsevier Australia. ACN 001 002 357
(a division of Reed International Books Australia Pty Ltd)
Tower 1, 475 Victoria Avenue, Chatswood, NSW 2067

ISBN: 978-0-7295-4427-6

National Library of Australia Cataloguing-in-Publication Data

 A catalogue record for this book is available from the National Library of Australia

Senior Content Strategist: Melinda McEvoy
Content Project Manager: Shruti Raj
Edited by Lynn Watt
Proofread by Tim Learner
Copyrights Coordinator: Gobinath Palanisamy
Cover by Natalie Bowra
Index by Innodata Indexing

Typeset by GW Tech

Printed in China by 1010 Printing International Limited

Last digit is the print number: 9 8 7 6 5 4 3 2 1

CONTENTS

ONLINE VIDEO—INTERVIEWS

This edition of *Introduction to Public Health* includes a suite of video interviews that are available on the Evolve site.

The video interviews further explore the themes and content within the chapters in the book, on topics such as public health advocacy, international health issues, climate change policy, Aboriginal and Torres Strait Islander health and refugee health, the prevention agenda and health futures. Below we include the questions asked of each presenter, and we identify the main chapters where topics are covered. One of the great things about the interviews is that the content of each interview also covers a broad contextual overview of public health now and in the future.

Structure of the Book
Section 1: Definitions, determinants and challenges—Chapters 1, 2, 3 and 4
Section 2: Policy, ethics and evidence—Chapters 5, 6, 7 and 8
Section 3: Public health strategies—Chapters 9, 10 and 11
Section 4: Contemporary issues—Chapters 12, 13, 14, 15 and 16.

Interview	Questions	Links to Chapter
Dr Amaya Gillespie Former Director in the United Nations; International Consultant, Career and Executive Coach	1. What are the lessons you have learned about working internationally, and what changes have you observed? 2. Why is it important to know about international developments in public health? 3. What are the public health differences and challenges between overseas countries and within Australia? 4. Why is it important for public health students to know something about international developments in public health? 5. Are there differences in health issues between Australia and overseas countries? 6. Are there developments and trends in public health internationally that influence what you might do in Australia? 7. How would you advise a public health graduate wanting to work overseas?	Chapters 1 and 2, 9–11, 14
Dr Melissa Stoneham Director, Public Health Advocacy Institute of Western Australia, based at Curtin University, Western Australia	1. What is the Public Health Advocacy Institute of Western Australia, and what are its major goals and objectives? 2. Western Australia has a long tradition of public health advocacy, so how has the Institute continued this tradition? 3. Your focus is on developing local networks and creating a state-wide umbrella organisation capable of influencing public health policy and political agendas. In that context, what is the Advocacy Institute focused on at the moment? 4. How do reactive and proactive advocacy differ, and where does the Institute focus its attention? 5. Where should the focus be for current public health advocacy efforts? 6. Has your advocacy work been successful in strengthening the evidence base for public health and health policy? 7. What are the top insights and skills you would recommend for public health graduates?	Chapters 1, 2, 5–7, 9–11, 14

Interview	Questions	Links to Chapter
Professor Karen Hussey Director, Centre for Policy Futures, University of Queensland; Councillor with the Climate Council	1. Tell us about your work in public policy and sustainable development. 2. In your role as a Councillor of the Climate Council, what have been the greatest challenges in the past 5 years? 3. What are the important points to think about in terms of the science behind climate change? 4. What role does politics play in the policy process at a national level? 5. How much progress do you think Australia has made on climate science to support the necessary changes to our environment in Australia? 6. What role do you think people studying public health and those in the workforce could have in advancing sustainable development in Australia and indeed in other countries?	Chapters 2, 5, 6, 11 and 16
Adrian Carson Chief Executive Officer, Institute of Urban Indigenous Health (IUIH) South East Queensland	1. What is the Institute for Urban Indigenous Health (IUIH)? 2. What is the IUIH model of care? 3. Can you describe some of your successes in using this model? 4. What are the issues for the Indigenous workforce in using this model of care? 5. What are the challenges facing Aboriginal and Torres Strait Islander health in Australia? 6. What are the big opportunities that will make a sustainable difference to the social determinants of health for Indigenous people?	Chapters 1, 2, 4, 6, 13 and 14
Donata Sackey Associate Director Mater/University of Queensland Centre for Integrated Care and Innovation	1. What experiences have you had working in the refugee sector and what is your current role? 2. What are the strengths that people from refugee backgrounds bring with them when they come to Australia? 3. What are the key barriers facing people from refugee backgrounds when accessing healthcare services? 4. What other issues can have an impact on the health and wellbeing of people from refugee backgrounds? 5. What factors and strategies contributed to the successful development of the first ever Queensland Refugee Health and Wellbeing Policy and Action Plan (2017–2020)? 6. Can you tell us a bit more about the Queensland Refugee Health Network and its role in the implementation of the Refugee Health and Wellbeing Policy and Action Plan? 7. How can the Australian community contribute to the health, wellbeing and settlement of people from refugee backgrounds? 8. What are three essential issues about refugee health that public health graduates need to know?	Chapters 1, 2, 6, 13 and 14

Continued

Interview	Questions	Links to Chapter
Professor Andrew Wilson Co-Director of the Menzies Centre for Health Policy at the University of Sydney; Director of the NHMRC Partnership Centre for Better Health 2013 (Systems perspectives on prevention of lifestyle-related chronic disease) NHMRC Partnership Centre for Better Health 2017. Strengthening systems for preventing lifestyle-related chronic diseases: insights from a multi-sectoral perspective	1. Through the Partnership Centre, what new ways have you uncovered of understanding what works to prevent lifestyle-related chronic health problems in Australia? 2. The Partnership Centre aims to provide health decision-makers with the best evidence to inform their policies, and programs and tools for a comprehensive systemic approach to preventing chronic health problems. Where have you had success? 3. You discuss bridging the knowledge translation gap through creating learning environments. Can you give us some examples of such learning environments? 4. Aside from the main lifestyle-related determinants of chronic disease risk, you clearly draw on relevant research and practice from other fields that can advance thinking. Are there success stories in this regard? 5. Is a stronger understanding of the business case for prevention about the economics of prevention? How well are we doing in understanding such a business case? 6. How far away do you think Australia is from an effective, efficient and equitable prevention system? 7. How hard do you think it is to identify and improve the next generation of a chronic disease prevention system for high-risk populations? 8. In the Centre's research on the community's perceptions of policies and programs to prevent lifestyle-related chronic disease, what did you uncover? How can this research be used to further inform practice? 9. From your work, what are the important areas of knowledge and skill for early-career public health graduates?	Chapters 1–4, 5, 8, 9–12
Dr Rob Grenfell Director Special Advisor Health CSIRO https://www.csiro.au/en/work-with-us/services/consultancy-strategic-advice-services/csiro-futures/health-and-biosecurity/future-of-health	1. How difficult is it to shift the focus of attention to the promotion of health, and what do you perceive the major barriers to be? 2. You identified five areas for attention in your *Future of Health Report 2018.* Do you see these priority areas as equally important? 3. Are there particular parts of the health workforce that are crucial to change, or is there a need to change the workforce profoundly to achieve a focus on the promotion of health? 4. Is the complexity and siloed nature of the healthcare system a major barrier to change and how can such an issue be overcome? 5. How far do you think the "system" needs to move to be able to achieve a level of safety, quality and clinical effectiveness? 6. Are cost-effectiveness, relevant financial models and payments systems major drivers to support the shift from illness care to health promotion? 7. The *Future of Health Report* discusses the need for a digitally supported healthcare system. Does this facilitate the entire system? 8. Do you think governments should play an even stronger role in enabling community-wide promotion initiatives? 9. What sector of the healthcare system has responsibility for the social determinants of health? 10. What advice would you give to public health students in relation to their role in the health workforce and in the promotion of health?	Chapters 1 and 2. Section 2 and 3 are generally relevant. Chapter 16 in particular. This video interview integrates many themes discussed throughout the textbook

Please see the inside front cover for the access instructions for these online resources.

INTRODUCTION

WHY IS PUBLIC HEALTH IMPORTANT?

Introduction to Public Health is about the discipline of public health, the nature and scope of public health activity and the challenges that face public health in the 21st century. The book is designed as an introductory text to the principles and practice of public health. This is a complex and multifaceted area. What we have tried to do is make public health easy to understand without making it simplistic. Public health is transdisciplinary in nature, and it is influenced by genetic, behavioural, social, cultural, economic and government and political determinants of health as well as climate change, other environments and social issues such as the needs of refugees and asylum seekers.

How do we define "public health", and what are the disciplines that contribute to public health? And how has the area changed over time? There are a range of health issues that change and challenge the focus of public health activity in the 21st century. We introduce you to these issues in the book.

How is public health shaped by the many health and other disciplines that contribute to it or influence its impact? How might an understanding of public health enable a range of health professionals to use the principles and practices of public health in their professional activities? These are the questions this book addresses. *Introduction to Public Health* leads the reader on a journey of discovery that concludes with an understanding of the nature and scope of public health and the challenges facing the field into the future.

The book is designed for a range of students undertaking health courses where there is a focus on advancing the health of the population. While it is imperative that people wanting to be public health professionals understand the theory and practice of public health, many other healthcare workers contribute to effective public health practice. This book would also be relevant to a range of students completing courses such as architecture, or to those in the "business of healthcare" and in engineering in robotics, artificial intelligence and technology for health, as examples.

Public health is an innately political process. As we discuss in this book, there is a clear relationship between disease and the way in which society is structured. Income distribution, the allocation of resources to ensure sufficient infrastructure for transport, housing and education, and how much political support there is to provide adequately for these fundamental services all impact on our health. They particularly impact on the health of certain groups within the population who do not have the financial, social and political resources to advocate for change. Why is it that we still have such disparities in health? In an egalitarian society such as Australia, which prides itself on a "fair go for all", should this be acceptable?

DEFINING AND UNDERSTANDING "PUBLIC HEALTH"

Defining "public health" is not an easy task. This is because not everyone who works in public health agrees on a single definition. Definitions also vary from country to country.

Public health is essentially both a science and an art, in that it relies on evidence, skill and judgment, it examines the contribution of a range of factors to improving population health, it addresses inequalities and it is based on partnerships.

These elements of public health will be discussed throughout the book, particularly in terms of their application to public health practice. We will be asking you to think about how you might define public health within the context of your own developing professional understanding.

To understand public health we also need to think about the contribution of both the "art" and the "science" of improving the health of the population.

The *science* of public health is about knowing the determinants of health, what works and in what circumstances. It is about using evidence as a basis for making decisions about selecting interventions that work with the hard-to-reach and the economically and socially isolated. The *art* of public health has more to do with the practice of public health, and how the science is interpreted and implemented according to population needs and circumstances. In the book we discuss public health approaches for "people", "place" and "environments" and wrap these approaches around the multiple determinants of health.

Health practitioners who work in public health also need a vision about what public health could look like in the future. As practitioners, we need to be vigilant to changing circumstances and issues. In addition, we need a set of values and ethics that underpins our practice to be brought to bear in all our public health dealings. Public health must take up the challenge of measuring its success in the short, medium and longer term in order to demonstrate its contribution to population health.

In summary, this book includes a conversation about the determinants of health and how they shape public health practice, it discusses the important role for evidence in underpinning public health practice and it looks into the future to describe the emerging epidemics, and the achievements and challenges facing public health in the 21st century.

We hope you enjoy the book!

ABOUT THE AUTHORS

LOUISE BALDWIN

Dr Louise Baldwin is a health promotion specialist, academic, researcher and consultant at the local, state and national level in Australia. She is the Global Vice President (Membership) for the International Union for Health Promotion and Education, Founder and Director, Health and Social Change Australia (consultancy), and is a passionate advocate for mentoring, capacity building and connecting health promoters across global disciplines. Her work has spanned all facets of health promotion disciplines and largely focuses on sustainable change across communities including capacity building; policy; systems shifting and built environments. She holds a Visiting Fellow role in the School of Public Health and Social Work and in the Design Lab, Faculty of Creative Industries and Australian Centre for Philanthropy and Non-profit Studies – Faculty of Business and Law at Queensland University of Technology, Education and Social Justice, Queensland University of Technology, Brisbane, Australia.

HILARY BAMBRICK

Professor Hilary Bambrick is Director of the National Centre for Epidemiology and Population Health at the Australian National University in Canberra. She is an environmental epidemiologist and bioanthropologist whose research focuses on the health impacts of climate variability and change and adaptation planning to improve health. Her research is largely based in Australia, Africa, Asia and the Pacific. She has published over 190 articles, editorials, articles, book chapters, reports and conference items. She consults for government (federal, state and international) and non-government organisations on climate change impacts and adaptation. In 2016 she was appointed to the Climate Council. She holds a PhD, BA(Hons), BSc and Grad Cert Higher Ed.

CATHERINE M. BENNETT

Professor Bennett's career in applied biostatistics and epidemiology cuts across health, university and government sectors, including working on outbreak preparedness and response with NSW Health and the Australian Government. After working as Olympic Public Health Coordinator for Northern Sydney in 2000, Catherine returned to academia and was Associate Professor in Epidemiology and Director of Population Health Practice with the Melbourne School of Population and Global Health before taking up the inaugural Chair in Epidemiology at Deakin in late 2009. Her research focuses on community transmission of infectious diseases, and Catherine is involved in a range of COVID-19 projects, including global analyses of excess deaths, public health risk communication, contact tracing methods and COVID-safe industry protocols. Catherine has been a leading public analyst during the COVID-19 response, keynote speaker, expert witness and advisor to industry, governments and institutions globally.

GERRY FITZGERALD

Gerry FitzGerald is Professor Emeritus in the School of Public Health and Social Work at Queensland University of Technology (QUT). Prior to his retirement he led Health Management programs at QUT. His particular research interests lie in the performance of emergency medical systems in response to both routine and disaster challenges. He holds medical specialist qualifications in Emergency Medicine and Medical Administration as well as a Bachelor of Medicine/Bachelor of Surgery degree, a Bachelor of Health Administration, and a Doctor of Medicine degree.

MARY LOUISE FLEMING

Professor Mary Louise Fleming is Public Health Consultant and Board Director, and Adjunct Professor, School of Public Health and Social Work at Queensland University of Technology. She has over 30 years' experience in teaching and research in higher education, in public health and health promotion. Her research experience is in action research; process, impact and outcome evaluation in health promotion; and public health intervention design, development and implementation. Mary Louise has worked as a consultant for the World Health Organization and for Commonwealth and state health departments, and has sat on National Health and Medical Research Council (NHMRC) public health project grant review panels. She is a member of the Board of Wesley Medical Research and the Metro North Hospital and Health Service in Queensland. She is widely published in the area of health promotion and public health. Her current role recognises the importance of value-based healthcare and the need for innovative solutions to the healthcare system of the future, and working with the healthcare system to realise gains in efficiency and effectiveness while focusing on the patient at the centre of care.

RICHARD FRANKLIN

Richard Franklin is Associate Professor Public Health in the Discipline of Public Health and Tropical Medicine, College of Public Health, Medical and Veterinary Sciences, James Cook University, Australia. Richard has been involved in working on developing a greater understanding of the risk and prevention strategies around disasters, with a focus on flooding and cyclones. He has worked in government, not-for-profit and university positions working to reduce the burden of injury. He holds a Doctor of Philosophy from Sydney University, a Master of Social Science (Health) and Bachelor of Science from The University of Queensland, and is a Fellow of the Public Health Association of Australia.

TRISH GOULD

Trish Gould is a contract health researcher and developmental editor. She has previously worked in the School of Public Health and Social Work at Queensland University of Technology. She has over 20 years' experience in public health and health promotion research, and project management and coordination. Trish has an MA in biological anthropology, and her interest areas include ethics, human rights and the health impacts of migration, acculturation, inequity and discrimination.

MELISSA HASWELL

Melissa Haswell is Professor of Practice (Environmental Wellbeing) within the Portfolio of the Deputy Vice Chancellor (Indigenous Strategy and Services) and Honorary Professor in the School of Geosciences at the University of Sydney. She is also Professor of Health, Safety and Environment at Queensland University of Technology. Melissa holds a Master of Science (Bacteriology and Immunology) and a PhD in Infectious Disease Epidemiology (Imperial College, London University). Melissa is a member of the University of Sydney's Indigenous Strategy and Services Leadership Team, Sustainability Strategy Committee and the Sydney Environment Institute Advisory Board. She is the Academic Lead of the transdisciplinary Service Learning in Indigenous Communities unit of study at University of Sydney and regularly guest lectures on environmental/planetary health and sustainability. Her teaching, research, advocacy and service work transects Aboriginal and Torres Strait Islander health, environmental health, toxicology and infectious disease epidemiology, mental health, social and emotional wellbeing, climate change adaptation and community empowerment.

PETER A. LEGGAT AM, ADC

Peter Leggat is Professor and Director of the World Safety Organization Collaborating Centre for Disaster Health, Resilience and Emergency Response, College of Public Health, Medical and Veterinary Sciences, James Cook University, Australia. He is also Adjunct Professor, Faculty of Law, Australian Centre for Health Law Research, Queensland University of Technology, and a member of Council of the Australasian Faculty of Public Health Medicine. He has more than 30 years' experience in teaching, research and leadership in public health and tropical medicine. A former Fulbright Scholar and Fulbright Ambassador, he has published more than 500 journal papers, more than 30 books and directories, and more than 100 book chapters. He holds a higher Doctorate in Medicine from The University of Queensland, a Doctorate in Philosophy from the University of South Australia, and a Doctorate in Public Health from James Cook University.

RAY MAHONEY

Ray Mahoney is Professor of Aboriginal and Torres Strait Islander Health and Discipline Lead of Population Health at College of Medicine and Public Health, Flinders University and Visiting Scientist, Australian eHealth Research Centre (AeHRC), CSIRO. Professor Mahoney, is a descendant of the Bidjara people of Central West Queensland. He has previously worked in health for the Queensland, New South Wales and Victorian state governments, and with the Aboriginal Community Controlled Health Service Sector in Victoria. Ray's career in Aboriginal and Torres Strait Islander health spans more than 20 years. He holds a Doctor of Health Science degree from Queensland University of Technology.

GREG MARSTON

Greg Marston is a Professor of Social Policy in the School of Social Science and Deputy Executive Dean of the Faculty of Humanities and Social Sciences at The University of Queensland. He also holds an adjunct appointment with the School of Public Health and Social Work at Queensland University of Technology. He has an extensive record in applied social policy research. He has led a number of Australian Research Council grant-funded projects on welfare conditionality, long-term unemployment, disability and employment services, and the fringe lending industry in Australia. His latest publications are a co-authored book on conditional welfare in Australia and New Zealand (published by Policy Press, 2022), a co-edited collection on basic income in Australia and New Zealand (published by Palgrave

Macmillan, 2016), the implementation of welfare-to-work in a variety of countries (published by Georgetown University Press, 2013) and another on who benefits from the Australian welfare state (published by Palgrave, 2013).

ELIZABETH PARKER

Elizabeth Parker was an Adjunct Associate Professor in the School of Public Health and Social Work at Queensland University of Technology. She has teaching and research experience in public health and health promotion in Australia. Elizabeth was formerly a senior manager in the Department of Public Health, Toronto, Canada. She is co-author, with Professor Mary Louise Fleming, of the book *Health Promotion: Principles and Practice in the Australian Context*. She holds a Doctor of Education degree from the University of Toronto.

ANKUR SINGH

Ankur Singh is an Australian Research Council Senior Research Fellow at the University of Melbourne (Australia). He holds a joint position between Melbourne School of Population and Global Health and Melbourne Dental School. Ankur has research training in social epidemiology and he applies a range of quantitative skills to quantify the impact of policy interventions on health inequalities. His research contributions are in the area of population oral health, tobacco control and social determinants of health. He holds leadership positions in Global Oral Health Inequalities Research Network (International Association of Dental Research), International Union for Health Promotion and Education and is an Adjunct Faculty at the Public Health Foundation of India.

ACKNOWLEDGEMENTS

Thank you to my family for their ongoing support and patience during the writing of the fifth edition of *Introduction to Public Health*. A special thank you to all of the authors who have contributed to the text. They make up the rich fabric that is public health. Long may this rich fabric continue! In the 21st century the challenges for public health are transdisciplinary in nature, and cut across the continuum of care from health advancement to a health promoting end of life. The public health community now finds itself refocusing on infectious diseases and dealing with the consequences of them as pandemics as well as continuing its efforts to advocate for health promotion and prevention and managing non-communicable diseases. We hope that this text gives you an understanding of public health into the future and encourages you to be one of the many advocates for "good health for all".

Mary Louise Fleming

Thank you for joining us in the public health profession through your study and career journey. We hope you enjoy this book and use it as a companion in your everyday practice. Health is truly everybody's business and without our health, we truly have nothing. Public health is a collaborative profession, working together across multiple sectors. This book is a testament to that collaborative nature where colleagues from far and wide have joined together to author chapters to provide a rich and insightful learning experience. Thank you to each and every author, to Mary Louise Fleming for inviting me to co-edit this edition and to Elizabeth Parker whose work in the first four editions laid the foundation for the legacy of this textbook. To my family, thank you and I hope this inspires you to do great things, give back and work towards what matters for a healthy, happy and sustainable future.

Louise Baldwin

REVIEWERS

Angela Sheedy, RN, BHSc, GCUTL, MPH
Senior Research Officer
CDU Menzies School of Medicine
Charles Darwin University
Darwin, Australia

Catharine Fleming, BSc (Poulation Health and Nutrition), PhD
Lecturer, Public Health
School of Health Science
Western Sydney University
Sydney Australia

Christine Roseveare, MPH, FHEA, Dip.Tchg
Lecturer, Public Health
School of Health Sciences
Massey University
Palmerston North, New Zealand

Colleen Van Lochem, RN, MN
Lecturer
School of Nursing and Midwifery
University of Notre Dame Australia
Fremantle, Australia

Lesley Andrew, PhD, MSc, BSc (Hons), RN, RHV
Senior Lecturer
School of Nursing and Midwifery
Edith Cowan University
Joondalup, Australia

Definitions, Determinants and Challenges

The first four chapters in Section 1 provide you with background information about how health, illness and public health are defined, and the major roles, responsibilities and challenges for public health. Throughout this edition we introduce you to the coronavirus disease (COVID-19) and the virus that caused it, severe acute respiratory syndrome coronavirus 2 (SARS-CoV-2). A virus and the diseases that cause it have different names. Viruses are named by the International Committee on Taxonomy of Viruses (ICTV), based on the virus's genetic structure, to enable the development of diagnostic tests, vaccines and medicines. Diseases, on the other hand, are named by the World Health Organization (WHO), using the International Classification of Diseases (ICD) to support discussion on disease prevention, transmissibility and spread, severity and treatment.

Chapter 1 covers the nature and scope of public health, considering various definitions of health, disease and illness, and examines the changing nature of public health definitions. We explore the core functions of public health, and the roles and responsibilities of public health practitioners. In the process, we discuss the ways in which public health practitioners do their job, and, in fact, who is the public health workforce and how broadly we might consider that definition. We look briefly at the roles and responsibilities of various levels of government in Australia, and we discuss the role of non-government organisations, associations, community organisations and advocacy groups.

Chapter 2 addresses the challenges for public health now and into the future. In this chapter we explore global threats to the environment, the re-emergence of infectious diseases and the globalisation of chronic disease and health inequalities. In addition, changing patterns of consumption and communication, along with accelerating social and demographic changes to work, to learning, family and community life, all influence health. We explore contemporary trends impacting on how we promote, protect and manage population health through the use of genetics, advancing personal and treatment technologies, the use of artificial intelligence and the impact of robotics on a number of levels in the health system. We ask the question, what is the public health workforce and what impact do many contemporary trends have on the workforce now and into the future? Of course, political will and actions are fraught with challenges and that is how we conclude this chapter with the grand challenges for public health into the future.

Chapter 3 examines epidemiology as the study of factors affecting the health and illness of populations. It serves as the foundation and logic for interventions made in the interests of public health and preventive medicine. It is considered a cornerstone methodology of public health research. The role of the epidemiologist is to investigate the occurrence of disease or other health-related conditions or events in defined populations. The control of disease in populations is often also considered to be a task for the epidemiologist. The COVID-19 epidemic will be centre stage in these discussions. In this chapter, we focus on the three main aims of epidemiology: describing disease patterns in human populations; identifying the causes of disease; and the provision of essential data to manage, evaluate and plan services for prevention, control and treatment of disease.

Chapter 4 Aboriginal and Torres Strait Islander health is an essential focus for public health. The chapter discusses the health status of Indigenous Australians, focuses attention on the important role of community-controlled health organisations and discusses many of the most important public health strategies used by Aboriginal and Torres Strait health workers. The chapter has a strong focus on advocacy at all levels of government to emphasise the importance of improving the health of Indigenous Australians. Importantly it provides evidence of more contemporary research activity based on ethics and protocols since the late 1990s. The ongoing challenges for Indigenous public health workers in Closing The Gap are considered.

These four chapters provide a foundation for the book, in that they define the nature and scope of health and illness and public health, examine its transdisciplinary and multisectoral elements, its place within the healthcare system, and the fundamental role for advancing Aboriginal and Torres Strait Islander health for and by Indigenous people.

Defining Health and Public Health

Mary Louise Fleming

LEARNING OBJECTIVES

After reading this chapter, you should be able to:
- Define the diverse terms used to describe "wellness", "health", "illness" and "disease".
- Analyse changing public health definitions, their development and implementation.
- Critique the principles of public health.

- Discuss the relationship between public health and other disciplines.
- Provide examples of public health in practice, as applied to your discipline.
- Discuss the changing roles of the public health workforce and the increasing complexity of public health work.

INTRODUCTION

What is health? How is it defined and described? What do you mean when you describe yourself as "healthy"? There are other words to describe "health" such as "wellness" and "wellbeing". How is "public health" defined? What are the fundamental principles of public health? How does public health interact with other disciplines? And how do we describe what public health workers do?

These are many of the questions that we consider in this chapter and this book, which are designed to help you become familiar with the principles and practices of public health. This book is about introductory principles and concepts of public health for students. It is also relevant for health workers from a range of disciplines whose focus ranges from clinical to population health, and who want to understand and incorporate public health principles into their work.

We begin our journey by discussing how the public define health. Complete Activity 1.1 to help you think about the range of factors influencing how people define health.

Defining Health and Illness

The World Health Organization (WHO) initially defined health as "a state of complete physical, social and emotional wellbeing and not merely the absence of disease or infirmity" (WHO, 1948). Contemporary definitions suggest the need for a diverse approach to a definition that depends on the scope of application (Leonardi, 2018).

Definitions of health by the public often have a singularity of description, such as a "healthy life" as being physically fit or having energy or vitality. Still others take "health" to mean social relationships—that is, relationships with other people—or see it as a function of the ability to do things, or as psychosocial wellbeing. However, Mendenhall and Weaver (2019) talk about "structural competence" that goes beyond the individual's ability to intervene in their health to a focus on culturally competent providers, whereas Trickett and Rauk (2019) use a socioecological model to argue the need for individuals to be seen by a broader set of influences, including social, economic, educational and ecological influences, as examples.

In Australia, Aboriginal and Torres Strait Islander peoples consider "health" to be the totality of their environment, including control over their physical environment, dignity, community self-esteem and justice (Australian Institute of Health and Welfare [AIHW], 2020a) and the social, emotional and cultural wellbeing of the whole community (Askew et al., 2020). These ideas reflect the connectedness among these factors and acknowledge the impact that social and cultural determinants have on health (AIHW, 2020b). See Chapter 4 for more detail.

Illness, on the other hand, is primarily about how an individual experiences disease, which itself represents a set of signs and symptoms and medically diagnosed pathological abnormalities. Illness can be culturally specific, and influenced by social, spiritual, supernatural and psychological factors (WHO, 2021).

ACTIVITY 1.1 Defining "Health"

- Ask five of your friends, fellow students or family members what 'health' means to each of them.
- What common themes have emerged among the five definitions?
- What was unique about the definitions?
- Do you think they might change over time? If so, why might they change?

Reflection

Keep these definitions in mind as you compare them with contemporary definitions. How do **you** think of the term "health"? Does it mean an absence of illness, or an ability to do all the things you want or must do every day? Does it have more of a religious, cultural or social significance? Are other terms used other than "health" to define a person's state of wellbeing? The term "health" is difficult to define. How an individual defines his or her health is sometimes different from how a professional might define health.

Most health workers see protection, improvements or return to a level of health as being central to their work and believe many people think so too. However, we know that without access to the basics in life, health is not a priority. Considering definitions of health as defined by people and professionals enables us to understand a component of the nature and scope of public health in our society.

How, then, is "public health" defined? There are books devoted to philosophical debates about how difficult it is to define public health. While these conversations are beyond the scope of this book, it is important to consider issues that identify the nature and scope of public health.

DEFINING "PUBLIC HEALTH": AN ART AND A SCIENCE?

Public health is based on scientific principles, and a range of disciplines such as epidemiology, biostatistics, biology and biomedical sciences. It relies heavily on environmental sciences and the social and behavioural sciences. Public health is also an art, in that it involves applying scientific knowledge to a range of practical settings. Furthermore, public health is impacted by social, cultural, political and economic issues. DeSalvo and colleagues (2017) suggest that public health is what we do together as a society to ensure the conditions in which everyone can be healthy.

The Public Health Association of Australia (PHAA) wants to drive better health outcomes "through increased knowledge, better access and equity, evidence informed policy and effective population-based practice in public health" (PHAA website, 2022).

Twenty-first-century health challenges require public health to deal with chronic illness and to manage the spread of infectious diseases, as well as be a part of a global effort to sustain the planet and its environment for generations to come through improving and promoting health for all (PHAA, 2022; WHO, 2021).

Contemporary definitions of public health still rely on organised effort to improve the health of the population as a whole, a sense of general public interest and a focus on the broader determinants of health as both risk and protective factors (Valles, 2018).

What are 'determinants' and how do they influence the public's health? Determinants are defined as "factors that influence how likely we are to stay healthy or to become ill or injured". An understanding of the key determinants of health suggest going beyond social determinants, biomedical and behavioural risk factors (AIHW, 2021), to encompass broader concepts such as environmental, political and economic factors that have an influence on health. The ways in which these determinants manifest themselves in each society depend on history, culture and politics (Valles, 2018). Determinants are the causes of, and risk and protective factors for, health events. This requires defining causal pathways such as socioeconomic, geopolitical and climatic determinants and plotting them to individual and collective health outcomes. It means including disciplines as diverse as environmental science, climatology, sociology, economics, politics, psychology and biomedicine (Kelly, 2011).

Consider Case Study 1.1, which looks at the contribution of public health to daily life.

Another way to think about addressing a public health problem might involve levels of prevention—primary, secondary and tertiary. Primary prevention focuses on maintaining health—for example, school health programs, seat belts in motor vehicles, anti-smoking campaigns and physical activity and nutrition programs. Secondary prevention aims to minimise the extent of a health problem by focusing on early intervention, such as prostate, bowel and breast screening. Tertiary intervention reduces disability and provides rehabilitation services, such as cardiac rehabilitation. Public health problems can also consider public health in terms of a chain of causation, involving an agent, a host and the environment. In this case, prevention is achieved by interrupting the chain of causation—for example, by providing immunisation, using antibiotics or purifying the water supply.

For you to gain a more comprehensive understanding of public health, it is vital that you appreciate its underlying vision, values and core components, as they provide the foundations upon which strategies are developed, implemented and evaluated.

PUBLIC HEALTH VISION AND VALUES

Having a vision of where you think public health is placed in the next 10 years is important for the discipline and your practice. Many factors impacting on health and public health

CASE STUDY 1.1 A Typical Morning

You get up in the morning, woken earlier than expected by the waste-disposal truck collecting rubbish on your street. Having completed your morning grooming routine (shower, toilet, etc.), you dress and check your phone. One of your friends has mentioned that it is Breast Cancer Awareness Week. You realise that you are running late for your first lecture at university and rush out the door to your car. You fasten your seat belt and pull out into the usual traffic chaos. As you approach McDonald's, the sign reminds you that you have not had breakfast yet. You drive through and pick up a Big Mac and a coffee. Across the road, at the local state school, you notice there are two ambulances on the oval, and that school students are climbing in and out of them. Finally arriving at university, you park your car as near as possible to the lecture theatre and walk quickly to your class.

Questions

1. From the scenario above, list the issues that you think are relevant to public health.
2. Did you consider any of the following issues?
   - Your access to clean water, sewerage and rubbish removal and disposal.
   - Your friend's mention of the breast cancer and screening media campaign, which raises your awareness of these issues.
   - Your safety on the road, such as legislation relating to the wearing of seat belts, traffic lights and the construction of roadways to maximise safety.
   - Your ability to drive on maintained roads for safe use.
   - Your purchase of food, which has been prepared according to standards of hygiene that protect your health.
   - The type of the food you consumed for breakfast.
   - The ambulance service visiting a school to discuss their role.
   - The fact that you parked your car close to the lecture theatre and walked a short distance to your class.

ACTIVITY 1.2 Vision and Values for Public Health

Write a vision statement for public health. What does this mean? A vision statement answers the question "Where do we want to go?" We might need to stop and consider who "we" are. Is it the Australian government? Is it a state or territory government, or a not-for-profit? Let us assume it is the Australian government. Where would you look to find such a vision for public health? Which websites would you use? Now consider what values you would like to inform your vision statement. List the values you think ought to complement your vision statement.

Reflection

Think back to the definitions of health, illness and public health discussed earlier in this chapter. Do these help you to define a vision for public health in Australia? Does the Australian Government's Department of Health have a vision statement for public health? Is there a vision for public health in the Australian Institute of Health and Welfare's most recent document on "Australia's health"? How are values defined? Look up the article by Lee and Zarowsky (2015) and summarise the values the authors consider most important. What has changed for public health between 2015 and 2023?

BOX 1.1 Roles and Functions of the Public Health Workforce

- Understanding the context for public health activity, and its role and functions
- Clarity around political impacts on public health
- Ability to apply a range of methodological approaches to understand data
- A theoretical understanding of the disciplines that underpin public health and their contribution to strategy selection
- Understanding a range of skills around the surveillance, prevention, promotion and restoration of the population's health
- Developing and analysing policy
- Planning, implementation and evaluation for a diverse range of the population including Aboriginal and Torres Strait Islander communities and Culturally and Linguistically Diverse communities
- Evidence-based practice
- Advocacy, communication and negotiation skills
- Working intersectorally and with transdisciplinary groups
- Ethical practice

will have a profound effect on the nature and scope of the discipline in the next decade.

There are, however, traditional values of public health that include using scientific evidence as a basis for action; focusing on health across sectors of the population; and emphasising a collective action dimension (Donaldson et al., 2017; see Activity 1.2). Using up-to-date scientific evidence is essential to good practice because it is based on research and its application in practice (see Chapter 8). Addressing health issues across population subgroups affirms the principles of equity and social justice, which are central to public health activity. A 'collective action' dimension varies according to the social and cultural aspects of the society in which we live. For example, in the United States there is still a very strong emphasis on individual rights and freedom. An example is gun legislation and the 'right to bear arms' as enshrined in the Constitution. By contrast, in Australia the community accepts laws and regulations that limit the individual. The roles and functions of the public health practitioner can be reviewed in Box 1.1. These are considered in terms of where you work, the nature of the position and the clients' needs, the organisational philosophy, the governance structure of the organisation and whether it is for-profit or not-for-profit, state-based or non-government.

ACTIVITY 1.3 Health in the Public Arena

The media often reports on public health issues, initiatives or health problems. Identify two sources from any social or mainstream media source that comments on a current public health issue. Write a brief review of each of your chosen media sources, using the following questions to frame your comments:

- Why is it a public health issue? Think about our discussion of definitions of public health.
- Is this an important public health issue? Use evidence to support your case. Where should this evidence come from?
- What population or subpopulation is involved?
- What strategies, if any, are implemented to address the issue or concern?
- What component or components of the public health system would take responsibility (e.g. the state health department or a non-government organisation [NGO])?
- What ramifications might there be in the future if it is not addressed?

Reflection

Media sources are an effective communication vehicle by which the public's awareness is raised about an issue or an event that directly, or indirectly, impacts on the public's health. Think about the pros and cons of social media in the context of public health. Can social media have a negative impact on the public's health? How? Consider the role of social media and mainstream media in the COVID-19 example.

BOX 1.2 WHO Leadership Priorities

1. Universal health coverage
2. The International Health Regulations (2015)—a global defence mechanism against shocks from the microbial world
3. Increasing access to medical products to everyone as a public health response
4. Social, economic and environmental determinants
5. Non-communicable diseases including disability, mental health, violence and injuries
6. Health-related Millennium Development Goals

Source: WHO, Leadership Priorities, v9, n.d.

Influences such as these impact on the nature and scope of the public health work you may be doing.

Stop here and complete Activity 1.3. Think about your understanding of what public health is, and its role and value in society. For public health to be effective, it must adopt a transdisciplinary approach, and collaborative efforts should engage with many organisations, both governmental and non-governmental. It is also important to apply ethics to inform our practice (see Chapter 7).

THE WORLD HEALTH ORGANIZATION AGENDA FOR PUBLIC HEALTH

(See https://www.who.int/news-room/feature-stories/detail/what-has-cop26-achieved-for-health.) The WHO has played a significant role in promoting public health, particularly the concept of 'health for all', which is embraced by countries throughout the world to underpin their health policies (WHO, 2021). Box 1.2 identifies the key areas in which the WHO is taking the lead.

Since the 1970s, the WHO and other substantial international players have had a focus on primary healthcare, prevention and promotion. This has been evident in policy that supports the advancement of promotion and prevention. For example, the WHO *Declaration of Alma-Ata* stressed the importance of the slogan, "Health for all by the year 2000" (WHO, 1978). This primary healthcare philosophy spoke about the principles of equity, social justice, intersectoral collaboration, community participation and empowerment. Later, in 1986, the WHO championed the Ottawa Charter for Health Promotion and its focus on health promotion and disease prevention (see Chapter 12).

In more recent times, globalisation and concern for ecosystem sustainability have emerged as prominent themes for public health action (see e.g. International HP Conferences including in Adelaide, Sundsvall, Jakarta, Bangkok, Nairobi, Helsinki, Shanghai, 1988–2016). The WHO focused its attention on 'Health for all by 2010', although some regions had targets dated to 2020. The emphasis is on sustainable development, collaboration, protection, prevention, resilience, adaptation, the emergence of chronic diseases and the re-emergence of infectious diseases. Social determinants of health became an important focus area for the WHO with the creation of the Commission on Social Determinants of Health (CSDH) (WHO CSDH website, 2008), which operated until May 2008. A lifetime of focus on social determinants of health gave Marmot (2017) the imprimatur to discuss six areas for reducing inequalities in health. They included a good start in life for every child, education and life-long learning, good employment and working conditions, sufficient income for a healthy life, healthy and sustainable environments in which to live and work and the social determinants approach to the prevention of ill health.

In concert with these activities, the United Nations (UN) member states agreed on eight Millennium Development Goals (MDGs), with targets to be achieved by 2015 (United Nations, 2013). In the same year, the 2030 Agenda for Sustainable Development (UN General Assembly, 2015) was introduced, with the Sustainable Development Goals (SDGs) being broader, deeper and far more ambitious in scope (UN, 2022; WHO, 2022).

These developments focus on the impact of globalisation, ecological sustainability and the social determinants of health.

This is because inequalities in health are seeded in the structures of society—economically, politically and culturally—and it will take collaborative efforts across sectors to bring good health within the reach of everyone (see Chapter 2). It is also important to remember that ecological sustainability impacts on all components of people's lives (see Chapter 11). It considers the impact that these factors have on the health of populations, or subgroups of populations, and that individuals are not entirely responsible for their own health status.

PUBLIC HEALTH IN THE AUSTRALIAN CONTEXT

In Australia, managing public health activity is multilayered and influenced by prevailing political thinking. Responsibility for public health occurs at all levels of government in Australia, from the Australian Government's Department of Health, to state and territory health departments, local government departments, non-government organisations, professional associations and a range of advocacy groups. For example, general practitioners and different health workers in community health centres undertake health protection and health promotion roles and responsibilities.

Many other organisations also play a role. The National Health and Medical Research Council (NHMRC) funds public health research and makes policy statements on health issues; the Australian Institute of Health and Welfare (AIHW) and the Australian Bureau of Statistics (ABS) monitor and report

on health data; and universities educate the health workforce and undertake research and consultancy activity in public health. Primary Health Networks have a focus on the efficiency and effectiveness of medical services for patients in local areas, particularly those at risk of poor health outcomes, and improving coordination of care to ensure patients receive the right care in the right place at the right time (Australian Government Department of Health, Primary Health Networks, 2022).

Australian Government Department of Health and Aged Care

The activities of the Department of Health are currently administered by three government ministers and a deputy minister (see the organisational chart, Australian Government Department of Health and Aged Care, 2022, at: https://www.health.gov.au/sites/default/files/documents/2022/02/department-of-health-organisational-chart_0.pdf). The complexity of the system, including funding arrangements, is illustrated in Figure 1.1. The primary purpose is to design, develop, implement and oversee policies and programs for health, aged care and sport to enable better health and ageing outcomes, have an affordable, quality health and aged care system and better outcomes for sport (Australian Government, Department of Health and Aged Care, 2021).

To build a prevention agenda in a health system that expends most of its funds on treatment is an ongoing challenge. In Australia, the costs of treatment continue to rise,

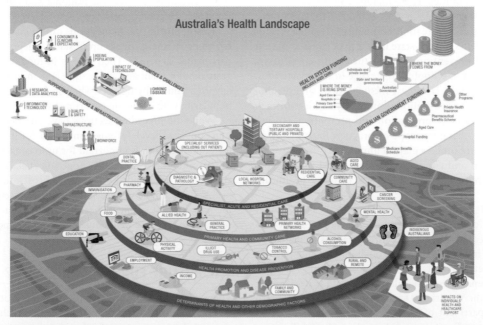

Fig. 1.1 Australian health landscape, updated 2019. (Source: Australian Government, Department of Health. Online. Available: https://www.health.gov.au/resources/publications/australias-health-landscape-infographic.)

the population is ageing and there are enhanced clinician and consumer expectations. These factors, combined with the impact of health technology, means that a focus on prevention has gained modest traction over the years. While chronic diseases still cause much illness and disease in Australia, the emergence of infectious disease, such as COVID-19, have seriously complicated the activities and financial costs of the Department (Australian Government Department of Health and Aged Care, 2021). Further, financial complexities between Health Departments/Territories and the Federal Government increase the difficulties of realising true collaboration across levels of Government.

State and Territory Departments of Health

Public health activity at state/territory levels involve:

- Managing public hospitals, community health services and mental health services
- Leadership and planning of public health
- Health surveillance
- Delivering breast cancer screening and immunisation programs
- Public dental services
- Ambulance and emergency services
- Local government regulation
- Health promotion, including working with non-government and other organisations.

Other roles and responsibilities of public health activity include that of the chief health officer, under whose authority many health activities are located, and who exercises statutory responsibilities. These include environmental protection, occupational health and safety, road and traffic authority, sport and recreation and consumer affairs. Education departments in each state have a major role to play in promotion and prevention through the health curriculum, health promotion in schools and a range of other activities, including *Sun Smart*, *Healthy Tuckshops*, drug and alcohol programs and driver education. Emergency services in each state also play a role in promotion and prevention. For example, with the changing scope of practice, health workers such as ambulance officers play an important role in providing information and education to the general public, and, in rural and remote communities, as primary healthcare workers.

States and Territories now focus on specific health activities as opposed to earlier including disability and aged care services. The success of any structural changes depends on political will, interdepartmental collaboration and positive interaction between all tiers of government (see e.g. Queensland Department of Health, New South Wales Department of Health, Victorian Department of Health, Western Australian Department of Health, Tasmania Department of Health, Northern Territory and Australian Capital Territory Departments of Health).

Local Government

Local government has a critical role to play in public health, especially in legislation and creating healthy communities, for example regulating, inspecting, licensing and monitoring health premises. Local governments' roles in public health activity vary across Australia, often including well-baby clinics, food safety, environmental protection, a strong role in cultural and recreational activities and community development and, importantly, local economic development.

Organisations, Associations and Public Health Advocacy Groups

There is a broad range of organisations and associations that support public health endeavours in Australia. That support comes in a variety of different forms. For example, large well-funded NGOs, such as the Cancer Council, the National Heart Foundation and Diabetes Australia, play a range of roles—including providing information and education, fundraising, advocacy, lobbying and research—in the promotion of health and the detection and treatment of specific health issues.

Other organisations, such as professional associations, are lobbyists, advocates and policy developers, and ongoing workforce educators through conferences and professional development activities. These associations include the PHAA, the Australian Health Promotion Association, the Australasian Epidemiology Association and the Australian Institute of Environmental Health.

A third group of organisations are those focused on advocacy and lobbying, including the Women's Health Network, the Consumer Health Forum and the National Aboriginal Community Controlled Health Organisation (NACCHO) (Baum, 2016).

Health promotion foundations can be integrated into state health departments or set up to stand independently of a departmental structure. Their role is in funding research, program development and application and, in some jurisdictions, advocacy and lobbying roles. They do, however, tend to vary in popularity with changing governments and policy foci.

While the preceding sections have outlined the structure, functions and levels of government in Australia responsible for public health it is important for us to consider what Baum (2019) and other researchers (Rogerson et al., 2020, Backholer et al., 2021) have said about a new approach to governing for health. They challenge prevailing policies asserting the need for policies that result in healthy, equitable and sustainable societies to enhance wellbeing, and that these policies need to be across sectors.

THE FUTURE FOR PUBLIC HEALTH?

There are a number of emerging challenges that public health faces in the 21st century. These challenges include the emergence and re-emergence of infectious diseases and a range of chronic diseases resulting from, for example, the impact of overweight and obesity influencing the population's health. Add to these issues the influence of global climate change and ecological sustainability, and you have a public health system stretched to capacity across a range of fronts.

Throughout the book, we return to these themes and issues as we explore the nature and scope of public health and as we examine alternative propositions for health governance.

A FINAL WORD

In this chapter, we have covered a broad range of issues that are reflective of elements of public health. We have defined wellness, health, illness and disease, and considered the definition, vision and values of public health. We have also examined the important role of health workers in public health.

We have discussed the place of the WHO in setting a global agenda for public health, and the specific role of governments at three levels in Australia. We introduced you to the range of other associations, community organisations and advocacy groups who all play important roles in improving the health of the population.

In conclusion, we briefly discussed public health issues emerging in the 21st century, and the challenges facing professionals working in the public health field if they are to deal with these issues. In the chapters that follow in this section, we examine public health challenges, epidemiology and Aboriginal and Torres Strait Islander health.

REVIEW QUESTIONS

1. What do you understand by the terms "wellness", "health", "illness", "disease" and "public health"?
2. Why should public health have a vision, and what values should public health workers espouse and put into practice?
3. Identify the core tasks of public health and think about how these might differ in the future.
4. Who is the public health practitioner, and what do you believe to be the core functions of a public health worker?
5. Make up a table of the three levels of government in Australia, and in each column describe their public health roles and responsibilities.
6. What role do NGOs play in public health?
7. List and briefly comment on the issues you believe will impact on public health in the next 10 years.
8. How have varying political agendas at state and federal levels impacted on public health funding and activity?

USEFUL WEBSITES

Australian Bureau of Statistics (ABS): http://www.abs.gov.au
Australian Government Department of Health and Aged Care: http://www.health.gov.au

Australian Institute of Health and Welfare: http://www.aihw.gov.au/
National Health and Medical Research Council: http://www.nhmrc.gov.au
Primary Health Networks: https://www.health.gov.au/initiatives-and-programs/phn/what-phns-do
United Nations: http://www.un.org/en
US Department of Health and Human Services: Healthy People 2030 Draft: https://health.gov/healthypeople
World Health Organization: http://www.who.int/en
WHO Transformation: 2020 progress report. World Health Organization, Geneva. ISBN 978-92-4-002666-7 (electronic version): https://www.who.int/publications/i/item/9789240026667

REFERENCES

Askew DA, Brady K, Mukandi B, et al 2020 Closing the gap between rhetoric and practice in strengths-based approaches to Indigenous public health: a qualitative study. *Australian and New Zealand Journal of Public Health* 44(2): 102–105

Australian Government, Department of Health and Aged Care 2021 What we do. Available: https://www.health.gov.au/about-us/what-we-do

Australian Government, Department of Health and Aged Care 2022 Primary Health Networks. Available: https://www.health.gov.au/initiatives-and-programs/phn/what-phns-are#why-phns-are-important-

Australian Government, Department of Health and Aged Care 2022 Health structure. Available: http://www.health.gov.au/internet/main/publishing.nsf/Content/health-struct.htm/

Australian Institute of Health and Welfare (AIHW) 2020a Available: https://www.aihw.gov.au/reports-statistics/behaviours-risk-factors/social-determinants/overview/.https://www.aihw.gov.au/reports-data/australias-health/australias-health-snapshots?section=indigenous

Australian Institute of Health and Welfare (AIHW) 2020b Australia's health 2020. Available: https://www.aihw.gov.au/reports-data/australias-health

Baum F, 2016 The New Public Health, 6th edn. South Melbourne: Oxford University Press

Baum F, 2019 Governing for Health. USA: Oxford University Press

Baum F, 2021 How can health promotion contribute to pulling humans back from the brink of disaster? *Global Health Promotion* 28(4): 64–72

Backholer K, Baum F, Finlay SM, et al 2021 Australia in 2030: what is our path to health for all? *The Medical Journal of Australia* 214(S8): S5–40. http://doi.org/10.5694/mja2.51020

DeSalvo KB, Wang YC, Harris A, et al 2017 Public health 3.0: a call to action for public health to meet the challenges of the 21st century. Discussion Paper, National Academy of Medicine. Available: https://nam.edu/public-health-3-0-call-action-public-health-meet-challenges-21st-century/

Donaldson LJ, et al 2017 Donaldson's Essential Public Health. Taylor & Francis Group, ProQuest Ebook Central. Available: https://ebookcentral.proquest.com/lib/qut/detail.action?docID=4912166

Leonardi F, 2018 The definition of health: towards new perspectives. *International Journal of Health Services*, 48(4): 735–748. doi:10.1177/0020731418782653

Lee LM, Zarowsky C, 2015 Foundational values for public health. *Public Health Reviews* 36(2): 1–9. doi:10.1186/s40985-015-0004-1

Marmot M, 2017 Closing the health gap. *Scandinavian Journal of Public Health* 45(7): 723–731. doi:10.1177/1403494817717433

Mendenhall E, Weaver LJ, 2019 Socially determined? Frameworks for thinking about health equity and wellness. In: Page-Reeves J (ed). *Well-being as a Multidimensional Concept: Understanding Connections Among Culture, Community, and Health*. Lanham: Lexington Books; pp 25–48

Public Health Association of Australia 2022. Available: http://www.phaa.net.au/

Rogerson B, Lindberg R, Baum F, et al 2020 Recent advances in health impact assessment and health in all policies implementation: lessons from an international convening in Barcelona. *International Journal of Environmental Research and Public Health* 17(21): 7714

Trickett EJ, Rauk L, 2019 Community wellbeing, community intervention, and community development: changing community ecology. In: Page-Reeves J (ed). *Wellbeing as Multidimensional Concept: Understanding Connections Among Culture, Community, and Health*. New York: Lexington Books, pp 97–98

United Nations (UN) 2013 The Millennium Development Goals Report 2013. New York: UN

United Nations General Assembly 2015 UN adopts new Global Goals, charting sustainable development for people and planet by 2030. Available: https://news.un.org/en/story/2015/09/509732-un-adopts-new-global-goals-charting-sustainable-development-people-and-planet/

United Nations (UN) 2022 Department of Economic and Social Affairs (UNDESA) The Sustainable Development Goals Report 2022. Available: https://sdgs.un.org/ (Accessed 29 Mar 2022)

Valles SA, 2018 Philosophy of Population Health Science: Philosophy for a New Public Health Era. Milton Park, Abingdon: Routledge

World Health Organization (WHO) 2022 The Global Health Observatory. Monitoring health for the SDGs. Available: http://www.who.int/sdg/en/ (Accessed 29 Mar 2022)

World Health Organization (WHO) 1948 Constitution. WHO. Available: http://www.who.int/governance/eb/who_constitution_en.pdf (Accessed 3 Apr 2014)

World Health Organization (WHO) 1978 Declaration of Alma-Ata. International Conference on Primary Health Care, Alma-Ata, USSR, 6–12 September. Available: http://www.who.int/publications/almaata_declaration_en.pdf (Accessed 3 Apr 2014)

World Health Organization (WHO) 1986 The Ottawa Charter for Health Promotion. First International Conference on Health Promotion, Ottawa, 21 November. Available: http://www.who.int/healthpromotion/conferences/previous/ottawa/en/ (Accessed 23 Feb 2022)

World Health Organization (WHO) 2008 Commission on Social Determinants of Health, 2005–2008. Available: http://www.who.int/social_determinants/thecommission/en/ (Accessed 3 Feb 2018)

World Health Organization (WHO) 2021 Newsroom. What has COP26 achieved for health? Available: https://www.who.int/news-room/feature-stories/detail/what-has-cop26-achieved-for-health (Accessed 18 Mar 2022)

World Health Organization (WHO) n.d. Leadership Priorities. Available: https://www.who.int/about/resources_planning/WHO_GPW12_leadership_priorities.pdf (Accessed 18 Mar 2022)

2

Public Health Challenges

Mary Louise Fleming

LEARNING OBJECTIVES

After reading this chapter, you should be able to:
- Describe the main challenges facing public health in the 21st century.
- Critique the relationship between these challenges and the capacity of the workforce to meet such challenges.
- Discuss the complexity of emerging infectious diseases and the continued growth of chronic illnesses.
- Learn about effective advocacy at various levels of government for public health.
- Analyse the importance of globalisation, ecological sustainability and climate change to the survival of the planet, and its impact on public health activity in the future.

INTRODUCTION

In the 20th century, substantial progress in public health occurred in Australia. Some of these improvements resulted from increasing knowledge about the natural history of disease, treatment and medical intervention. However, other factors have made substantial changes, such as legislative measures for protecting health and improved promotion and prevention strategies as well as general improvement in social and economic conditions. Other factors influencing determinants of the public's health at the start of the 21st century look further afield to the impacts of globalisation, an infectious disease pandemic (Holst, 2020) and a war between two European countries. The same could not be said for developing countries nor for sub-population groups in developed countries like Australia. For example, in sub-Saharan Africa, analysis reveals the challenging context of mitigating the spread of the COVID-19 pandemic, given the disparities in health and the socioeconomic conditions in which they arise (Okoia & Bwawb, 2020).

In Australia, a focus on strengths and successes told through Aboriginal and Torres Strait Islander voices counters deficit narratives of Aboriginal and Torres Strait Islander health. *The 2021 Close the Gap Campaign Report* focuses on the leadership of Aboriginal and Torres Strait Islander peoples, communities and organisations, and how strengths-based approaches are the most effective way to improve health outcomes for Australia's First Peoples (Lowitja Institute, 2021, p. 6). Aboriginal and Torres Strait Islander approaches to health are canvassed extensively in Chapter 4.

The 10 most significant public health achievements in Australia are listed in Box 2.1 (PHA, 2018). While these achievements are substantial, they do not mention the climate imperative or ecological sustainability. However, sustainability is an issue that is firmly on the public health agenda, globally and in Australia, for action in the 21st century (see Chapter 11).

The WHO key global health issues are listed in Box 2.2, providing both ongoing health challenges as well as climate and humanitarian issues (Whiting, 2022).

Challenges for public health include global threats to the environment, the globalisation of chronic disease, global infectious disease pandemics and epidemics and health inequalities. In addition, changing patterns of consumption and communication, along with accelerating social and demographic changes to work, learning, family and community life, all impact on health (Parkes et al, 2020).

> ### BOX 2.1   10 Public Health Achievements in Australia 2018
>
> - Folate: we reduced neural tube defects
> - Immunisation and eliminating disease
> - We contained the spread of HPV and its related cancers
> - Oral health: we reduced dental decay
> - Slip! Slop! Slap!: we reduced the incidence of skin cancer in young adults
> - Fewer people are dying due to smoking
> - We brought down our road death and injury toll
> - Gun control: we reduced gun deaths in Australia
> - HIV: we contained the spread
> - Finding cancer early: we prevented deaths from bowel and breast cancer

Data from Public Health Association of Australia., 2018. Top 10 public health successes over the last 20 years. PHAA Monograph Series No. 2. Canberra: Public Health Association of Australia.

> ### BOX 2.2   World Health Organization Key Global Health Moments
>
> - COVID-19 vaccine and inequities
> - Humanitarian crisis in Afghanistan
> - Universal health coverage
> - Tobacco use in decline
> - Violence against women
> - Malaria vaccine
> - Diabetes in the spotlight
> - The state of dementia
> - Health and climate change

Data from Whiting K 2022 Year in review: 2021's key global health moments, according to the World Health Organization. January 6, 2022 by World Economic Forum.

GLOBALISATION AND HEALTH

A global agenda for public health is a major challenge for health practitioners, public health advocacy groups and governments.

Globalisation is about increasing international interdependence in important areas of life such as politics, economy, culture and environment. The promotion and acceleration of globalisation has come about by factors such as, "the internationalisation and liberalisation of production and trade, increasing digitisation, new means of communication, growing migration pressure due to population growth, protracted conflicts and ecological challenges" (Holst, 2020, p. 4).

Governments are often caught up in arguments about free trade, mobility of capital and the deregulation of labour conditions. Such issues do contribute to socioeconomic inequalities and environmental challenges (McInnes et al, 2020). Climate change, biodiversity loss, persisting poverty, the growing obesity epidemic and food insecurity are all examples of complex problems (Walls, 2018). A major contribution from public health must be the creation of sustainable environments and social conditions that result in equitable and enduring improvements in population health (Holst, 2020).

Health systems are also under stress globally. Many countries are confronting the challenges of ageing populations and the growing burden of chronic illness, which now accounts for 70% of deaths globally as well as the impact of COVID-19. The need for universal health care remains central to building human capital and an effective response and recovery from the COVID-19 pandemic. Strong primary health care services are also essential to preventing, detecting and managing diseases, as well as the promotion of health (World Bank, 2020). At the same time, there are issues such as malnutrition, unmet need for sexual and reproductive health services and maternal mortality across the globe (World Bank, 2020). The World Bank acknowledges that inequalities are a substantial barrier to prosperity and growth, and that there is a need for strong government leadership, an active trade union movement and greater equality in developing countries. Pressures from vested interests, such as the tobacco industry and the food industry, put pressure on the World Health Organization (WHO) to modify their position on contentious issues (Donaldson & Rutter, 2017). Strong and consistent leadership will be required for the WHO and other organisations in the 21st century in order to adopt a sustainable development agenda to end poverty, protect the planet and ensure prosperity for all (UN, 2022).

To further understand how globalisation impacts on public health, complete Activity 2.1.

To be effective, public health must consider global issues and take on a strong advocacy role to deal with global inequalities and inequities within countries. We set the scene by discussing Australia's population growth and the factors contributing to that growth.

Population Growth

Australia's population growth is being affected by the coronavirus disease 2019 (COVID-19) pandemic, and the measures taken to limit its spread. The closure of international borders has already led to negative net overseas migration and the lowest rate of population growth in more than 100 years (Australian Government, Centre for Population, 2021).

Longer-term trends continue to affect the size and distribution of the population. These trends are the ongoing decline in the fertility rate, the decline in the rate of internal migration and the slower rate of mortality improvement observed in recent years (ABS, 2022). Changes to Australia's demographic profile, in particular population ageing, have implications for

ACTIVITY 2.1 Why is Globalisation Important to Public Health?

Read the following article:

Patrick R, Armstrong F, Capon A, et al (2021) Health promotion in the Anthropocene: the ecological determinants of health. *Med J Aust.*, 214 (8 Suppl), S22–6.

In this article the Anthropocene is described as a mid-20th century geological epoch focused on industrialisation where humans are seen as the major disrupter of the planet by impacting the climate system and damaging earth systems.

Make a list of the ways in which human activities are driving ecosystem decline. What are the human health impacts of the Anthropocene? Develop a table that identifies the four priority directions. Then list the potential opportunities that can make a difference to each of the priority areas.

Reflection

We need to understand that health concerns are influenced not only by the physical determinants of health, but also by global climate and social and economic determinants. Opportunities exist to make changes to how we live and how we treat our planet. These factors include planetary health, climate resilient development, ecological economics, leadership and workforce development, as examples.

the economy and living standards, as set out in the 2021 Intergenerational Report (Australian Government, Centre for Population, 2021).

PUBLIC HEALTH CHALLENGES IN AUSTRALIA

We now discuss the major Australian public health challenges in the 21st century. These challenges continue the themes of diet and physical activity, population ageing and mental health and the rise of infectious diseases. They also include technological advances, ecological challenges and, particularly, climate change.

Dietary Imbalance, Physical Inactivity and Sedentary Behaviour

The Australian Bureau of Statistics said that two-thirds (67.0%) of Australian adults were overweight or obese (12.5 million people) (ABS, 2018). This was an increase from 63.4% in 2014–15 produced by an increase in the proportion of adults categorised as obese from 27.9% to 31.3%. There was a large increase for those aged 18–24 years, with 38.9% overweight or obese in 2014–15 compared with 46.0% in 2017–18. More men than women, 18 years or older, were overweight or obese with 74.5% and 59.7%, respectively. For children aged 5–17 years, 24.9% were overweight or obese in 2017–2018. These rates were similar for boys and girls and have remained stable over the previous ten years (ABS, 2018).

The conditions in which people live and work are closely linked to their health. For example, living in a rural or remote community, lower socioeconomic populations, people with disability and Aboriginal and Torres Strait Islander people experience higher rates of illness, hospitalisation and death than other Australians (Australian Institute of Health and Welfare [AIHW], 2020). In addition, food insecurity in Australia, described as limited and uncertain availability or ability to acquire nutritionally adequate and safe foods (Bowden, 2020), negatively impacts the physical, mental and social health of adults and children (Bowden, 2020).

Participation in physical activity is an important protective factor for health (AIHW, 2020). Evidence suggests that having a high level of sedentary behaviour negatively impacts on health independently of other factors, including body weight and diet (Dempsey et al, 2020). Caballero (2019) argues that no country has reversed its obesity epidemic despite a growing body of evidence about the effectiveness of available solutions. Reasons for this failure include vested economic interests, debates about the responsibility resting with the individual or the collective, government regulation versus industry self-regulation and prevention versus treatment priorities (Walls, 2018). Additionally, policy and environmental changes are needed to support the marketing of appropriate food choices to children, and to make healthy choices easier, thus creating more opportunities for children to achieve a healthy weight (Sainsbury et al, 2018).

The contribution of both the lack of physical activity and the overconsumption of food has a strong association with cardiovascular risk factors, obesity and diabetes. It also compounds the risks when associated with smoking, alcohol consumption and poor nutrition (AIHW, 2020). One solution gaining much traction is city planning and its impacts on health. Giles-Corti and colleagues (2020) argue for interventions that create healthier and more sustainable compact cities, which reduce the environmental, social and behavioural risk factors that affect lifestyle choices, levels of traffic, environmental pollution, noise and crime. Health professionals, working in collaboration with governments, architects and builders, need to reorganise living spaces to facilitate physical activity. True multisector collaboration for enhancing health is likely to be a central strategy for public health into the future. Consider now Activity 2.2 to develop a deeper understanding of the contribution of the physical environment to public health.

Population Ageing

Older Australians account for an increasing share of the population. Table 2.1 demonstrates the changing demographics.

Major health issues facing Australians 65 years and over include chronic disease, with the over-85 age group more likely to experience multiple long-term conditions that impact on daily functional capacity, overweight and obesity, pain management, frailty, falls, memory loss, dementia and other

ACTIVITY 2.2   Creating Healthy and Sustainable Urban Development

Tonne and colleagues (2021) argue that goals and pathways to achieve sustainable urban development are linked to human health and wellbeing. The paper:

- defines the process of urbanisation and its relationship to heath research
- reviews the evidence linking health with urbanisation, urbanicity and cities, and identifies the relationship between urban systems and health.

Working in a group, can you identify what the authors suggest as specific actions to promote health through sustainable urban development. The article can be found here: Tonne C., Adair L., Adlakha D., et al, 2021 Defining pathways to healthy sustainable urban development. Environment International, 146, 106236, https://doi.org/10.1016/j.envint.2020.106236

Reflection

What are the main points addressed in the article? Your attention should focus on, (1) demography and the implications for health; (2) climate change and health; (3) food systems, diet and health; (4) land use and transport; (5) air pollution; (6) noise; and (7) green space. Look at Figure 3 in particular.

TABLE 2.1   Population Projections, Australians 65 years and Older

	65 Years and Older	85 Years and Older
2017 (actual)	3.9 million (15%)	439,600 (2%)
2066 (projected)	8.3 million (21%–23%)	Over 1 million (3.4–3.6%)

Sources: ABS 2018, AIHW 2022

neurological conditions. Some of these health concerns are due to the ageing process, where physiological changes, such as increased frailty, reduced mobility and progressive loss of vision and hearing, are more evident. Common risk factors can exacerbate the impact of these changes.

The quality and safety of many aged care services has come under the spotlight in Australia. The final report of the Royal Commission into Aged Care Quality and Safety was handed down in February 2021 (https://agedcare.royalcommission.gov.au/publications/final-report). It marked many failures in governance of quality and safety across the country in aged care facilities (see Government response at https://www.health.gov.au/resources/publications/australian-government-response-to-the-final-report-of-the-royal-commission-into-aged-care-quality-and-safety).

Maintaining good health among older Australians helps to moderate the demand for health and aged-care services, which is important as Australia's population ages over the coming decades (AIHW, 2020). Importantly, social connectedness and appropriate living conditions impact on the health and wellbeing of older Australians (Thompson et al, 2022)

Mental Health

Mental health is a state of wellbeing in which an individual realises his or her own potential, can cope with the normal stresses of life, can work productively and fruitfully and is able to make a contribution to her or his community (WHO, 2018). Globally, mental health is recognised as playing an important role in achieving global development goals, as illustrated by the inclusion of mental health in the Sustainable Development Goals (WHO, 2022).

Many Australians enjoy good mental health; however, a significant proportion of the population will experience mental illness during their lives. A mental illness will affect how they think, behave and interact with those around them (AIHW, 2016). It was expected that some 4 million people experienced a common mental illness in 2015, and some $9 million was spent on mental health in 2015/2016 (AIHW, 2018). Reform of the mental health and suicide prevention strategy is based on five pillars:

1. Prevention and early intervention
2. Suicide prevention
3. Treatment
4. Supporting vulnerable Australians
5. Workforce and governance (Commonwealth of Australia, 2021).

Considerable research has examined the links between mental health and COVID-19 (Newby et al, 2020), the school context (Teesson et al, 2020) and the mental health issues impacting farmers, such as social, environmental and economic factors (Daghagh Yazd, 2019). Australian migrant and refugee populations are often considered together in mental health policy and planning. However, mental health strategies and initiatives must be based on the evidence related to migration and resettlement, which act as social determinants of mental health (Sullivan et al, 2020). The work of Awaworyi Churchill and colleagues (Awaworyi Churchill et al, 2019) suggests policy development is needed that promotes social inclusion in multicultural societies and builds trust between heterogeneous ethnic groups as a vehicle to improve mental health.

Youth suicide is a significant public health problem. In 2011, suicide was the leading cause of death in young Australians aged 15–24 (AIHW, 2016). In the National Health Survey (2017–18) overall, 15–24-year-olds had the highest proportion of mental or behavioural conditions (26%) (ABS, 2018). However, there is a need for better ways to screen for mental health problems in the community (Centre for Mental Health Research, ANU, 2018).

Screening for mental health problems can increase help-seeking behaviour and link individuals with appropriate services (Australian Government Department of Prime Minister and Cabinet, 2021). It is important that people can speak freely about their feelings of stress and psychological needs, in order to be supported in seeking help (Aguirre Velasco, 2020).

Sustainable Ecological Public Health

Accomplishing sustainable social, economic and environmental conditions underpins achieving population health in Australia, while environmental changes, including climate change, loss of biodiversity, productivity downturns in land and oceans and freshwater depletion, all add to possible serious health risks (Hickel, 2020). It is likely that the highly contested nature of climate change and multiple interest groups and opinions will pose major policy governance challenges for the Australian government and stakeholders in grappling with climate adaptation (see Chapter 11).

The current WHO-endorsed work plan on climate change and health addresses four main areas that need attention: advocacy and partnerships; supporting countries to protect human health from climate change; monitoring science and evidence; and building capacity on climate change and human health. These aspects are discussed in Box 2.3. Complete Activity 2.3 to consider the key principles of the WHO work plan on climate change and how they apply in the Australian context.

There have been some positive signs regarding climate change initiatives, in particular with the development of alternative energy sources such as solar energy and wind power.

BOX 2.3 WHO Work Plan on Climate Change and Health, 2022

Advocacy and Partnerships—to coordinate with partner agencies within the UN system, and ensure that health is properly represented in the climate change agenda. To provide and disseminate information on the threats that climate change presents to human health, and opportunities to promote health while cutting carbon emissions.

Monitoring science and evidence—to coordinate reviews of the scientific evidence on the links between climate change and health, and to assess country's preparedness and needs in the face of climate change. To develop a global research agenda.

Supporting countries to protect human health from climate change—strengthening national capacities and improving the resilience and adaptive capacity of health systems to deal with the adverse health effects of climate change.

Building capacity on climate change and health—to assist countries to build capacity to reduce health vulnerability to climate change, and promote health while reducing carbon emissions.

(Source: WHO 2022)

ACTIVITY 2.3 Climate Change and Public Health in Australia

Consider each of the four main points outlined in the WHO Work Plan, 2017—advocacy and partnerships; monitoring science and evidence; building capacity on climate change and human health; supporting countries to protect human health from climate change—as they might apply in the Australian context.

Reflection

Think about who best to partner with in Australia to ensure that climate change is on the agenda. How would you approach that organisation, and how might they help you? How would you provide and disseminate information about climate change so that the community is aware and supportive of such strategies? Obtain some evidence about climate change from a reputable source—what would a reputable source be? Look at public health responses to date. Where might you find these, and how might you consider which ones you choose?

The creation of an environment that is conducive to renewable energy production will enable sustainable growth of energy utilisation in Australia with renewable energy becoming the dominant energy source of the future (Li et al, 2020). The clearest signal to date is evidenced by a transitioning to a low-carbon environment.

Emerging and Re-emerging Infections

The re-emergence of infectious diseases is a major challenge for public health in Australia. A number of infectious diseases such as Zika virus, Ebola, swine flu, severe acute respiratory syndrome (SARS), avian influenza ('bird flu'), Australian bat lyssavirus (ABLV) and Hendra virus have emerged in recent years, associated with mobility, shifts in the ecology of human living, technologies and economic activity.

COVID-19 and the many variants have travelled across the planet creating a pandemic that exemplifies the differing impact of the disease on people from different parts of the world where there are social, cultural, economic and political diversity, in particular where the healthcare system is non-existent or unable to cope with the veracity of the disease (World Economic Forum, 2022). It should be said that even in developed countries healthcare systems have been stretched to breaking point.

More recently Monkeypox (MPX) has appeared in Australia and in other countries. The Monkeypox virus (MPXV) is a disease with symptoms similar to smallpox. It is spread through close contact with an infected person or animals, or with contaminated material (Australian Government, Department of Health and Aged Care, 2022). Other infectious diseases are appearing at an alarming rate! What are some of these?

A variety of factors influence the range, burden and risk of infectious diseases, including increased population density, persistent poverty and the vulnerability of younger population groups, as well as many environmental, political and social factors. These causes are compounded by gender, economic and structural inequalities, and by political denial, vaccine obstacles and the mismatch between health resource distribution and major causes of illness (Nkengasong, 2021).

All of these infectious diseases underscore the importance of comprehensive and ongoing public health strategies along a continuum of care from advancing wellbeing to treatment, rehabilitation and long-COVID recovery. In particular, Webster and colleagues (2022) suggests that over time the long-term effects of COVID-19 on "public health governance—or broader political economic systems" (p. 3683) will emerge but will vary widely.

The health of people is closely connected to animal health and the shared environment. One Health, while not a new concept, has become important because of the many factors that have modified the interactions between people, animals, plants and our environment (CDC, 2022). The prevention and control of infections in humans and animals is an essential step in tackling antimicrobial resistance. The affordability of, and access to, existing and new antibiotics and vaccines are important considerations (Shafiq et al, 2021).

Genetics, Technology, Artificial Intelligence and Robotics

Molecular and genetic approaches to controlling diseases are well developed in Australia. A major focus of these approaches is to ensure the appropriate use of such technology to heal the sick, to prevent disease now and in the future and to alter traits that are not related to health issues. Molecular and genetic approaches to controlling disease, such as the use of genome editing to promote human health, raise important questions about scientific, ethical and social issues, as well as about the capability of systems to ensure the responsible development and use of these technologies (Claussnitzer et al, 2020). Ramaswami and colleagues (2018) argue that public health practitioners will have to take a critical and sceptical view of genetic technology, questioning its potential for impact on population health status and the impact of its availability on equity and access.

Technology potentially raises both ethical and legal issues, which will need to be resolved through public debate and difficult policy choices. Included among them are genetic engineering, cloning, stem cell research and slowing of the ageing process. The bottom line with respect to biotechnology is not that these advances might occur; the ultimate challenge to public health is the cost of these innovations, and the limited resources available to pay for them (Schneider & Schneider, 2021).

Advances in information technology have led to improvements in public health surveillance capabilities. However, as technology has improved, ethical and legal questions have arisen around information privacy, as well as ensuring that important public information remains available. The rise of the internet as a source of information and commerce also poses many challenges for consumers, including appropriate evaluation of information, and for governments and policymakers about how to protect consumers from inappropriate advice and information (Schneider & Schneider, 2021).

The use of artificial intelligence (AI) and robotics also poses questions of a legal, ethical and social nature. Consider these issues as you progress through Case Study 2.1.

The Public Health Workforce: Skills for a Complex Future

The ability of the public health workforce to deal with the complexity of health and wellbeing issues is essential to advancing public health activity into the 21st century. In Australia there has been ongoing debate in the profession about the extent to which health professionals can be considered public health experts. There is a need for strong political and institutional support and leadership for public health education and training, to ensure that present and future health issues are dealt with effectively in a multisectoral way.

Health professionals need an understanding of, and an ability to utilise, core competencies of public health practice, and a clear appreciation of the complexity of the task and the multiple drivers of population health patterns, including regulatory strategies. The development of competencies for public health and health promotion has been well researched in Australia. In addition, issues of access and equity, broad issues around ecological sustainability and globalisation, skills in risk identification and management and the re-emergence of infectious diseases are central areas of focus for the promotion of population health in Australia.

Political Will and Action for Public Health

As Walls (2018) suggests, political commitment is essential to advance the public's health. This is in the face of documented industry strategies to create debate and confusion, influence country positions and delay government regulatory responses (Walls, 2018). In countries like Australia, political support for public health has waxed and waned as big industry groups have countered or proposed alternative positions about the evidence supporting various public health solutions. Governments in Australia now face dealing with an ever-increasing range of chronic diseases with limited financial ability to respond through medical intervention. As well, a pandemic has meant that politics and public health have intersected in many positive and some less positive ways to focus public health interventions across a continuum of care. The need for planning and coordination of public health activities is, as ever, the

CASE STUDY 2.1 Health Care in 2070: a Wellness-centric Model of Care?

Will we see a shift to a wellness-centric model of health care? This model will be driven by mass personalisation and design-heavy, proactive healthcare interventions. Many educated individuals are becoming more informed about health and wellness through on-demand access to data, and more empowered through the greater availability of service options, such as GP clinics, home doctors and online video consultations.

Data and digital solutions have begun to be introduced in response to these population trends and in an effort to create a more seamless health and wellness experience. We have seen this through the implementation of Electronic Medical Record solutions and My Health Records.

Despite these advancements, we are only just beginning to scrape the surface of the benefits offered by technology in delivering enhanced health outcomes. With the exponential rise of robotics and artificial intelligence (AI), routine tasks are increasingly being automated to release capacity for health and wellness providers to deliver high-value services. Constraints hindering the uptake of these technologies include cost and workforce readiness.

In the future, we envisage people-driven healthcare that is seamless, flexible and tailored, and puts the patient at the centre of decision-making. We will observe a shift from bricks-and-mortar services to community-based, mobile services. Easily accessible, AI-operated emergency care hubs located across Australia will provide individuals with instant treatment and health advice, relieving pressure on hospital Emergency Departments. Advanced technologies will enable the genetic profiling of people to eliminate genetic mutations that are harmful to health.

Questions
1. Do you think that such levels of connectivity will widen the gap between people's expectations and the existing service offering?
2. Can we see a shift in healthcare priorities towards prevention, wellness and maintenance, as opposed to current healthcare based on a medical model of intervention and treatment?
3. What will be the first step in this decentralisation of our healthcare system, which will ultimately shift services out of the hospital and into the community and the home?
4. What impact will these advancements in technology have on the human element of doctor-to-patient care?
5. Will individuals have the choice to opt out of interacting with health technologies? Can you see some people being excluded from such technologies, and why might they be excluded?
6. How are the social determinants of health impacted if at all? Discuss your group responses with the class. Are there different points of view, and, if so, why is that the case?

Source: Imarisio 2017

underlying priority for advancing a national public health agenda in Australia. Public health is as much about democracy, empowerment, accountability, transparency and communication as it is about professional skill sets.

The introduction of Sustainable Development Goals (SDGs) was set to be inclusive and aims to deal with the multiple underlying issues that impact on health, including the elimination of poverty, and an emphasis on equality and sustainability (Stewart, 2015). For such issues to be achieved, the goals must be interpreted and committed to at a national level, the underlying economic structures that can reduce inequality must be addressed and (most importantly) the sustainability goals must be integrated with economic goals (Yiu & Saner, 2014). However, Naidoo and Fisher (2020) talk about the need for a reset as a result of COVID-19, because of the lack of funding or attention available now to reduce poverty and inequality, to focus on a vision of healthcare for all, to enhance biodiversity and reduce the climate emergency by 2030. They argue for screening of every goal and target to examine: (1) is it a priority, post-COVID-19; (2) is it about development not growth; and (3) is its achievement resilient to global disruptions?

Leadership and Public Health: Establishing a Research Agenda

Most recently, there has been increased attention in Australia on translating public health research into practice (Brownson, 2018). However, there are a number of factors that limit the application and dissemination of basic scientific research into health policy and community and institutional practice, and the ability of practice to inform the evidence base (see Chapter 8). These factors include the lack of an evaluation culture, ethical and programmatic difficulties in designing evaluations, the selection of appropriate outcome measures, the poor design and implementation of current interventions and the reality that policymaking is based on more than evidence alone (Shelton et al, 2018). The challenge for researchers, practitioners and advocates is to provide timely access to information, and to employ improved techniques for communicating and managing public health program evaluation results that begin when the project is being designed. (See Chapter 3 for research and evaluation techniques.)

GRAND CHALLENGES FOR PUBLIC HEALTH: WHAT IS THE FUTURE?

A number of forces beyond the health arena will have an impact on health. These factors include globalisation (Sparke, 2018), a potential major financial crisis and armed conflicts and deteriorating security situations, leading to large displacements and migration of populations. Public health workers have lost their lives while doing humanitarian work, and climate change has led to severe and changeable weather conditions. A way forward to deal with many of these issues remains contested.

A pandemic has challenged global and national economic systems, healthcare capacity and political and social determinants of health. All of these factors have had a major impact on the health and wellbeing of nation states and local communities, particularly those in the poorest parts of the world (Keshky, 2020).

The progress that was made in public health during the 20th century has been remarkable in many respects, particularly in developed countries. However, progress in the health of subpopulations, such as Indigenous peoples in Australia, remains a major challenge for public health amidst the need for and importance of Indigenous self-determination.

A FINAL WORD

Public health faces many challenges. Ecological sustainability, inequitable resource distribution and political conditions all impact on health. There is often limited political will to restructure resources and infrastructure to ensure the equitable distribution of the means to support health in our society. In addition, we face issues of social isolation, an ageing population, problems of overweight and obesity and mental health, particularly among young Australians. Not to mention the complexities of dealing with chronic illness together with new and emerging infectious disease pandemics.

However, despite these many overarching issues, the future of public health is an exciting one. Health professionals of the future will need to use transdisciplinary approaches, and be multiskilled, flexible and adaptable if they are to meet the challenges they will face. Challenges in public health are there to be met, and overcome, in order to make a difference to the health of the population.

REVIEW QUESTIONS

1. Draw a diagram of your choice that displays developments that have advanced the health of the Australian population in the 21st century.
2. What are the main challenges facing public health? For example, is overconsumption a problem across the world? What other issues are important considerations?
3. How do these challenges differ for developed countries compared with developing countries?
4. Has globalisation played a part in emerging patterns of mortality and morbidity in the 21st century?
5. How important is ecological sustainability and climate change in terms of impact on health?
6. What skills and expertise do the health workforce of the 21st century need that might not have been as important in the previous century?
7. How likely are the examples found in Case Study 2.1? What factors might make these changes possible, and what challenges might there be to their realisation?

USEFUL WEBSITES

Australian Bureau of Statistics: http://www.abs.gov.au/

Australian Government Department of Aged Care. Coronavirus (COVID-19) Pandemic: https://www.health.gov.au/health-alerts/covid-19

Australian Institute of Health and Welfare. Report on Australia's health: https://www.aihw.gov.au/reports/australias-health/australias-health-2020-in-brief/summary

Australian Institute of Health and Welfare website on chronic diseases: https://www.aihw.gov.au/reports-statistics/health-conditions-disability-deaths/chronic-disease/reports

The World Bank home page covering research, data and topics of interest relating to health: https://www.worldbank.org/en/home

United Nations website on the Sustainable Development Goals: https://www.un.org/sustainabledevelopment/sustainable-development-goals/

World Health Organization's Global Health Data Observatory: http://www.who.int/gho/en/

REFERENCES

Aguirre Velasco A, Cruz ISS, Billings J, Jimenez M, Rowe S, 2020 What are the barriers, facilitators and interventions targeting help-seeking behaviours for common mental health problems in adolescents? A systematic review. *BMC Psychiatry* 20(1): 293

Australian Bureau of Statistics (ABS) 2018 Mental health services in Australia. Web report. Canberra: AIHW. Available: https://www.aihw.gov.au/reports/mental-health-services/mental-health-services-in-australia/report-contents/summary. Last updated: 2 February 2018

Australian Bureau of Statistics (ABS) 2022 Population. Available: https://www.abs.gov.au/statistics/people/population#:~:text=Australia's%20population%20was%2025%2C750%2C198%20people,net%20overseas%20migration%20was%20%2D67%2C300

Australian Bureau of Statistics 2018 Population Projections, Australia. Available: https://www.abs.gov.au/statistics/people/population/population-projections-australia/2017-base-2066

Australian Government, Centre for Population 2021 Population Statement, Commonwealth of Australia, Canberra. https://www.aihw.gov.au/reports/australias-welfare/profile-of-australias-population

Australian Government, Department of Health and Aged Care 2022 Monkeypox (MKX). Available: https://www.health.gov.au/diseases/monkeypox-mpx

Australian Government, Department of Health and Aged Care 2021 National Mental Health and Suicide Prevention Plan. Available: https://www.health.gov.au/resources/publications/the-australian-governments-national-mental-health-and-suicide-prevention-plan

Australian Institute of Health and Welfare (AIHW) 2016 Australia's health 2016. Australia's health series no. 15. Canberra: AIHW

Australian Institute of Health and Welfare (AIHW) 2018 Australia's health 2018: in brief. Cat. no. AUS 222. Canberra: AIHW

Australian Institute of Health and Welfare (AIHW) 2020 Australia's health 2020. Available: https://www.aihw.gov.au/reports/australias-health/australias-health-2020-in-brief/summary

Awaworyi Churchill S, Farrell L, Smyth R, 2019 Neighborhood ethnic diversity and mental health in Australia. *Health Economics* 28(9): 1075–87

Bowden M, 2020 Understanding food insecurity in Australia. Canberra: Australian Institute of Family Studies

Brownson RC, Eyler AA, Harris JK, Moore JB, Tabak RG, 2018 Getting the word out: new approaches for disseminating public health science. *Journal of Public Health Management and Practice: JPHMP* 24(2): 102–11.

Caballero B, 2019 Humans against obesity: who will win? *Advances in Nutrition*, 10(suppl_1): S4–9. https://doi.org/10.1093/advances/nmy055

Centre for Mental Health Research, Australian National University (ANU) 2018 Assessing mental health survey. Canberra: ANU

Claussnitzer M, Cho JH, Collins R, et al 2020 A brief history of human disease genetics. *Nature* 577(7789): 179–89

Commonwealth of Australia 2021 Intergenerational Report. Australia over the next 40 years. Available: https://treasury.gov.au/sites/default/files/2021-06/p2021_182464.pdf

Daghagh Yazd S, Wheeler SA, Zuo A 2019 Key risk factors affecting farmers' mental health: a systematic review. *International Journal of Environmental Research and Public Health* 16(23): 4849

Dempsey PC, Biddle SJH, Buman MP, et al 2020 New global guidelines on sedentary behaviour and health for adults: broadening the behavioural targets. *International Journal of Environmental Research and Public Health* 17(151). Available: https://doi.org/10.1186/s12966-020-01044-0

Donaldson LJ, Rutter PD 2017 Donaldsons' essential public health. Boca Raton: CRC Press

Holst J 2020 Global Health – emergence, hegemonic trends and biomedical reductionism. *Globalization and Health* 16(1): 42

Giles-Corti B, Lowe M, Arundel J 2020 Achieving the SDGs: evaluating indicators to be used to benchmark and monitor progress towards creating healthy and sustainable cities. *Health Policy (Amsterdam)* 124(6): 581–90

Hickel J, 2020 The sustainable development index: measuring the ecological efficiency of human development in the anthropocene. *Ecological Economics* 167: 106331

Imarisio M, 2017 Extract from the QUT PwC Chair in Digital Economy and QUT Faculty of Health. Health 5.0 event. Brisbane: PricewaterhouseCoopers Brisbane Office, 23 November

El Keshky MES, Basyouni SS, Al Sabban AM, Al Sabban AM, 2020 Getting through COVID-19: the pandemic's impact on the psychology of sustainability, quality of life, and the global economy– A systematic review. *Frontiers in Psychology* 11, 585897

Li HX, Edwards DJ, Hosseini MR, Costin GP, 2020 A review on renewable energy transition in Australia: an updated depiction. *Journal of Cleaner Production* 242: 118475

Lowitja Institute 2021 Leadership and legacy through crises: keeping our mob safe. Close the Gap Campaign Report 2021. Close the Gap Campaign Steering Committee for Indigenous Health Equality

McInnes C, Lee K, Youde J, 2020 The Oxford Handbook of Global Health Politics. Oxford: Oxford University Press

Naidoo R, Fisher B, 2020 Sustainable Development Goals: pandemic reset. *Nature* 583: 198–201

Newby JM, O'Moore K, Tang S, Christensen H, Faasse K, 2020 Acute mental health responses during the COVID-19 pandemic in Australia. *PLoS ONE* 15(7): e0236562

Nkengasong JN, 2021 COVID-19: unprecedented but expected. *Nature Medicine* 27(3), 364. Available: https://www.nature.com/articles/s41591-021-01269-x.pdf

Okoia O, Bwawab T, 2020 How health inequality affect responses to the COVID-19 pandemic in Sub-Saharan Africa. *World Dev* 135, 105067. Published online 2020 Jul 10. doi:10.1016/j.worlddev.2020.105067

Parkes MW, Poland B, Allison S, et al 2020 Preparing for the future of public health: ecological determinants of health and the call for an eco-social approach to public health education. *Canadian Journal of Public Health* 111: 60–4. https://doi.org/10.17269/s41997-019-00263-8

Patrick R, Armstrong F, Capon A, et al 2021 Health promotion in the Anthropocene: the ecological determinants of health. *The Medical Journal of Australia* 214(suppl_8): S22–6

Public Health Association of Australia 2018 Top 10 public health successes over the last 20 years. PHAA Monograph Series No. 2. Canberra: Public Health Association of Australia

Ramaswami R, Bayer R, Galea S, 2018 Precision medicine from a public health perspective. *Annual Review of Public Health* 39: 153–68

Sainsbury E, Hendy C, Magnusson R, et al 2018 Public support for government regulatory interventions for overweight and obesity in Australia. *BMC Public Health* 18, 513. https://doi.org/10.1186/s12889-018-5455-0

Schneider MJ, Schneider HS, 2021 Introduction to public health, 6th edn. Burlington: MA Jones and Bartlett Learning

Shafiq N, Pandey AK, Malhotra S, et al 2021 Shortage of essential antimicrobials: a major challenge to global health security. *BMJ Global Health* 6(11): e006961

Shelton RC, Cooper BR, Stirman SW, 2018 The sustainability of evidence-based interventions and practices in public health and health care. *Annual Review of Public Health* 39: 55–76

Sparke M, 2018 Globalisation and the politics of global health. In Sparke M (ed). *Globalisation and the Politics of Global Health*. Oxford: Oxford University Press, Ch 3: pp. 37–58

Stewart F, 2015 The sustainable development goals: a comment. *Journal of Global Ethics* 11(3): 288–93

Sullivan C, Vaughan C, Wright J, 2020 Migrant and refugee women's mental health in Australia: a literature review. Melbourne: School of Population and Global Health, University of Melbourne

Teesson M, Newton NC, Slade T, et al 2020 Combined prevention for substance use, depression, and anxiety in adolescence: a cluster-randomised controlled trial of a digital online intervention. *The Lancet Digital Health* 2(2): e74-84. https://doi.org/10.1016/S2589-7500(19)30213-4

Thompson C, Morris D, Bird S, 2022 Evaluation of the improving social connectedness of older Australians project pilot: informing future policy considerations. Wollongong: Centre for Health Service Development, Australian Health Services Research Institute, University of Wollongong

Tonne C, Adair L, Adlakha D, et al 2021 Defining pathways to healthy sustainable urban development. *Environment International* 146: 106236. https://doi.org/10.1016/j.envint.2020.106236

United Nations (UN) 2022 Sustainable Development Goals. 17 goals to transform our world. Available: https://www.sdgsinaction.com (Accessed 10 February 2022)

Walls HL, 2018 Commentary. Wicked problems and a 'wicked' solution. *Globalization and Health* 14, 34. Available: https://doi.org/10.1186/s12992-018-0353-x/

Webster DG, Aytur SA, Axelrod M, et al 2022 Learning from the past: pandemics and the governance treadmill. *Sustainability* 14(6): 3683

Whiting K, 2022 Year in review: 2021's key global health moments, according to the WHO. January 6, 2022 by World Economic Forum

World Economic Forum. Available: https://www.weforum.org/agenda/2022/01/health-stories-2021-covid19/

World Bank 2020 Health context. Available: https://www.worldbank.org/en/topic/health/overview#1 (Accessed 5 February 2020)

World Health Organization (WHO) 2018 Mental health: strengthening our response. Available: https://www.who.int/news-room/fact-sheets/detail/mental-health-strengthening-our-response

World Health Organization (WHO) 2022 Climate change and health. Fact Sheet. Available: https://www.who.int/health-topics/climate-change#tab=tab_2

Yiu LS, Saner R, 2014 Sustainable development goals and millennium development goals: an analysis of the shaping and negotiation process. *Asia Pacific Journal of Public Administration* 36(2): 89–107. Available: https://doi.org/10.1080/23276665.2014.911487

3

Epidemiology

Catherine M. Bennett

LEARNING OBJECTIVES

After reading this chapter, you should be able to:
- Appreciate the role of epidemiology in public health.
- Understand exposure and outcome measures.
- Identify the main types of epidemiological study design.
- Report and interpret measures of association between exposures and health outcomes.
- Discuss the concepts of chance, bias and confounding.

INTRODUCTION

This chapter will provide you with a basic understanding of epidemiology, and introduce you to some of the epidemiological concepts and methods used by researchers and practitioners working in public health. Epidemiologists, often described as "disease detectives", play a key role in identifying and presenting the evidence that underpins policy and practice in both the clinical and the public health settings. The ultimate goals of epidemiology are to contribute to the prevention of disease and disability, promote health and delay mortality.

Epidemiology is fundamental to evidence-based medicine and to public health policy and practice. Rather than examine health and illness on an individual level, as clinicians do, epidemiologists focus on communities and populations, where important information and insights can be gained regarding the health of populations, the distribution of disease and injury and the determinants of these conditions, as well as the effectiveness of health interventions.

But why do we need epidemiology and this population-level understanding of health? Our health, risk of disease and chance of having an injury are all determined by a complex interaction between multiple factors related to our family history, and where and how we live. These factors can be difficult to tease apart unless we have a systematic way of studying them and determining real causal associations. Only then can we determine the best ways to treat or prevent poor health outcomes. Epidemiology is a structured, logical framework for thinking about and unravelling complex causal pathways, and piecing together the best evidence available. Epidemiology therefore provides the basis for evidence-based clinical practice, strategic planning, prioritising health issues and evaluating health services and prevention programs.

This example of an association between an exposure of interest and a health outcome will help you to understand how epidemiology works and how it is useful in public health. Australia has the highest incidence of asthma in the world; it is commonly found that people who own cats are less likely to have asthma. Does this mean that owning a cat protects you from developing asthma? Or that people with asthma tend not to own cats, as it exacerbates their asthma? Or is it possibly a bit of both? Should doctors tell women with a family history of asthma to get rid of their cat, if they are planning to get pregnant; or to get a cat if they are thinking of getting pregnant, to reduce the chances of their child having asthma? We will come back to this example at different times in the chapter to illustrate different aspects of epidemiological concepts and methods.

DEFINING EPIDEMIOLOGY

Epidemiology can be defined as "the study of the *occurrence* and *distribution* of health-related events, states or processes in specified populations, including the *determinants* influencing such processes, and the *application* of this knowledge to control relevant health problems" (emphasis added) (Porta 2014, p. 95). This definition succeeds in capturing the scope of epidemiology in a clear and concise manner. Look carefully at each of the italicised words.

Occurrence and *distribution* refer to the frequency and pattern of health events by person (*who* gets affected), place (*where* it happens) and time (*when* it happens). We will expand on this when we consider "person, place and time" in more detail, together with the ways we capture and measure health outcomes. *Determinant* refers to both the causes of, and risk factors for, health events. These can include any aspect of the environment we live in (e.g. biological, physical, cultural, social), including living organisms (e.g. viruses and bacteria), physical entities (e.g. radiation, pollution and dangerous machinery), lifestyle (e.g. stress and diet), social factors (e.g. poverty) and genetic factors (e.g. inherited or changed genes that cause genetic diseases or genetically determined immune response to infections). We will revisit health determinants when we consider how to measure these exposures when trying to understand the patterns of disease and health in populations. The World Health Organization defines *health* as "a state of complete physical, mental, and social wellbeing and not merely the absence of disease or infirmity" (WHO, 1948).

OBJECTIVES OF EPIDEMIOLOGICAL STUDIES

Epidemiological studies can fulfil three primary roles: description, analysis and intervention. Depending on the study design, the descriptive information may then be used to look for relationships between possible causal factors and health outcomes, by means of statistical analysis. This analysis can help determine whether certain population or individual factors are associated with certain health outcomes (e.g. the inverse relationship between asthma and cat ownership). Finally, the outcomes of analytical studies can be used to develop and justify the implementation of further analytical studies to explore these associations (e.g. clarifying what is cause and what is effect), or there may be sufficient information to drive interventions, such as introducing new treatments or health promotion programs. Epidemiological approaches are also integral to the evaluation of the effectiveness of interventions. Complete Activity 3.1 by providing an example of the relationship between public health and epidemiology.

ACTIVITY 3.1 **Application of Epidemiology to Public Health Issues**

Think of a public health issue relevant to your area of interest. Write a paragraph to explain how epidemiology could contribute to better understanding or quantifying the issue.

Reflection

This activity requires you to apply your understanding of epidemiology and its objectives. What resources will you use to investigate the public health issue? Try using the definition of "epidemiology" above to help you.

MEASURING THE OCCURRENCE OF EXPOSURES OF INTEREST AND OF HEALTH OUTCOMES

Measuring the health of populations can help to answer some fairly simple, yet crucial, questions. For example, how much disease is present? How quickly are new cases occurring? How long do people remain ill? How does the rate of disease or death differ over time within this population, or compared with another? Who does the disease affect? Where and when are they getting sick? What strategies are effective at reducing the occurrence of a certain disease or condition? *Health indicators* are measurable characteristics of a person, population or environment that are indicative of one or more aspects of a population's health (e.g. infant mortality rate).

Case definitions are fundamental in epidemiology; they must be unambiguous and consistently applied across populations and time in order to allow reliable reporting and comparison of health data. This is equally true of health outcome data, as well as exposures of interest. (See Example 3.1 about measuring asthma exposure and outcome.)

Epidemiologists can *count* disease events or, more usually, calculate rates and proportions, so that comparisons of health status can be made between populations and over time. Several measures of disease frequency are employed. The simplest quantitative measure is a count—the number of people in a certain health state, or who die or become ill or injured from a specified cause. However, these data have limited value without information about the population size or the number of people at risk.

Example 3.2 identifies the issues you need to consider in counting and reporting cases.

A *ratio* describes the magnitude in one group relative to another. For example, if, of 20 people who died from a COVID-19 infection, 12 were men and eight were women,

---

EXAMPLE 3.1 **Measuring Exposure and Outcome**

Asthma data can be collected in a variety of ways. Asthma may be self-reported from symptoms (Have you ever had a persistent wheezing cough?), from a doctor's diagnosis of asthma (Have you ever been diagnosed by a doctor as having asthma?), from medication typically associated with asthma (Have you ever used a preventer or reliever puffer?) or directly from medical records. You can see that these measures might have varying degrees of reliability, and you would not want to compare the frequency of asthma between groups based on different measures. If the exposure of interest is "cats", we must be equally careful to define whether this includes any cat ownership, or whether only "indoor cats" will be counted. The timing of exposure is also important, and so you also need to know the timing of the cat exposure (Did you own a cat before you developed asthma?).

EXAMPLE 3.2 Counting and Reporting Cases

The COVID-19 pandemic resulted in excess deaths in many countries across the globe (Achilleos et al, 2021). The challenge in reporting and comparing COVID-19 related deaths was due to differences in case definitions on what constituted a COVID-19 death—a person might die who tested positive for the virus, but the infection was incidental and did not contribute to the death, and some countries removed these from counts. To compare the impact of COVID-19 across countries, you also need to take into account both the deaths and the risk of infection. We had reliable tests for COVID-19, but not all cases were tested, especially in the first waves, so we were limited to deaths per "reported case' instead of deaths per infection. What is more, the proportion of cases that were reported can vary over time and across countries. The numbers were reported and held great public interest, but few people understood the complexities.

EXAMPLE 3.3 Calculating Prevalence

We discover that a COVID-19 case attended a wedding reception while infectious 5 days ago with 200 other attendees. We test all people who were present to calculate the prevalence of infections in this group. If eight test positive, the prevalence of infection is eight out of 200 attendees at that point in time. That is 4% of the cohort (or 40 cases per 1000 attendees). This is point prevalence.

then the sex ratio would be 3:2 male to female. Another commonly used measure is a *rate*, which is a measure of the frequency of occurrence of an event. A rate differs from a proportion in that it involves units of time in its calculation (e.g. the number of COVID-19 cases in a given year). Two of the most widely used measures of *risk* calculated from the frequency of a health outcome (e.g. asthma) or exposure (e.g. cat ownership) are prevalence and incidence. *Prevalence* refers to the number of people in a defined population who have a specific disease, condition or exposure at a certain point in time (e.g. at the time the data were collected in a health survey). Measuring prevalence involves counting cases and dividing the count by the total number of people in the population from which the cases arose (e.g. the number of people who completed the survey). Prevalence can directly refer either to a specific point in time (point prevalence) or to a period of time (period prevalence). For example, we might count the number of motor vehicle accidents occurring on 31 December, or the number of accidents that occurred between 1 January and 31 December in a given year.

Prevalence is calculated using the following equation:

$$\text{Prevalence} = \frac{\text{Number of people with the disease/condition at a specific time}}{\text{Number of people in the population at risk at the specified time}} \times 10^n$$

Multiplying by 10^n allows you to adjust the reporting units so that prevalence is expressed in the same standard units for comparison across populations or time. It also allows you to report very low prevalence as cases per 100,000 (e.g. 13 cases of meningococcal disease per 100,000).

If we ask students in the same class to put up their hands if they had experienced a headache at any time during the past week, this would be *period prevalence*. If 15 students reported

that they had experienced a headache during the past week, the period prevalence is 15 cases out of 200 students over a 1-week period = 7.5% of the class per week (or 75 per 1000 students per week). Note that period prevalence will include those with the condition at the start of the specified time period, and also all the new cases (incident cases) that develop the condition over that specified time period.

Example 3.3 describes how to calculate prevalence.

Incidence refers to the number of *new* cases of disease, injury or death in a population during a specified time period. For chronic diseases that are not that common and can last a lifetime (e.g. tuberculosis), there may be a large difference between incidence and prevalence, as there are few new, or incident, cases but many persistent ones. However, for acute diseases where all cases are incident cases of short duration (e.g. influenza), there will be little difference between incidence and prevalence estimates.

Unlike prevalence, incidence is a true rate, as it always specifies a unit of time in its calculation. There are two main measures of incidence: incidence rate and cumulative incidence. *Incidence rate* is a more precise measure that describes the rate at which new cases occur in a population over a specified period of time (see Example 3.4). *Cumulative*

EXAMPLE 3.4 When to Use Incidence Rate

Many epidemiological studies follow people over time to see who develops certain health outcomes in a population deemed to be "at risk". Not everyone will be followed for the full study period (some drop out of the study, die from other causes, etc.), and we need to take this into account so that we do not underestimate disease incidence relative to time at risk. For example, let's say that in a group of 100 people who have had a coronary artery bypass graft, 24 have had a myocardial infarction (MI) after 2 years. This gives a 2-year incidence risk of 24%. This could also be expressed as a risk of *12 MIs per 100 person-years*. However, that figure assumes that everyone was followed up for the full 2 years. If, instead, you find that the average follow-up time was actually only 18 months, this should then be reported as 12 MIs per 150 person-years (which is the same as saying *16 MIs per 100 person-years*). So, you can see that we may underestimate the disease incidence, or disease risk, if we do not take into account the variation in the individual follow-up periods.

incidence is a simpler measure of the occurrence of disease or death, and tells us the proportion of a population at risk that develops a disease during a specified time period. As with prevalence, cumulative incidence can be expressed as a proportion, a percentage or the number of cases per population. Incidence rate and cumulative incidence are calculated using the following equations:

$$\text{Incidence rate} = \frac{\begin{array}{c}\text{Number of new people with disease}\\\text{or condition in specified period}\end{array}}{\begin{array}{c}\text{Total "person-time" at risk}\\\text{during specified period}\end{array}} \times 10^n$$

Note: "Person-time" represents the sum of each participant's individual time at risk (i.e. duration of follow-up) and can be expressed in any time unit, depending on the context—for example, person-years, person-months or person-days.

$$\text{Cumulative incidence} = \frac{\begin{array}{c}\text{Number of new people with the disease}\\\text{or condition in specified period}\end{array}}{\begin{array}{c}\text{Number of people in the population}\\\text{at risk during specified period}\end{array}} \times 10^n$$

(For further information on the concept of person-time, see Webb et al, 2011 pp. 41–5.)

See Box 3.1 for an illustration of the calculation of incidence rate.

Mortality rates and life expectancy are important health indicators. In Australia, a major public health effort is focused on "Closing the Gap", to reduce inequalities between Indigenous and non-Indigenous Australians. However, progress is slow, and the discrepancy in the average age at death in 2018 of about a decade remains an important policy driver. Mortality patterns can be described using crude rates, or rates that are age-specific, sex-specific or cause-specific (deaths attributed to a certain disease). Crude mortality rates (CMRs) are derived from the equation:

$$\text{CMR} = \frac{\text{Number of deaths in a specified period}}{\text{Total population}} \times 10^n$$

Comparing CMRs can be misleading. CMRs are affected by a number of population characteristics, particularly age structure. For example, in 1990, Sweden's annual death rate was 11 per 1000. This rate was higher than that of Guatemala (8 per 1000), even though life expectancy in Sweden (78 years) was greater than in Guatemala (63 years). The difference in CMRs between the two countries was due mainly to differences in age structure: 18% of Sweden's population was aged over 65 years, compared with only 3% of Guatemala's population. The differences in the age structure of a population, together with the fact that risk of mortality varies with age, can cause misleading conclusions about comparative health status.

A range of approaches are used to take age structure into account when comparing populations:

- *Age-specific mortality rates (ASMRs):* Calculated as for CMR, but both cases and the population denominator are restricted to a specific age group—for example, infant mortality rates (IMR) (birth to 1 year of age).
- *Direct age-standardised rates:* Adjusts for age differences between comparison populations. The age-specific rates from the two populations are applied to one standard population of known age structure to allow the overall adjusted mortality rates to be compared independently of age structure.
- *Indirect age-standardised rates:* Used when age-specific rates are not available for the populations being compared: the total observed death rate in each of the populations of interest is compared with the deaths expected from applying age-specific rates from a reference population to the

---

BOX 3.1   Incidence of Hearing Loss Among Workers in Heavy Industry

Imagine you are studying the incidence of hearing loss in 16,000 workers in heavy industry in Victoria, Australia. There are 750 new cases of hearing loss over a 10-year period. During those 10 years, the employees completed a total of 116,000 years of work (calculated by adding up all the years of employment during the specified 10-year period for all 16,000 workers). The average employment was 7.25 years over that 10-year period.

What was the incidence rate of hearing loss in workers in heavy industry in Victoria over the 10-year period (expressed in 1000 person-years)?

$$\text{Total person-years exposed} = \frac{750}{116,000}$$
$$= 6.47 \text{ per 1000 person-years}$$

This figure can be compared with the incidence of hearing loss in people working in light industry (1.22 per 1000 person-years). Hearing loss among workers in heavy industry occurs more frequently than in workers in light industry.

What is the cumulative incidence of hearing loss in these workers?

$$\text{Total number of people at risk during 10 years} = \frac{750}{16,000}$$
$$= 0.047 \text{ over 10 years}$$

You conclude that, among workers exposed to noise in heavy industry over a 10-year period, 4.7% developed hearing loss. This can be further interpreted as a risk statement: if workers are exposed to noise in heavy industry, they have a 4.7% chance of developing hearing loss within a 10-year period. However, it is more correct to report these findings in person-years (6.47 per 1000 person-years), as the risk is actually higher when you take into account the fact that not all workers were exposed for a full 10-year period.

given age structure of each population being compared. If the number of observed deaths in one population is higher than in the other, then one or more of the age-specific rates in that population must also be higher, but in this case you don't know which age band(s) are involved without further study. (If you are interested in reading further about these measures, see AIHW, 2011.)

EPIDEMIOLOGICAL STUDY DESIGN

Different types of epidemiological study design are used to answer different research questions. Each has advantages and disadvantages in terms of the costs involved in carrying out the study, the quality of data the study generates and the strength of the conclusions that can be drawn. Table 3.1 summarises these advantages and disadvantages.

Studies can be classified as either observational or experimental, and the distinction is an important one. *Observational studies* allow nature to take its course, and the investigator simply observes events in different populations/groups. The investigator then seeks information about the patterns of diseases and potential risk factors, or exposures of interest. In contrast, in *experimental (intervention) studies*, the investigator actively manipulates an exposure to judge its effect on a health outcome. This is a powerful study design for isolating the effects of an exposure and making causal inferences about the relationship between the exposure under study and the health outcome of interest (see Figure 3.1).

Studies can also be classified as descriptive or analytical, but they can also be both. *Descriptive* studies are used to describe and measure health indicators or the burden of disease within a population, whereas *analytical studies* are performed to evaluate the association between one or more exposures and the development of a particular disease or health state, or a number of health outcomes.

OBSERVATIONAL EPIDEMIOLOGY

For ethical reasons, many factors thought to influence disease, or protect against it, cannot be imposed on a study population. Instead, researchers make use of naturally occurring situations, and observe and measure exposures and patterns of health in naturally occurring groups. The investigator does not intervene.

Ecological Studies

Studies built on an ecological design are quick and cheap to run and are usually based on the examination of existing data. For example, with the roll out of COVID-19 vaccines, the impact on infection rates was studied by looking at the association between vaccination rate and reported case numbers (Cerio, 2021). The research found that there was an association between the proportion of people vaccinated according to

number of doses and disease rates per 100,000 in the counties studied in the USA, with the two-dose vaccination rate a significant negative predictor of cases per 100,000 population. This is population-level data, so the next step is to access more detailed case data including vaccination status to determine whether infection rates were lower in those individuals who had received two doses.

Cross-sectional Studies

Cross-sectional (prevalence) studies are one of the most common study designs used in descriptive epidemiology. Many health surveys in which people are interviewed are cross-sectional—that is, they collect data about both exposure and outcomes from an individual at one point in time.

The study group is usually selected in a way that makes them arguably representative of the whole population. For example, a questionnaire is going to provide more generalisable data if it is completed by a sample of 1000 people, based on randomly selected phone numbers, rather than by 10 people visiting a particular shopping centre. This design is particularly useful for studies investigating the impact of multiple exposures on health, including personal characteristics such as socioeconomic status, country of birth and age.

An example is an Australian cross-sectional study designed to explore the experiences of people from culturally and linguistically diverse (CALD) backgrounds in Greater Western Sydney, Australia, during the first year of the COVID-19 pandemic (Mude et al, 2021). A cross-sectional survey was used to collect data between 25 August and 30 September 2020, including information on experiences in housing, finances, safety, accessing social services and activities, finding work, food, clothing and relationships during COVID-19, as well as the perceived impact of the pandemic on their lives. The survey of 198 people found high levels of resilience, but also highlighted the need for policy and interventions to be designed to meet CALD community needs. These are important recommendations, but unfortunately this work was not published until after the Delta outbreak of 2021, which disproportionately impacted this part of Sydney. Activity 3.2 provides an example of inconsistencies between cross-sectional studies when examining cat ownership and asthma.

Case-control Studies

Case-control studies are useful when investigating the causes of rare conditions or diseases. Like cross-sectional studies, the information on case status and history of exposure is collected at a single point in time, so these studies can be quite economical to run and can yield results quite quickly, which is particularly important if investigating rapidly evolving disease outbreaks.

The case-control study design recruits a group of people with the disease/outcome (cases) and a comparison group who do not have the disease (controls). The design allows us to selectively recruit cases (e.g. identified through a disease

Text continued on page 30

TABLE 3.1   Epidemiological Study Designs: Advantages and Disadvantages

Study Type	Study Design	Timeframe	Basis for Recruitment	Basic Design	Strengths	Practical Challenges	Inference
Observational	Ecological	Information on exposures and outcomes is collected at the population level, and may be collected independently and at different time points	No recruitment as such; uses existing population-level data collected for other purposes	Data on exposures and outcomes of interest collected in the same population to see if there is an association between the prevalence of exposures and outcomes	Can include the whole population or the subset for whom data are available. Low cost relative to efficiency	Making sure that data from different sources are comparable in population coverage, and are concurrent	A useful way to see whether there is an association between a certain exposure and outcome at the population level. However, even if an association is observed, you cannot confirm that it holds true at the person level—i.e. were those individuals with the outcome the same people who also reported higher exposure?
Observational	Cross-sectional	Information on case status and history of exposure is collected at a single point in time	Approach often used in large-scale surveys, so entire populations or a random subsample may be targeted	One-time data collection, often via a survey or questionnaire if large-scale	Can reach thousands of people through large-scale surveys. Cheap compared with other forms of data collection, low cost relative to efficiency. Allows examination of multiple exposures, including personal and social characteristics where demographic information is also collected	Difficult to tease out the timing and sequence of exposures and outcomes. There is a risk of bias if people's exposure history is altered by the occurrence of the disease outcome, e.g. diet being modified after a diagnosis. People with long-term disease might be overrepresented compared with those with disease of short duration	**Descriptive studies** (prevalence surveys, etc.) involve simple presentation of facts. As not selecting participants on either exposure or outcome, the prevalence of both exposures and outcomes can be measured. **Analytical studies** set inferences about associations that can be explored statistically. Where studies are prone to bias and confounding, associations observed between the presence of exposures and outcomes cannot be interpreted as evidence of causation

Observational	Case-control	Cases are recruited on the basis of their disease status, and then information on their exposure history is collected retrospectively A group of controls selected at the same time, usually from the same population, is also asked about their exposure history	Disease or health outcome: the study sample comprises people with the disease/outcome (cases) and a comparison group at the same risk, but who don't have the disease (controls)	Allows estimation of the odds of having been exposed to specific risk factor(s) given current disease/case status	Useful for rare diseases Can examine multiple risk factors at once Low cost relative to efficiency	Analyses are restricted to the outcome that cases were selected on Finding a suitable group of controls who must be like the cases in every way and have the same potential opportunity for the outcome Recall error—inaccurate information may be reported about exposures occurring some time ago Recall bias—where someone's memory of their exposure history is distorted by the fact that they have developed the outcome Identifying and measuring confounders that you may have to adjust for	As for cross-sectional studies, with a particular risk of recall bias for cases who are selected on the presence of the disease outcome, and who may have an altered or distorted memory of their own exposure driven by their understanding of the possible causes of their own disease
Observational	Cohort	Sampled on exposure status and outcome information collected prospectively You may see retrospective cohort studies using existing data (e.g. medical records) to determine past exposures and the subsequent incidence of outcomes	People are recruited on the basis of their potential for exposure (e.g. asbestos workers) and/or may be population-based (a particular birth-cohort followed over time)	Allows estimation of the risk of disease in those exposed to specific risk factor(s) compared with those who are not	Exposure status ascertained before the outcome appears Incidence rates can be computed and compared for people with and without exposure	Requires follow-up to monitor for disease development; expensive and difficult to prevent loss to follow-up Need to measure all possible confounders, so can adjust statistically	As for other observational studies; however, for prospective cohort studies there is less risk of bias, as exposure information is recorded before disease outcomes present

Continued

TABLE 3.1 **Epidemiological Study Designs: Advantages and Disadvantages—cont'd**

Study Type	Study Design	Timeframe	Basis for Recruitment	Basic Design	Strengths	Practical Challenges	Inference
Experimental	Clinical trials	Prospective, with exposure allocated and follow-up to determine outcomes	Recruitment is aimed at including people who would be exposed to that intervention/ treatment if rolled out in real life Some clinical trials can have very restrictive inclusion and exclusion criteria to minimise adverse outcomes	As for cohort studies; however, here the exposure is allocated randomly to balance the presence of possible confounders between the different study arms so that they don't interfere with the estimation of the effect of the exposure under study	If well designed and conducted, can minimise all forms of bias and confounding, allowing the researcher to isolate the true impact of the intervention under study	Expensive to run and difficult to protect against various forms of selection and information bias, especially where the participants and researchers cannot be blinded to the arm of the study they are in Can only study the exposure that was randomised Participants studied may not be representative of the general population—need to look at both inclusion and exclusion criteria to ascertain potential selection bias	This is the only study design where there is the potential to make direct inference about causation If there has been selection bias, even if just by chance alone in smaller trials, then care must be taken to adjust for the impact this might have on the effect being estimated

Community intervention	Prospective with exposure allocated, and follow-up to determine outcomes	Unlike standard trials where the intervention is applied at the individual level, here a whole subpopulation (district or school, for example) is randomised to receive an intervention or not	As for other trials, only here the exposure is allocated randomly at subpopulation level to balance the presence of possible confounders between the different groups across study arms	Allows the trialling of community-based interventions and, as the whole local population is allocated together into the one study arm, it removes the risk of cross-contamination where people not allocated an intervention might learn about it from those who were, which may allow them to adopt some of the changes, thereby reducing their validity as a control arm member	There are often relatively fewer population groups than there are individuals in regular trials; therefore, it is harder for the randomisation process alone to ensure that each arm contains similar populations. Analysis can also be quite complicated in these trials	The outcomes measured are at population level, just as the intervention was allocated at this level; therefore, causation should strictly be inferred at the population level. For example, an education program may be shown to lift vaccine uptake in one population compared with another control population where there was no education campaign. Individual data on whether a person who was vaccinated had actually been exposed to the intervention itself may not be known

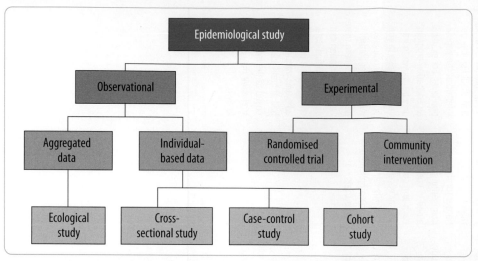

Fig. 3.1 Main types of epidemiological study design.

register, a doctor or laboratory diagnosis). The challenge is often in finding a suitable group of controls, who must be like the cases in every way with the same potential for exposure to risks, but without the disease in question. Case-control studies determine the proportion of cases that were exposed to the exposure(s) of interest, and compare this with the proportion of cases that were not exposed. The proportions of the controls that were or were not exposed to the same exposure(s) are also determined. The objective is to see whether there are differences in the odds of exposure between the two groups of people. We anticipate that if the exposure (e.g. cat ownership) is related to a disease outcome (e.g. asthma), then the prevalence

of a history of exposure will be significantly different in cases compared with controls: either greater if the exposure increases risk of disease, or less if the exposure is protective. Like cross-sectional studies, case-control studies are asking about past exposures and are susceptible to errors in recall, thus making the data less reliable (see Box 3.2). Moreover, there is an additional challenge with case-control studies: ensuring the appropriateness of the control group.

Cohort Studies

Cohort studies are generally considered to be the most robust of the observational designs. In this type of study design, we

BOX 3.3 A Longitudinal Cohort Study

Long COVID is the name given to long-term persistent effects from COVID-19 infection, some persisting for many months. The best way to fully understand chronic conditions and disease progression is through longitudinal studies that follow a population over time. Huang and colleagues commenced one of the first longitudinal studies in the world into long COVID, commencing in January 2020, and continued to follow these people, reporting on their 2-year follow-up (Huang et al, 2022).

By following this cohort, they were able to report on both the range and the duration of symptoms. The proportion of the 1149 COVID-19 survivors they followed who had at least one persistent symptom decreased significantly from 68% at 6 months to 55% at 2 years, with fatigue or muscle weakness always being the most frequent symptoms, but the burden remained high. COVID-19 survivors still had lower health status than the general population after 2 years. The study highlighted the need for further research into the pathogenesis of long COVID and interventions to reduce the risk of long COVID.

Based on Abaluck J, Kwong LH, Styczynski A, et al 2022 Impact of community masking on COVID-19: a cluster-randomized trial in Bangladesh. Science 375(6577):eabi9069. https://doi.org/doi:10.1126/science.abi9069

ACTIVITY 3.3 Observational Study Designs

Identify the type of observational study design applied in each of the following studies on the effect of raspberry leaf tea on the length of labour.

Design 1: 300 women were surveyed after they had delivered at the local maternity hospital. They were asked about their use of raspberry leaf tea and other herbal supplements in the preceding year. Data on length of labour were also collected from existing hospital medical charts upon discharge.

Design 2: 226 women giving birth and classified by length of labour (usual labour vs. long labour) were asked whether or not they had used raspberry leaf tea during their pregnancy.

Design 3: 457 pregnant women were followed from first antenatal visit to delivery. At each follow-up visit, they were given a questionnaire covering current complementary medicine usage at each time/visit. Women were classified according to whether or not they used raspberry leaf tea at all, and their length of labour was compared once they had delivered.

Reflection

In your assessment of each type of study, did you consider whether the exposure and outcome data were collected at one point in time, or if the study required participant follow-up? This is one of the first things to consider when identifying observational study types. Exposure and outcome collected at the same time signals either a cross-sectional study or a case-control. Were women recruited on the outcome measure? Did any of the studies compare cases and controls? Asking these questions helps you to distinguish between cross-sectional and case-control studies. For cohort studies (whether retrospective or prospective), the identifying design feature is that women are recruited based on their exposure.

investigate groups of people who have no apparent symptoms of the disease under study at recruitment. A critical feature of a cohort study is that the study population is observed over a period of time so that the rate of disease occurrence among people exposed to a suspected causal agent can be compared with that among unexposed people. Importantly, the measures of exposure and outcome are usually calculated prospectively (forthcoming) through time, so there is less chance of recall error. However, cohort studies are often large and expensive, because the participants have to be followed up over time, often years, to allow sufficient time for the disease outcomes of interest to present. (See Box 3.3 for an example.)

Consider the observational study designs discussed above, and then complete Activity 3.3.

EXPERIMENTAL EPIDEMIOLOGY

Experimental designs are used in clinical epidemiology where medical interventions are evaluated, and increasingly to evaluate the health impacts of population health interventions. The essence of experimental designs is comparing outcomes among exposed and non-exposed groups where the exposure of interest is under the control of the investigator, therefore isolating its effects. This is the only study design that is considered to provide direct evidence of causation.

There are also limitations to consider in experimental design and conduct. They are often very expensive to run (given

the control required for the exposure under examination, they may have to run for a long time if the disease development or prevention runs a slow course), and they can focus on only one or a few exposures and outcomes, and only those that are designed into the study in the first place.

Randomised Controlled Trials

Randomised controlled trials (RCTs) are a type of experimental study in which the participants are individually randomly assigned to either experimental or treatment groups, or a control group. (Sometimes more than one intervention is tested in the one trial.) The experimental groups receive the treatment/intervention, and the control group receives either no treatment/intervention or, preferably, a placebo treatment/intervention (something that appears similar to the real treatment, but is not active, such as a pill of the same colour, size and shape but with no active ingredients).

Randomisation ensures that each participant has the same chance of receiving an intervention or entering the control group as the next person, which helps to ensure that the study groups (intervention and control) are the same from the start. Any differences between the groups may then be attributed to the intervention. RCTs are, therefore, thought to give the best quality of evidence out of all of the epidemiological study designs. An RCT has five important elements:

- The investigator controls the exposure for each group of people to study the effect on an outcome.
- The investigator has control over all elements of the research, including selecting the participants or subjects, measuring the exposure and the outcome, and setting the conditions within which the experiment is conducted.
- Participants are randomly allocated to intervention or control groups.
- The effects of the intervention (exposure) are measured by comparing the outcome in the experimental group with that in a control group.
- The investigators and the participants should ideally be unaware of the group to which they are allocated. ('Double-blind' describes where both investigators and participants are unaware.)

RCTs present challenges as well. For example, one of the most controversial proposed treatments and prevention measures in the COVID-19 pandemic was the use of ivermectin, an existing antiparasitic drug that showed some anti-inflammatory properties in the laboratory that pointed to it being a candidate worth looking in to. However, after a run of studies, including RCTs, the results were very inconsistent (Kory, 2021). Some of this may have been because of the small size of many of the trials, but other biases may have been introduced. For example, when a trial is open label, the participants are aware that they are being given ivermectin. Do you think this might have influenced the results? Imagine if half the participants who didn't get ivermectin left the study before its completion. How might this change the results? Consider another example. Could an RCT be designed to answer our questions about cat ownership and asthma? Would it be ethical to remove a pet cat or to impose cat ownership on families? If we restricted the RCT to only those who currently did not own a cat but would be willing to do so if assigned to the intervention group, would these participants be representative of the wider population?

Community Trials

Community trials, or field trials, are conducted at a population level rather than at an individual level. For example, early in the COVID-19 pandemic, it was not known how effective mask wearing by the general public could be in reducing infection. Given the advice about mask wearing and how the culture change needed to get people to adopt masks works at the community level, it makes sense to investigate this using field

---

or community trial (Abaluck et al, 2022). They were able to show that wearing of masks was associated with reduced infection rates, and that surgical masks had the strongest association. They also found that the uptake was higher in older members of the populations studied.

Consider the epidemiological study designs discussed above, and then complete Activity 3.4.

Measures of Association

Most epidemiological studies look for associations between different exposures and a particular health outcome. Measuring the occurrence of disease in a population (e.g. prevalence or incidence) describes the health of the population, but it does not tell us anything about possible causes of disease. The frequencies of disease or exposures in each group can be compared in a *measure of the association* between an exposure and the risk of developing the disease. The two-by-two table is a simple way of presenting data, and can be helpful when starting to look for patterns in disease incidence or risk (see Table 3.2).

Relative Risk

In RCTs and cohort studies, the objective is to determine whether there is an increased or a reduced risk of a particular health outcome associated with a particular exposure—in

TABLE 3.2 Two-by-two Table

		DISEASE		
		Yes	No	Total
Exposure	Yes	a	b	a + b
	No	c	d	c + d
Total		a + c	b + d	a + b + c + d

Note: The cells containing *a, b, c* and *d* each represent the number of individuals with a particular combination of disease and exposure: *a* = number of people who are exposed and who have the disease; *b* = number of people who are exposed and who do not have the disease; *c* = number of people who are not exposed and who have the disease; and *d* = number of people who are not exposed and who do not have the disease.

other words, whether there is an association between a specific risk factor and the disease. This objective allows researchers to calculate, and then compare, the incidence rates in the exposed and unexposed groups to produce a measure called the *relative risk (RR)*. RR is calculated by dividing the incidence of disease in the group of exposed people by the incidence of disease in a group of people who are not exposed to the same factor.

$$RR = \frac{\text{Incidence in exposed people}}{\text{Incidence in unexposed people}}$$

Or alternatively, using the two-by-two table:

$$RR = \frac{a/(a+b)}{c/(c+d)}$$

RRs range in value from 0 upwards. To interpret the RR, you should consider the following:

- If RR is near to or equals 1, there is no or little association. (Risk in exposed people equals risk in non-exposed people.)
- If RR >1, there is a positive association. (Risk in exposed people is greater than risk in non-exposed people.)
- If RR <1, there is a negative or inverse association. (Risk in exposed people is less than risk in non-exposed people.)

RR values close to 1 may also be unimportant from a public health perspective. An RR of 1.2 means that there is a 20% higher risk of developing the health outcome in the exposed group than the unexposed group; however, if the disease is very rare, this might not be important. An RR of 2.0 means that the exposed group is twice as likely—or 100% more likely—than the unexposed group to develop the health outcome. If the health outcome is positive (e.g. weight loss), then this may be sufficient evidence to justify expensive interventions being put in place. If the health outcome being measured is negative (increased likelihood of disease), then this is evidence against the intervention. An RR of 0.5 means that the exposed group is half as likely to develop the outcome as the unexposed group. If the outcome is a disease, then we say that the intervention is protective.

Consider a comparison of death from coronary heart disease (outcome) between males and females (gender = exposure). One thousand women and one thousand men were recruited into a cohort study and followed over 1 year. Sixteen of the women and 20 of the men died from coronary heart disease within that year. The rate of death from coronary heart disease among females was 16 per 1000 person-years of observation, and the rate among males was 20 per 1000 person-years of observation. RR and a two-by-two table for this scenario are shown in Tables 3.3 and 3.4.

To calculate the RR in this example:

$$RR = \frac{a/(a+b)}{c/(c+d)}$$

$$RR = \frac{20/(20+980)}{16/(16+984)}$$

$$= 1.25$$

This result is interpreted as meaning that, compared with females (referent group), males have a 25% increased risk of dying from coronary heart disease.

Odds Ratios

Relative risk requires knowledge of the disease incidence in the groups being compared; however, this is not available in case-control studies, where we actively seek out cases and compare them with a set number of controls. Therefore, the number of cases in the study is not indicative of the disease incidence in the population. In this situation, researchers need to use another measure of association, known as an *odds ratio (OR)*.

TABLE 3.3 The Relative Risk for Coronary Heart Disease (CHD) Mortality

		DEATHS FROM CHD		
		Yes	No	Total
Sex	M	20	980	1000
	F	16	984	1000
Total		36	1964	2000

TABLE 3.4 Two-by-two Table for a Case-control Study

		DISEASE	
		Yes (Cases)	No (Controls)
Past exposure	Yes (exposed)	a	b
	No (not exposed)	c	d
Total		a + c	b + d

The OR asks: "What are the odds that a case was exposed relative to the odds that a control was exposed?" Two-by-two tables are also helpful when calculating ORs (see Table 3.4).

To calculate an odds ratio:

$$OR = \frac{\text{Odds that a case was exposed}}{\text{Odds that a control was exposed}} = \frac{a/c}{b/d} = \frac{ad}{bc}$$

As with RR, ORs indicate the strength of the association between the disease and exposure. Odds ratios range in value from 0 to infinity. To interpret the odds ratio, consider the following:

- If OR is near or equal to 1, there is no or little association (and therefore the exposure is not related to the disease).
- If OR >1, there is a positive association (and therefore the exposure is associated with an increased risk of the disease).
- If OR <1, there is a negative or inverse association.

The way ORs are interpreted is similar to RRs; however, now you should talk in terms of the odds of exposure, rather than the risk of disease. When the disease incidence is rare (present in less than 10% of the population), the OR approximates the relative risk, and then the OR can be reported in terms of disease risk.

SOURCES OF ERROR IN EPIDEMIOLOGICAL STUDIES

A primary aim of good research design is to minimise problems, such as error and bias, which may otherwise alter the outcomes of a study. There are two main types of error: *random error* (or chance error) and *systematic error* (or bias). Random error can occur when there is random sampling variation and/or random measurement error.

Random Error

If we sample a population, most of the time the characteristics of the people included in our study will be similar to the population as a whole. However, it is always possible that, by chance, the sample selected is not actually representative. This *random sampling variation* is more likely when small samples are used (less than 30), and can affect the generalisability of a study. There is no guaranteed way of preventing random sampling error, but the likelihood of it occurring is reduced when the sample size increases. Whenever possible, you should check for random sampling error if you have information on your target population (e.g. census data) against which to compare your sample.

Random measurement error refers to the random variation in measurement of key exposure or outcome variables. When you take measurements, there is a chance that there may be some sloppiness in the measurements and the data collected may vary by chance. For example, if you ask someone to recall whether they owned a pet 10 years ago, they may find it hard to recall accurately unless they have always or never had one.

Random variability in measurement can be minimised by the careful training of data collectors, and the use of standard protocols and routinely tested equipment.

Confidence intervals: we won't take you through the full range of statistical techniques that are used; however, we will introduce you to the confidence interval (CI), as each of the frequency estimates and measures of association described in this chapter should always be reported and interpreted with its associated confidence interval. The CI takes into account the random error that may be present based on the sample size and the variability in the measurements taken. It indicates the precision of your estimate of the true population parameter (e.g. RR) you are interested in.

The interval itself represents the range of statistically plausible values for the measure that is being estimated. A 95% CI is usually employed, meaning that 95% of the intervals computed with the appropriate formula will include the true value for the parameter you are estimating (RR, incidence, etc.). Always look at the full range of plausible values when interpreting a CI, not just the point estimate on its own.

Activity 3.5 discusses the introduction of error when using a self-reporting measure for data collection.

Systematic Error

Systematic error is a much more serious problem than random error in epidemiology. Because this error can be directional, we refer to it as *bias*. There are two types of bias to consider: *selection bias* and *information bias*. Bias can lead to incorrect results and, consequently, to incorrect conclusions about the association between the exposure and the outcome under

---

ACTIVITY 3.5 Issues Around Self-reporting

An investigator wants to measure daily fat intake among adolescents, and asks each participant to keep a food diary that will be used to assess their intake. Write a paragraph to describe how using a food diary might introduce error into the information the investigator is collecting.

Reflection

Did you consider that, even if all the adolescents are motivated and honest, and keep an accurate record of what they have eaten over the past week, it is very difficult to convert this diary into an accurate estimate of fat intake? For example, if a participant records the evening meal as spaghetti bolognaise, we don't know how large the portion was, or if the cook used lean mince or added extra oil in the cooking. We have to make estimates about the fat content of an "average" spaghetti bolognaise when converting the participant's food diary into estimated fat intake. In doing so, we could easily underestimate or overestimate fat intake, so the potential for random measurement error in this instrument (the food diary) is high.

investigation. Another type of error we need to consider is *confounding*, where factors other than those we are studying are acting to distort the study findings and can lead to incorrect conclusions.

Selection Bias

Selection bias arises when there are systematic differences between people involved in a study and those who are not involved in a study, or people assigned to a particular arm in an intervention study. This difference could be reflected in the way the sample was selected (*sampling bias*), or by the disproportionate representation of certain types of individuals who decide to participate after being selected by the investigators (commonly known as *participation bias*), or not to continue to participate in a longitudinal or cohort study (known as "loss to follow-up" or *attrition bias*). Sampling bias cannot be reduced by increasing the size of a sample; nor can it be measured using statistical tests. This form of bias arises when the identification of individuals for the sample is not truly random and so can affect the generalisability of the results.

Information Bias

Information bias (also known as *measurement bias*) occurs when either outcomes or exposures are systematically measured incorrectly. This can also be referred to as *misclassification* when the error in measuring exposures or outcomes results in assigning study participants to the wrong group or category within a study. The researcher may have incorrectly classified a person as being exposed to a risk factor when in fact they were not exposed; the data may incorrectly measure the amount of exposure; a person may be classified as having a disease when they don't, or as not having a disease when they do. Getting the grouping wrong in a cohort (based on exposure) or case-control study (based on case status) can result in the obscuring of important associations. If the errors are directional (e.g. the exposures are consistently under- or over-measured), then this might lead to completely spurious results that are hard to predict and impossible to detect.

Recall bias occurs when individuals with a disease are more likely to overestimate or underestimate their exposure than those without the disease. Recall bias is particularly an issue in retrospective studies, which ask participants for information about things that occurred sometime prior to the interview or survey. It is particularly an issue if the person is aware that they have the outcome of interest at the time they are recalling the exposure information (as in a cross-sectional study or a case-control study).

Interviewer bias, or *observer bias*, occurs when the interviewer asks questions or records information in a different way for different groups being compared. Systematic error in observation, measurement, analysis and interpretation can be controlled to some extent by using only one interviewer for the whole study, making the investigator/interviewer unaware of the study participant's exposure status ('blinding'), by training the interviewer, or with structured questionnaires or interviews and electronically recording interviews.

Confounding

Confounding can be an important source of error in epidemiological studies if it is not identified and addressed. Confounding occurs when a non-causal association between a given exposure and outcome is observed as a result of a third factor. Case Study 3.1 examines the issue of confounding factors.

Another example of confounding can be seen in Activity 3.6.

Finally, every study will be affected by some degree of error, and, while strategies can be implemented to reduce chance fluctuation and bias, in practice it is impossible to eliminate all sources of error. Therefore, it is important to always consider the effects that error may have on the results of any epidemiological study. Have you ever considered alternative explanations when you have heard media reports of new scientific discoveries? Next time you watch the news, or read a news report about some new discovery, stop to consider whether the

---

CASE STUDY 3.1 Confounding Factors

Let us consider our cat and asthma problem. Figure 3.2 shows this diagrammatically. Let us call the cat X (the exposure) and asthma Y (the outcome), and A is the confounder (some other factor that is associated with both the exposure and the outcome of interest that may be clouding the picture). Pollen is another known trigger for asthma. Many cats spend time outdoors as well as indoors; therefore, it might not be the cat itself that is associated with asthma, but the pollen it brings into the house on its fur. In order to rule out the confounding effect of pollen exposure when looking at the association between cats and asthma, you would have to measure pollen exposure and adjust for that statistically, so that you could then look at cat exposure independent of the confounding effects of pollen. Figure 3.2 illustrates the relationship between: (a) exposure X, disease Y and confounder A; (b) exposure X, disease Y and non-confounding factor on causal path A.

For a factor to be a confounder, it must meet the following criteria: it must be a definite risk factor for the disease (Y); it must be associated with the exposure of interest (X) under study; and it must not be an intermediate step between exposure (X) and the disease (Y). For example, obesity $\rightarrow$ hypertension $\rightarrow$ heart disease. Hypertension could be part of the causal chain, rather than a confounder.

Reflection

Why are confounding and error important to an epidemiologist? Confounding bias can undermine research by leading to an over- or underestimation of association between exposure and disease. In fact, it can completely mask an association within a study or even reverse the direction of a true association. It is therefore essential to anticipate potential sources of confounding.

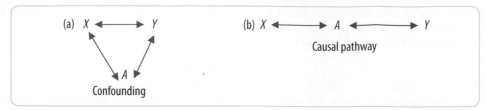

Fig. 3.2 Relationship between exposure, disease and confounder.

ACTIVITY 3.6   Evaluating Study Results

Is vitamin D deficiency associated with higher hospitalisation rates in people with COVID-19? A study conducted in north-west England of 80,670 people who had their vitamin D levels checked between April 2020 and January 2021 reported that hospital admissions for COVID-19 were 2.3 to 2.4 times higher in those people who had recorded a deficiency (Jude, 2021). Is this proof that vitamin D prevents serious COVID-19 illness? What else would you want to know about this study and the study participants before you reach any conclusions?

Reflection

Did you consider whether there might be other factors that could explain the apparent association? For example, were those people with normal vitamin D levels healthier and more health-conscious, and therefore less likely to have comorbidities that we know are associated with disease severity in COVID-19?

researchers have considered potential confounders. Refer to Table 3.1 for a review of experimental studies and their main components.

SUMMING IT UP

Epidemiology examines health at a population level, rather than at an individual level. Current developments in epidemiology focus on the contribution of intra-individual factors (e.g. inherited genetic susceptibility) and higher-level factors (e.g. social policy and climate change). Clinical medicine is excellent for examining health issues within the confines of known aspects of the human body, but it is not equipped to infer cause in the absence of well-controlled experiments. Olsen and colleagues, (2001, p. 15) wrote:

> *In its historical evolution epidemiology's successes have largely derived from its working as the investigative component of public health, studying the distribution and determinants of health and diseases in populations. This essence should continue to be preserved in the foreseeable future by incorporating into epidemiological research the new opportunities currently arising in particular fields of genetics, environmental sciences, medicine, and health care.*

In order to prevent disease effectively, epidemiologists have a responsibility not only to use appropriate methods, but also to translate their findings into something of benefit to both the local and the global communities.

The end of the cat and asthma story is still being unravelled, partly because of the difficulties in designing the perfect study that we have alluded to throughout this chapter. Cat fur and dander are proven triggers for asthma attacks in those with asthma. There is some evidence that those with asthma do give up their cat(s), but this is not considered to be as large an issue as previously thought, and may not fully account for the inverse associations we see between cat exposure and asthma (see below). The latest studies indicate that being exposed to a cat before developing asthma may indeed help some children develop tolerance and have a protective effect. One of the pivotal papers in this field of research is by Cecile Svanes and colleagues (Svanes et al, 2006), and you can look up more of this author's work if you are interested in following the story.

A FINAL WORD

This chapter has provided an introduction to some basic epidemiological concepts. As practising epidemiologists, we need to build on these concepts and consider more complex methods of assessing evidence, taking into account various measures of association and causal inference.

REVIEW QUESTIONS

1. Define the term "epidemiology" in your own words.
2. Describe how epidemiology differs from clinical medicine.
3. Describe two measures of disease frequency.
4. Discuss the differences between prevalence and incidence.
5. Explain the differences between observational and experimental study designs, giving examples of each.
6. What do relative risk and odds ratio measure?
7. What is the technical term used by epidemiologists when a third factor influences the relationship between an exposure of interest and a disease? Give examples.
8. Describe two types of systematic bias that epidemiologists should consider.
9. How might you use epidemiology in your future profession?

ACKNOWLEDGEMENTS

The author would like to acknowledge those who assisted with the development of early components of this chapter: Michelle Cook, Mary-Anne Kedda, Bonnie Macfarlane and Beth Newman, formerly of the School of Public Health, QUT; Diana Battistutta, Michael Dunne and Kate Halton, of the School of Public Health and Social Work, QUT; and Christopher Stevenson, School of Health and Social Development, Deakin University.

USEFUL WEBSITES

Centers for Disease Control and Prevention: http://www.cdc.gov/ophss/csels/dsepd/SS1978/Glossary.html

Epidemiology Supercourse: http://www.pitt.edu/~super1

John Snow—a historical giant in epidemiology: http://www.ph.ucla.edu/epi/snow.html

The James Lind Library: http://www.jameslindlibrary.org

REFERENCES

Abaluck J, Kwong LH, Styczynski A, et al 2022 Impact of community masking on COVID-19: A cluster-randomized trial in Bangladesh. *Science* 375(6577): eabi9069. https://doi.org/doi:10.1126/science.abi9069

Achilleos S, Quattrocchi A, Gabel J, et al 2021 Excess all-cause mortality and COVID-19-related mortality: a temporal analysis in 22 countries, from January until August 2020. *International Journal of Epidemiology* 51(1): 35–53. doi:10.1093/ije/dyab123

Australian Institute of Health and Welfare 2011 Principles on the use of direct age-standardisation in administrative data collections. For measuring the gap between Indigenous and non-Indigenous Australians. Canberra. Available: https://www.aihw.gov.au/getmedia/95237794-4b77-4683-9f00-77c4d33e0e7c/13406.pdf.aspx?inline=true#:~:text=Age%2Dstandardisation%20is%20a%20technique,between%20the%20populations%20being%20compared

Cerio H, Schad LA, Stewart TM, et al 2021 Relationship between COVID-19 cases and vaccination rates in New York State counties. *PRiMER* 5: 35. https://doi.org/10.22454/PRiMER.2021.432215

Huang L, Li X, Gu X, et al 2022 Health outcomes in people 2 years after surviving hospitalisation with COVID-19: a longitudinal cohort study. *The Lancet Respiratory Medicine*. https://doi.org/10.1016/S2213-2600(22)00126-6

Jude EB, Ling SF, Allcock R, et al 2021 Vitamin D deficiency is associated with higher hospitalization risk from COVID-19: a retrospective case-control study. *The Journal of Clinical Endocrinology and Metabolism* 106(11): e4708–15. doi:10.1210/clinem/dgab439.

Kory P, Meduri GU, Varon J, et al 2021 Review of the emerging evidence demonstrating the efficacy of ivermectin in the prophylaxis and treatment of COVID-19. *American Journal of Therapeutics* 28(3): e299–318. doi:10.1097/MJT.0000000000001377

Mude W, Meru C, Njue C, et al 2021 A cross-sectional study of COVID-19 impacts in culturally and linguistically diverse communities in greater Western Sydney, Australia. *BMC Public Health* 21, 2081. https://doi.org/10.1186/s12889-021-12172-y

Olsen JR, Saracci R, Trichopoulos D, 2001 Teaching epidemiology: a guide for teachers in epidemiology, public health and clinical medicine. Oxford: Oxford University Press

Porta M, 2014 A Dictionary of epidemiology. Oxford: Oxford University Press. https://doi.org/10.1093/acref/9780195314496.001.0001

Rodriguez-Lopez M, Parra B, Vergara E, et al 2021 A case-control study of factors associated with SARS-CoV-2 infection among healthcare workers in Colombia. *BMC Infectious Diseases* 21, 878. https://doi.org/10.1186/s12879-021-06581-y

Svanes C, Zock JP, Antó J, et al 2006 Does asthma and allergy influence subsequent pet keeping? An analysis of childhood and adulthood. *Journal of Allergy and Clinical Immunology* 118(3): 691–8

World Health Organization (WHO) 1948 Preamble to the Constitution of the World Health Organization as adopted by the International Health Conference, New York, 19–22 June 1946; signed on 22 July 1946 by the representatives of 61 States and entered into force on 7 April 1948. http://www.who.int/about/definition/en/print.html

4

Aboriginal and Torres Strait Islander Health

*Ray Mahoney**

LEARNING OBJECTIVES

After reading this chapter, you should be able to:

- Outline the role and importance of Aboriginal and Torres Strait Islander community-controlled health organisations.
- Provide an overview of the issues associated with research with Aboriginal and Torres Strait Islander peoples.

- Describe why Aboriginal and Torres Strait Islander Australians experience poorer health status than other Australians.
- Discuss some of the public health strategies being utilised to address health disparities in Australia.
- Advocate for extra emphasis and effort in improving the health of Aboriginal and Torres Strait Islander peoples.

INTRODUCTION

Aboriginal and Torres Strait Islander peoples are recognised as the Traditional Custodians of the lands and waters of Australia. Aboriginal and Torres Strait Islander peoples have a long and enduring connection to our lands and waters and celebrate this through spirit, language and culture. As the original inhabitants of Australia our continuing cultural connection to this land has been estimated to be more than 65,000 years, the world's oldest living continuous culture. Aboriginal and Torres Strait Islander people are our first educators, healers, scientists and researchers.

This chapter will detail contemporary health policies and practices and explore the impact of European colonisation on the health and wellbeing of Aboriginal and Torres Strait Islander people. It presents contemporary public health challenges and approaches to address health disparities through codesign, and is developed, delivered and led by Aboriginal and Torres Strait Islander people. There are similar disparities across all social, economic and health indicators. Specific public health approaches are needed to address these disparities and improve both the health status and the wellbeing of Aboriginal and Torres Strait Islander peoples. This chapter focuses on Aboriginal and Torres Strait Islander health within

Australia. It complements the content relating to Aboriginal and Torres Strait Islander peoples found in the other chapters in this book.

WHO ARE ABORIGINAL AND TORRES STRAIT ISLANDER PEOPLES?

Aboriginal and Torres Strait Islander peoples are the Indigenous peoples of Australia. Aboriginal peoples are indigenous to mainland Australia, and Torres Strait Islanders are indigenous to the islands between the Australian mainland and New Guinea. Australia and New Guinea annexed the Torres Strait Islands in the 1800s. Archaeological evidence from Northern Australia found the world's oldest-known edge-ground hatchets, demonstrating that Aboriginal people have lived in Australia for at least 65,000 years (Clarkson et al, 2017). Aboriginal peoples belonged (and still belong) to specific geographical areas, known as "Country". "Country" refers to a specific clan, tribal group or nation of Aboriginal people, and encompasses all the knowledge, cultural norms, values, stories and resources within that area. It is estimated that before European settlement there were 250–300 languages, with 600 dialects, spoken by Aboriginal and Torres Strait Islander peoples (Australian Institute of Aboriginal and Torres Strait Islander Studies [AIATSIS], 1994).

The notion of Country is central to Australian Aboriginal identity, and contributes to overall health and wellbeing. Torres Strait Islander people identify particular islands or island

---

*In the third edition, this chapter was written by Bronwyn Fredericks, Vanessa Lee, Mick Adams and Ray Mahoney.

groups as the areas to which they belong. While Aboriginal and Torres Strait Islander peoples are generally grouped under one banner, there are significant differences in social, cultural and linguistic customs between different clan groups (AIATSIS, 1994).

Prior to colonisation, Aboriginal and Torres Strait Islander peoples had complex societies and self-determining lives, with control over all of life's aspects, including ceremony, spiritual practices, medicine, birthing, child-rearing, relationships, management of land and organisational systems and law. People had a healthy diet of protein and plants that contained adequate minerals and vitamins. They ate very little fat, sugar and salt (Flood, 2006). They looked after their individual, family and community health and wellbeing, with most treatment provided by traditional spiritual healers and self-care, using traditional remedies (Couzos & Murray, 2008). Aboriginal people were active with fishing, hunting, food-gathering, land management, ceremonies and visiting other nations on their Country. They were physically fit (Dudgeon et al, 2010).

Evidence like that relating to the Gunditjmara people continues to emerge, which demonstrates that Aboriginal communities had all the characteristics of a 'modern complex' society. The Gunditjmara people are the traditional owners and nation of a specific geographical area in Victoria known as 'Gunditjmara Country', which extends from Portland in the south, around the coast to Port Fairy and Warrnambool, and inland to Camperdown. Gunditjmara people maintained a complex eel aquaculture system that produced a valuable and highly nutritious resource with seasonal abundance, and had the ability to preserve it for storage and trading. This resource specialisation was supported by permanent settlement of the area, and by an infrastructure associated with high productivity and the means to feed large numbers of people (Builth, 2005).

Accounts from early colonisers present evidence that, at the time of colonisation, Aboriginal people who survived infancy were fairly disease-free, fit and healthy. For example, James Cook outlined on several occasions the health and physical status of the Aboriginal peoples he observed. Cook stated that they were 'of middle Stature straight bodied slender-limb'd the Colour of Wood soot or of dark chocolate… Their features are far from disagreeable' (Cook in Clark 1966, p. 51). Eyre, an early European explorer writing on the Murray River area, described the Aboriginal people of that area as 'almost free from diseases and well-shaped in body and limb' (quoted in Cleland, 1928). Prior to the arrival of the British in 1788, Aboriginal Australian peoples experienced a relatively healthy lifestyle and quality of life (Saggers & Gray, 1991, p. 59).

Colonisation had a profound impact on Australia's Aboriginal and Torres Strait Islander peoples. The establishment of the British penal colony at Botany Bay began a parallel destruction of Aboriginal lifestyles and cultures. It involved massacres and the removal of children from their mothers, families, peoples and lands (Blainey, 1994; Evans et al, 1975; Rintoul, 1993).

ACTIVITY 4.1 Aboriginal Pre- and Post-colonisation Experience

Answer the following questions:
- Aboriginal people in Australia are often referred to as 'the oldest living culture on the planet'. Why do you think they are described as such?
- What do you think would be the kind of knowledge that Aboriginal people would have needed to sustain their health and wellbeing for such a long time?
- Why did colonisation have such an impact on the health and wellbeing of Aboriginal and Torres Strait Islander peoples? How might some of these events and issues from the past affect the health and wellbeing of Aboriginal and Torres Strait Islander peoples today?

Reflection

Reflect on your own background and your family's history. What is your culture? Where are your family from? What has been your family's history over the past 200 years? How have government and institutional policies directed, and impacted on, your family's health and wellbeing? How can you draw on your own family's history and culture to gain an understanding of how Aboriginal and Torres Strait Islander peoples might feel about their experiences?

Colonisation brought with it infectious diseases, such as smallpox, to which Aboriginal people had little immunity. The ill health of Aboriginal and Torres Strait Islander peoples today continues to exceed that of any other sector of Australian society across all measures of health inequality (Australian Institute of Health and Welfare [AIHW], 2018; National Aboriginal and Torres Strait Islander Health Council [NATSIHC], 2001). Since colonisation, Aboriginal and Torres Strait Islander peoples have been subjected to intense levels of discrimination and systemic disadvantage experienced over many decades (Mazel, 2018). The causes of the continued health inequality can be partly attributed to the continuing devastating impact of colonisation and the subsequent cultural devastation, facilitated by the assimilation, racism, trauma, poverty and social exclusion experienced by Aboriginal and Torres Strait Islander peoples (Dudgeon et al, 2014; Mazel, 2018). Activity 4.1 asks you to consider these issues.

GOVERNMENT POLICY

From the time of colonisation, policy decisions made by non-Indigenous people about Aboriginal and Torres Strait Islander peoples have influenced their health and wellbeing. The modern history of Aboriginal and Torres Strait Islander peoples is one of control by government and institutions. Policies were (and are) made by federal, state and territory governments, by churches and other institutions. A range of people, including health professionals, police officers and church and government administrators, have helped to implement the policies (and, in some instances, have carried out questionable practices). Phillips (2003, p. 93) explains that a range of people 'operated in concert to suppress local Aboriginal sovereignty, steal their lands, and destroy their languages, cultures and social cohesion'. An obvious example is the practice of removing children from their families. This practice continued through the 1950s and 1960s under child welfare legislation in most states, and allowed missionaries, government officials and others to restrict contact between Aboriginal children and their parents and culture (Beresford & Omaji, 1998, p. 96). Other government policies prevented Aboriginal and Torres Strait Islander peoples from enjoying the rights that other Australians exercised, such as buying a home, voting, moving from one town to another, receiving wages for work and going to school or university. These policies were implemented in the living memories of today's Aboriginal and Torres Strait Islander peoples, families and communities. They contribute to the attitudes held today by Aboriginal and Torres Strait Islander peoples towards health professionals, healthcare delivery, religious people, teachers, law-and-order workers and government officials. Some of the practices resulted in *situational traumatisation*, which has 'produced cumulative trauma as a result of shame and self-hate, and intergenerational trauma as a result of unresolved and unaddressed grief and loss' (Phillips, 2003, p. 23).

THE NATIONAL ABORIGINAL HEALTH STRATEGY 1987

In recent times, a concerted effort has been made by governments and institutions to address the poor health of Aboriginal and Torres Strait Islander peoples. The National Aboriginal Health Strategy Working Party, established in 1987, produced the *National Aboriginal Health Strategy* (NAHS) (NAHS, 1989). The NAHS was an important milestone, being the first time that representatives from Aboriginal and Torres Strait Islander communities, the Commonwealth, and the state and territory governments had collaborated on a national policy for Aboriginal and Torres Strait Islander peoples and embedded an Aboriginal and Torres Strait Islander concept of health in a national document:

> *Health is not just the physical wellbeing of the individual but the social, emotional, and cultural wellbeing of the whole community. This is a whole-of-life view and it also includes the cyclical concept of life–death–life (NAHS, 1989, p. ix)*

This statement has been widely adopted by Aboriginal and Torres Strait Islander peoples themselves, and in various government and academic documents. It has been used by Aboriginal and Torres Strait Islander peoples to work with governments to deliver more comprehensive health services and primary healthcare services. However, despite the efforts of many people, the NAHS was never fully funded. It is important to understand the significance of this document in relation to the history of Aboriginal and Torres Strait Islander health, including public health, in Australia.

CONTEMPORARY HEALTH POLICY

In July 2020, the Australian Government launched the new National Agreement on Closing the Gap. While NAHS will always be recognised as a significant milestone as the beginning of consultation with Aboriginal and Torres Strait Islander peoples in the development of health policy, this new Agreement is seen as the first National policy for Aboriginal and Torres Strait Islander peoples developed and negotiated between governments and Aboriginal and Torres Strait Islander representatives (Commonwealth of Australia, 2020).

This achievement is the result of many years of strong advocacy by the *Close the Gap* campaign for Aboriginal and Torres Strait Islander health equality. This human rights-based campaign was publicly launched in April 2007 and was initiated following the Aboriginal and Torres Strait Islander Social Justice Commissioner's *Social Justice Report 2005*. Australia's peak Aboriginal and Torres Strait Islander and non-Indigenous health bodies, non-government organisations (NGOs) and human rights organisations first met as the Close the Gap Steering Committee (CTGSC) in March 2006 (National Aboriginal Community Controlled Health Organisation [NACCHO] & Oxfam, 2007). The steering committee was led by its Aboriginal and Torres Strait Islander members.

The goal of the campaign is to close the gap by 2030: to raise the health and life expectancy of Aboriginal and Torres Strait Islander peoples so that within one generation they are on par with those of the non-Indigenous population (CTGSC, 2011, p. 2; Human Rights and Equal Opportunity Commission [HREOC], 2008, p. 5).

The terms 'Close the Gap' and 'Closing the Gap' are used interchangeably to describe a wide range of events, initiatives and government-led policy aiming to reduce the health and life expectancy gap between Aboriginal and Torres Strait Islander peoples and non-Indigenous peoples in Australia.

The National Agreement on Closing the Gap supports the need to address the social and cultural factors that influence the gap, including housing, community safety and security, justice, education, culture, language, community development and other issues that influence the health and wellbeing of Aboriginal and Torres Strait Islander peoples. These issues are often referred to as the *social determinants of health* (discussed in particular in Chapters 1, 2, 3 and 6), and they have specific relevance in addressing the health of Aboriginal and Torres Strait Islander peoples, who have lower levels of education, employment and income, and poorer-quality housing, than non-Indigenous Australians (AIHW, 2022; Fisher et al, 2019).

Each year since 2009, the Prime Minister has reported to federal parliament on progress in closing the gap; and each year since 2010, the *Australian Human Rights Commission (AHRC) Close the Gap Steering Committee Report* has published a 'shadow' report that is an assessment of the Australian Government's progress (CTGSC, 2016).

In 2020, the Close the Gap Campaign Report changed to a strengths-based analysis of good health through an Aboriginal and Torres Strait Islander narrative in the context of continuing to 'critique' Government Policy. The key message in the 2022 Report is the continuing missed opportunity by Governments and mainstream organisations in failing to recognise and invest in Aboriginal and Torres Strait Islander leadership and capacity. The 2022 Report highlights that this lack of investment continues to slow progress on addressing and eliminating racism, providing equal and equitable access to essential infrastructure and achieving true gender and climate justice (Lowitja Institute, 2022).

Following the signing of the National Agreement on Closing the Gap in 2020, in 2021 the Australian Government released the National Aboriginal and Torres Strait Islander Health Plan 2021–2031. This new policy framework commits State, Territory and National Government to the National Agreement on Closing the Gap, to improve health outcomes for Aboriginal and Torres Strait Islander people with a focus on the following Priority Reforms:

- Prioritising the Aboriginal and Torres Strait Islander community-controlled health sector.
- Actions to address racism.
- Mainstream health services are responsive and accountable to Aboriginal and Torres Strait Islander people and communities (Department of Health and Ageing, 2021).

Only time will tell if the aspirations of the Coalition of Peaks (Box 4.1), as representatives of the Nations community-controlled organisations, entrusted with the responsibility

---

ACTIVITY 4.2 Profile and Culture of Aboriginal and Torres Strait Islander Peoples

Answer the following questions:
- How many Aboriginal and Torres Strait Islander peoples live in the area in which you live?
- What are some of the Aboriginal and Torres Strait Islander organisations in your area or region? What do they do? Who goes there? Who works there? Have you noticed them before? Why/why not?
- Look at the local news reports in your city or regional area and analyse the way in which Aboriginal and Torres Strait Islander peoples and cultures are written about.

Reflection

What are some of the stressors you might experience being an Aboriginal or Torres Strait Islander person living in the city? How would you cope?

---

of negotiating on behalf of all Aboriginal and Torres Strait Islander people, will deliver true reform under this new Agreement.

Evidence of the impact of racism on the health of Aboriginal and Torres Strait Islander peoples continues to mount; in many cases, racism is considered an additional social determinant of health. The 2020 Australian Reconciliation Barometer found that racism is on the rise, with 60% of Aboriginal and Torres Strait Islander people now agreeing that Australia is a racist country, compared with 51% in 2018 in the same survey. Unfortunately this worrying trend continues with 52% of Aboriginal and Torres Strait Islander people experiencing at least one form of racial prejudice in the past 6 months compared with 43% in 2018 (ARB, 2020). Complete Activity 4.2 for a greater understanding of racism.

A 2012 survey, entitled The Mental Health Impacts of Racial Discrimination in Victorian Aboriginal Communities: The Localities Embracing and Accepting Diversity (LEAD) Experiences of Racism, found that 97% of respondents reported at least one racist incident in the past 12 months, and that Aboriginal and Torres Strait Islander people experienced racism in settings for key social determinants of health: education (51%), employment (42%), housing (35%) and health (29%) (Ferdinand et al, 2012).

ABORIGINAL AND TORRES STRAIT ISLANDER PEOPLES TODAY

In the 2021 Australian Census, Australia's Aboriginal and Torres Strait Islander population was reported to be 812,728 people, or 3.2% of the total Australian population of

---

BOX 4.1 Coalition of Peaks

The Partnership Agreement on Closing the Gap between the Coalition of Peaks and Council of Australian Governments details the agreed arrangements for shared decision-making on the design, implementation, monitoring and review of Closing the Gap strategy for the next 10 years.

The Coalition of Peaks is a representative body of over 70 Aboriginal and Torres Strait Islander community-controlled peak organisations and members. This Coalition came together as an act of self-determination to be formal partners with Australian governments on Closing the Gap.

The Coalition of Peaks are accountable to their communities, with a long history of advocacy, service delivery and leadership to ensure the full involvement of Aboriginal and Torres Strait Islander peoples in shared decision-making.

The formal partnership agreement defines the responsibility of the agreement as:
- Joint Council on Closing The Gap.
- Review the National Indigenous Reform Agreement.
- Three-yearly Indigenous-led Evaluation of Closing the Gap.
- Support for Aboriginal and Torres Strait Islander Partnership participation.
- Partnership Governance & Status.

More detail on their web site: https://coalitionofpeaks.org.au/

25,422,788 people (Australian Bureau of Statistics [ABS], 2022). Of the total Aboriginal and Torres Strait Islander population, 81% live in major cities and non-remote areas (ABS, 2018). This is in contrast to perceptions held by many Australians, and to the images shown by the Australian media that show Aboriginal and Torres Strait Islanders in Very Remote and/or Remote regions that make up 19% of the total population. There are large urban populations in some areas; for example, the ABS estimated that for 2018, 221,276 Aboriginal and Torres Strait Islander peoples (or 27.7% of Australia's total Aboriginal and Torres Strait Islander population) live in Queensland (ABS, 2018). Some Aboriginal and Torres Strait Islander peoples are now second-, third- or multi-generation urban dwellers, while others may travel to and from cities and big urban centres and their home communities. When Aboriginal and Torres Strait Islander peoples migrate into capital cities, they tend to move to areas where there are already concentrations of Aboriginal and Torres Strait Islander peoples—generally areas of low socioeconomic status (Taylor, 2006).

Living in urban areas is as much a part of reality for Aboriginal and Torres Strait Islander peoples as living in discrete Aboriginal rural, regional or isolated communities, or on one of the Torres Strait islands (Fredericks, 2004; Rowse, 2006). The Aboriginal and Torres Strait Islander population is also much younger than the non-Indigenous Australian population. In 2016, the median age of Aboriginal and Torres Strait Islander people was 23 years, compared with 38 years for the non-Indigenous population, with 53.1% of the Aboriginal and Torres Strait Islander population under the age of 25 (ABS, 2018).

Australia ranks lowest among the first-world wealthy nations in working to improve the health and life expectancy of its Indigenous peoples, while internationally life expectancy for non-Indigenous peoples has improved significantly over the past few decades (Australian Health Ministers Advisory Council, 2017). Life expectancy for Australia's Aboriginal and Torres Strait Islander peoples continues to lag behind that of non-Indigenous Australians with the gap in life expectancy remaining at approximately 10 years less. Aboriginal and Torres Strait Islander males have a life expectancy of 71.6 years compared with 81.2 for non-Indigenous males, and for Aboriginal and Torres Strait Islander females life expectancy is 75.6 years compared with 85.3 for non-Indigenous females (Australian Institute of Health and Welfare, 2022).

COMMUNITY-CONTROLLED HEALTH SERVICE SECTOR

Aboriginal Community Controlled Health Organisations (ACCHOs) are now found in every state and territory of Australia. The first such service, the Redfern Aboriginal Medical Service, was established by Aboriginal people in 1971 in the Sydney suburb of Redfern as a community response to the poor health services that Aboriginal people received. The aim of the service was to deliver holistic, comprehensive and culturally appropriate health care (NATSIHC, 2001). There are now 144 ACCHOs in urban, regional and remote Australia (NACCHO website). They range from large multi-functional services providing a wide range of medical, social and community services to small services made up of Aboriginal Health Workers and/or nurses delivering high quality primary care services, with a preventive, health education focus. See Case Study 4.1 and answer the accompanying questions to enhance your understanding of comprehensive care for Aboriginal people.

Community-controlled health services diagnose and treat illness, provide referrals to specialists and other providers, refer to allied health services (sometimes with visiting programs such as optometry and podiatry), provide counselling and support, and undertake broader community advocacy. They may also undertake research, support the development of culturally appropriate materials and provide training for health professionals. Most ACCHOs are run by a board of directors or a management committee that is elected by its members. The local Aboriginal and Torres Strait Islander populations become members of the Aboriginal Community Controlled Health Service (ACCHS). Accountability is through the board, annual general meetings, annual reports and reports to funding bodies (NATSIHC, 2001). The board sets the overall direction of the ACCHS and formally employs the staff.

The ACCHSs have a national representative organisation— the National Aboriginal Community Controlled Health Organisation (NACCHO). There are also state- and territory-based representative organisations. NACCHO and its state- and territory-based affiliates provide a representative voice for Aboriginal and Torres Strait Islander communities on health-related issues. They also have work areas that focus specifically on public health and research.

ACCHSs play an important role in providing primary healthcare services for Aboriginal and Torres Strait Islander people that are planned and managed by the communities themselves (Activity 4.3).

RESEARCH

There is a long history of research conducted on Aboriginal and Torres Strait Islander peoples, and on First Nations peoples throughout the world. Tuhiwai Smith (1999, p. 3) suggests that Aboriginal and Torres Strait Islander people 'are the most researched people in the world'. Historically, the vast majority of this research was carried out by non-Indigenous people. Often, research intrudes into Aboriginal and Torres Strait Islander peoples' lives and communities. For many years,

CASE STUDY 4.1 St George Community Wellbeing Centre

Goondir Aboriginal and Torres Strait Islander Corporation for Health Services is an Aboriginal Medical Service providing holistic healthcare since the mid 1990s with extensive community engagement within Goondir's service region. Predominantly these services cater to the Aboriginal and Torres Strait Islander people across an area of approximately 72,000 square km, from Oakey in South East Queensland to St George in far South East Queensland. Goondir's operations include medical centres at Dalby, Oakey and St George as well as a Mobile Service using a clinical van to cover the communities of Dirranbandi, Jandowae, Surat, Thallon, Chinchilla, Miles, Tara and surrounding regions.

In 2018, Goondir purchased the St George Returned and Services League (RSL) building with a view of refurbishing and establishing the St George Community Wellbeing Centre.

Community consultation revealed that there was no single facility or service that provided accessible holistic health and wellbeing services within the St George community. Existing providers operated independently on smaller scales given the community's reluctance to accessing such services within a clinical setting.

Goondir established partnerships with organisations operating in and around the St George community to collectively host over 30 programs and activities within the Community Wellbeing Centre (CWBC) targeted at the social determinants of health for Aboriginal and Torres Strait Islander health and wellbeing.

As a remote rural community of 3130 people with the Aboriginal and Torres Strait Islander population comprising 22% of the St George population, it faces issues similar to rural communities across Australia—high incidence of chronic disease, youth disengagement, domestic and family violence, mental health issues stemming from intergenerational trauma, unemployment, high rates of criminal offences, substance abuse and youth suicide.

The CWBC and its activities seeks to address these challenges in a holistic manner, using evidence-based approaches to strategically incorporate reform into everyday activities. They span across health and social-emotional wellbeing services, cultural development, youth engagement and empowerment, women empowerment, training and education, exercise and fitness, food security, nutrition and healthy lifestyle intervention and social support and enterprise.

Facilities within the St George CWBC support and host these specific programs:
- Big Buddy Youth Program (Youth empowerment).
- Cultural Development Program (Binna Thinna Tharrka) (connection to culture/SEWB through art and artefact workshops).
- Healthy Body and Mind.
- Food Distribution Program (addressing nutrition and food insecurity needs).
- Wandir Gunde Playgroup (early childhood development).
- Gira Gira Women's Group (social activity, safe yarning space).
- Suga Shakers Diabetes Group (healthy lifestyle promotion).
- Elders' Groups.

All these activities collectively address health, social and emotional wellbeing and the social determinants of health impacting the St George community. Goondir will also work with leading education and research institutions to perform a medium- to long-term evaluation of the collective impact the CWBC's programs and activities have on the health and social determinants of health within the St George community.

Questions

1. What might have been the catalyst for the Goondir Health Service to establish the Wellbeing Centre in St George? What evidence and/or sources would you access to support your case if you were establishing this initiative?
2. What would you consider to be the health risk factors relevant to this cohort of people, and what may need to be considered in developing public health responses for Aboriginal and Torres Strait Islander people in these communities?
3. What might be some of the barriers to accessing services to address social determinants of health for people living in rural and remote areas? Are there any barriers that only Aboriginal and Torres Strait Islander people may face? Would these be different in urban settings?
4. Consider some of the challenges facing Aboriginal and Torres Strait Islander people living in rural and remote communities across Queensland. How might the definition of Aboriginal health, the history of colonisation and past policies of administration (discussed earlier in this chapter) affect the way you approach delivering services as a non-Indigenous health practitioner?

Aboriginal and Torres Strait Islander peoples questioned research: how non-Indigenous people have wrongfully assumed ownership of Aboriginal and Torres Strait Islander knowledge; how museums and libraries have misappropriated precious objects and ancestral remains; and why numerous non-Indigenous people have gained qualifications, assumed 'expert' status over and above Aboriginal and Torres Strait Islander people and secured career advancement and increased salaries, while the communities that are 'researched' have been left with very little.

Over the past 20 years, there have been considerable changes in the way research is conducted with Aboriginal and Torres Strait Islander populations. Even the *Medical Journal of Australia* raised concerns about the 'dearth of interventional studies' being published, due to a perceived deficit-focused research conducted by authors seeking publication (Thomas et al, 2014). Since 1997, the Lowitja Institute, Australia's national institute for Aboriginal and Torres Strait Islander health research, has led a substantial reform agenda in health research by working with communities, researchers and policymakers,

ACTIVITY 4.3 Aboriginal and Torres Strait Islander Health Services

Access a few of the following organisational websites:

Aboriginal and Torres Strait Islander Community Health Service Brisbane Ltd: http://www.atsichsbrisbane.org.au/

Danila Dilba Health Service, Biluru (Aboriginal and Torres Strait Islander) people in the Yilli Rreung (greater Darwin) region of the Northern Territory: https://ddhs.org.au/

HealthInfoNet: https://healthinfonet.ecu.edu.au/

National Aboriginal Community Controlled Health Organisation (NACCHO): http://www.naccho.org.au/

Queensland Aboriginal and Islander Health Council (QAIHC): http://www.qaihc.com.au/

Victorian Aboriginal Community Controlled Health Organisation (VACCHO): http://www.vaccho.org.au/

Victorian Aboriginal Health Service: http://www.vahs.org.au/

Wuchopperen Health Service: http://www.wuchopperen.com/

Questions

- What are the aims of Aboriginal and Torres Strait Islander health services? What kinds of services do they offer?
- Who are the websites designed for? How are they structured and presented? Is their structure different to other health websites?
- What are five key messages you have gained about the community-controlled health service sector?
- What are some of the issues they might face in the future?

Reflection

Think about why Aboriginal and Torres Strait Islander peoples established their own health services, and why they still exist today. A number of them have been going for over 40 years, showing great sustainability and strength in organisational management. Think about the changes in policy they have experienced along the way. Try to imagine what some of the challenges and benefits might be in working in an Aboriginal community-controlled health organisation on a day-to-day and week-to-week basis.

with Aboriginal and Torres Strait Islander people setting the agenda and driving the outcomes. Several publications on ethics and protocols in Aboriginal and Torres Strait Islander health research have been developed since the 1990s. The National Health and Medical Research Council (NHMRC) has produced and regularly updated research guidelines for all health research and contains a chapter specifically for Aboriginal and Torres Strait Islander research (see the National Statement on Ethical Conduct in Human Research (2007) – Updated 2018, Chapter 4.7: Aboriginal and Torres Strait Islander peoples: https://www.nhmrc.gov.au/about-us/publications/national-statement-ethical-conduct-human-research-2007-updated-2018#toc__1428).

The NHMRC is Australia's largest health research funding body and mandates that researchers respond to the Indigenous research excellence priorities:

- Community engagement.
- Benefit.
- Sustainability and transferability
- Building capability.

In December 2020 the Australian Institute of Aboriginal and Torres Strait Islander Studies (AIATSIS) released the updated *AIATSIS Code of Ethics for Aboriginal and Torres Strait Islander Research* and *A Guide to applying The AIATSIS Code of Ethics for Aboriginal and Torres Strait Islander Research*. These documents recognise that Aboriginal and Torres Strait Islander peoples have the right to control and maintain their culture and heritage, and that means benefiting from research undertaken by, with and about them. The four major principles of the AIATSIS research ethics framework are:

- Indigenous self-determination.
- Indigenous leadership.
- Impact and value.
- Sustainability and accountability.

Researchers in Australia now have access to extensive guidelines to assist and support the development and delivery of health research that protects and supports Aboriginal and Torres Strait Islander people (AIATSIS, 2022: https://aiatsis.gov.au/research/ethical-research).

Indigenous Data Sovereignty and Governance has become an important priority for Aboriginal and Torres Strait Islander people. Indigenous Data Sovereignty and Governance advocates for Aboriginal and Torres Strait Islander people to be informed when, how and why their data are gathered, analysed, accessed and used; and ensuring Indigenous data reflects Aboriginal and Torres Strait Islander peoples' priorities, values, culture, lifeworlds and diversity.

To support researchers navigate Indigenous Data Sovereignty and Governance, in 2021, the Lowitja Institute released the Indigenous Data Sovereignty Readiness Assessment and Evaluation Toolkit (Lowitja Institute, 2021). This guide was developed to evaluate Indigenous Data Sovereignty (ID-SOV) principles and practices in action within research and academic organisations, and as a resource for Aboriginal and Torres Strait Islander communities and organisations to identify ID-SOV in practice. The goal of the ID-SOV Toolkit is to improve the capabilities and processes of individuals through a whole-of-organisation approach to embedding ID-SOV in practice.

A FINAL WORD

Within the Australian population, Aboriginal and Torres Strait Islander peoples have the poorest health status and are considered the most socially and economically disadvantaged. The reasons for this are complex, and include a range of factors that influence health and wellbeing, such as housing, community safety and security, justice, education, culture, language, employment and income, locality, community development and discrimination based on race. In order for public health to make a difference to the health and wellbeing of Aboriginal and Torres Strait Islander peoples, it needs to recognise, understand and work across the historical, cultural, social, physiological, psychosocial, economic, environmental and political contexts of individuals, groups and communities (Dune et al, 2021). The poor health and wellbeing of Aboriginal and Torres Strait Islander peoples presents many challenges for public health workers, researchers, policy makers and clinicians. As the subpopulation with the greatest need, it is also the area where you can make the greatest difference.

REVIEW QUESTIONS

1. How has colonisation impacted on Aboriginal and Torres Strait Islander peoples' health and wellbeing?
2. What are some of the present-day health and wellbeing concerns of Aboriginal and Torres Strait Islander peoples?
3. What might you need to consider when working with Aboriginal and Torres Strait Islander peoples in improving their health and wellbeing?
4. What do you understand to be the social determinants of health, and how do they impact on the health and wellbeing of Aboriginal and Torres Strait Islander peoples?
5. What are the differences between the 'Close the Gap' campaign and the 'Closing the Gap' policy?
6. What are some of the settings where Aboriginal and Torres Strait Islander people may experience racism?

USEFUL WEBSITES

Australian Bureau of Statistics (ABS): http://www.abs.gov.au/

Aboriginal and Torres Strait Islander Peoples: http://www.abs.gov.au/Aboriginal-and-Torres-Strait-Islander-Peoples

Australian Indigenous HealthInfoNet: http://www.healthinfonet.ecu.edu.au/

Australian Institute of Health and Welfare (AIHW): Indigenous Australians: https://www.aihw.gov.au/reports-statistics/population-groups/indigenous-australians/overview

AIHW: Indigenous Australians and the Health System https://www.aihw.gov.au/reports/australias-health/indigenous-australians-use-of-health-services

Common Ground: https://www.commonground.org.au/learn

AIATSIS Code of Ethics for Aboriginal and Torres Strait Islander Research: https://aiatsis.gov.au/research/ethical-research

Overview of Aboriginal and Torres Strait Islander health status 2021 (2022): http://www.healthinfonet.ecu.edu.au/health-facts/overviews

Summary of Aboriginal and Torres Strait Islander health: https://healthinfonet.ecu.edu.au/key-resources/publications/44569/?title=Summary+of+Aboriginal+and+Torres+Strait+Islander+health+status+-+selected+topics+2021&contentid=44569_1

Maiam nayri Wingara Aboriginal and Torres Strait Islander Data Sovereignty Collective: https://www.maiamnayriwingara.org/projects-1

National Aboriginal Community Controlled Health Organisation (NACCHO): https://www.naccho.org.au/

Wardliparingga SAHMRI: https://sahmri.org.au/research/themes/aboriginal-health

REFERENCES

Australian Bureau of Statistics 2022 Australian Census 2021 Aboriginal and/or Torres Strait Islander Quick Stats. Available: https://www.abs.gov.au/census/2021-census-data-release-plans/2021-census-product-release-guide#quickstats (Accessed 10 July 2022)

Australian Bureau of Statistics (ABS) 2018 Census of Population and Housing: Reflecting Australia—Stories from the Census, 2016. ABS Cat. No. 2071.0. Canberra: ABS

Australian Health Ministers' Advisory Council 2017 Aboriginal and Torres Strait Islander Health Performance Framework 2017 Report. Canberra: AHMAC

Australian Institute of Aboriginal and Torres Strait Islander Studies (AIATSIS) 1994 Ethical Research. Canberra: Encyclopaedia of Aboriginal Australia. Aboriginal Studies Press

Australian Institute of Aboriginal and Torres Strait Islander Studies (AIATSIS) 2022 Ethical research. Available: https://aiatsis.gov.au/research/ethical-research (Accessed 10 August 2022)

Australian Institute of Health and Welfare (AIHW) 2018 Australia's health 2018: in brief. AIHW Cat. No. AUS 222. Canberra: AIHW

Australian Institute of Health and Welfare (AIHW) 2022 Australia's health 2022: in brief. Canberra: AIHW

Beresford Q, Omaji P 1998 Our state of mind: racial planning and the stolen generations. South Fremantle: Fremantle Arts Centre Press

Blainey G 1994 Triumph of the nomads: a history of ancient Australia. South Melbourne: Macmillan

Builth H 2005 What we can learn from Lake Condah about sustainable living. Local–Global: Identity, Security, Community 1: 16–22

Clark M 1966 Sources of Australian history. New York: Mentor

Clarkson C, Jacobs Z, Marwick B, et al 2017 Human occupation of northern Australia by 65,000 years ago. *Nature* 547: 306

Cleland JB 1928 Disease amongst the Australian Aborigines. *Journal of Tropical Medicine and Hygiene 31*, pp. 53–70, 125–130, 141–145, 157–160, 173–177, 196–198, 202–206, 216–220, 232–235, 262–266, 281–282, 290–294, 307–313, 326–330 (series of articles across same volume, different editions, available at University of Queensland)

Close the Gap Campaign Steering Committee 2016 Progress and Priorities Report 2016. Australian Human Rights Commission. Sydney: Oxfam Australia

Close the Gap Steering Committee 2011 Shadow report: On Australian governments' progress towards closing the gap in life expectancy between Indigenous and non-Indigenous Australians. Canberra: Close the Gap Campaign Steering Committee

Commonwealth of Australia 2020 Closing the Gap – Prime Minister's Report 2020. Canberra: Australian Government

Couzos S, Murray R 2008 Aboriginal primary health care: an evidence-based approach. South Melbourne: Oxford University Press

Department of Health and Ageing 2013 National Aboriginal and Torres Strait Islander Health Plan 2013–2023. Canberra: Australian Government Department of Health and Ageing

Department of Health and Ageing 2015 Implementation Plan for the National Aboriginal and Torres Strait Islander Health Plan 2013–2023. Canberra: Australian Government Department of Health and Ageing

Department of Health and Ageing 2021 National Aboriginal and Torres Strait Islander Health Plan 2021-2031. Canberra: Commonwealth of Australia

Dudgeon P, Milroy H, Walker R 2014 Aboriginal and Torres Strait Islander Mental Health and Wellbeing Principles and Practice. Perth: Australian Government Department of the Prime Minister and Cabinet. Available: https://www.telethonkids.org.au/our-research/early-environment/developmental-origins-of-child-health/expired-projects/working-together-second-edition/

Dudgeon P, Wright M, Paradies Y et al 2010 The social, cultural and historical context of Aboriginal and Torres Strait Islander Australians. In: Purdie N, Dudgeon P, Walker R (eds). *Working Together: Aboriginal and Torres Strait Islander Mental Health and Wellbeing Principles and Practice*. Canberra: AIHW, pp. 25–42

Dune T, McLeod K, Williams R (eds) 2021 Culture, diversity and health in Australia: towards culturally safe health care. UK: Routledge

Evans R, Cronin K, Saunders K (eds) 1975 Exclusion, exploitation and extermination: race relations in colonial Queensland. Sydney: Australia and New Zealand Book Company

Ferdinand A, Paradies Y, Kelaher M 2012 Mental health impacts of racial discrimination in Victorian aboriginal communities: the localities embracing and accepting diversity (LEAD) experiences of racism survey. Melbourne: The Lowitja Institute

Fisher M, Battams S, Mcdermott D, et al 2019 How the social determinants of Indigenous health became policy reality for Australia's National Aboriginal and Torres Strait Islander Health Plan. *Journal of Social Policy* 48(1): 169–89

Flood J 2006 The original Australians: story of the Aboriginal people. Sydney: Allen & Unwin

Fredericks B 2004 Urban identity. *Eureka Street* 14(10): 30–1

Human Rights and Equal Opportunity Commission (HREOC) 2008 Close the gap: national indigenous health equality targets. Sydney: HREOC

Lowitja Institute 2022 Close the Gap Campaign Report 2022 – Transforming power: voices for generational change. Close the Gap Steering Committee

Lowitja Institute 2021 Indigenous Data Sovereignty Readiness Assessment and Evaluation Toolkit. Available: https://www.lowitja.org.au/page/services/tools/indigenous-data-sovereignty-readiness-assessment-and-evaluation-toolkit (Accessed 10 August 2022)

Mazel O 2018 Indigenous health and human rights: a reflection on law and culture. *International Journal of Environmental Research and Public Health* 15(4) doi:10.3390/ijerph15040789

National Aboriginal Community Controlled Health Organisation (NACCHO) website. Available: https://www.naccho.org.au/acchos/ (Accessed 10 August 2022)

National Aboriginal Community Controlled Health Organisation (NACCHO) and Oxfam Australia 2007 Close the Gap: Solutions to the Indigenous Health Crisis Facing Australia. Braddon, ACT: NACCHO and Oxfam Australia

National Aboriginal Health Strategy (NAHS) Working Party 1989 A National Aboriginal Health Strategy. Canberra: AGPS

National Aboriginal and Torres Strait Islander Health Council (NATSIHC) 2001 National Aboriginal and Torres Strait Islander Health Strategy: consultation draft. Canberra: NATSIHC

Phillips G 2003 Addictions and healing in aboriginal country. Canberra: Aboriginal Studies Press

Reconciliation Australia 2020 Australian Reconciliation Barometer. Available: https://www.reconciliation.org.au/reconciliation/australian-reconciliation-barometer/ (Accessed 10 August 2020)

Rintoul S 1993 The wailing: a national black oral history. Port Melbourne: William Heinemann

Rowse T 2006 Transforming the notion of the urban Aborigine. *Urban Policy and Research* 18(2): 171–90

Saggers S, Gray D 1991 Aboriginal Health and Society: The Traditional and Contemporary Aboriginal Struggle for Better Health. Sydney: Allen & Unwin

Smith LT 1999 Decolonising methodologies research and indigenous peoples. London: Zed Books

Taylor J 2006 Population and diversity: policy implications of emerging Indigenous demographic trends. Discussion Paper No. 283/2006. Canberra: Centre for Aboriginal Economic Research

Thomas DP, Bainbridge R, Tsey K 2014 Changing discourses in Aboriginal and Torres Strait Islander health research, 1914–2014. *Medical Journal of Australia* 201(Suppl 1): S15–18

SECTION 2

Policy, Ethics and Evidence

The first four chapters in Section 2 of the book introduce you to the important role of public policy and public health policy as it impacts on the provision of public healthcare, care of an ageing population and the provision of social services such as the national Disability Insurance Scheme. This section also contains two important chapters on the role of ethics in public health practice and the use of evidence-based practice.

Chapter 5 examines contemporary public health policy, and we present you with information about public health policy and the relationship between public health and the broader health system. We define terms such as 'policy', 'public policy' and 'health policy', and the role that values and politics play in policy-making. We discuss the basic structure and financing of the health system in Australia, and the role of public health within that context. Discussions take place regarding Australia's national public health priorities and the policy implications as the chapter examines and discusses influences on Australia's health and the implications for contemporary professional practice. The chapter recognises contemporary international developments in public health, and their impact on policymaking in Australia and the health of Australians. We discuss Australia's National Strategic Framework on Chronic Conditions as a public health policy priority.

Chapter 6 introduces you to social policy and the implications for public health. We contextualise this discussion around the sociology of health and a conversation about social justice, liberal-democracy and public versus private providers. The chapter describes the history of universal health in Australia and how this system compares with other countries. It examines what is meant by the term 'neo-liberalism' and how it is influencing the design of health services. There is a discussion on the difference between a health and welfare system that has a high degree of commodification (market-based provision) and a health and welfare system that has a high degree of direct government provision and universal-based health services. It explains how other areas of social policy, such as employment, income support and housing policy impact on population health and wellbeing. It concludes with a discussion about the potential benefits of the National Disability Insurance Scheme.

Chapter 7 begins with a conversation about why ethics are at the very core of public health, as well as recognising that the term 'ethics' is often defined and applied in different ways. It provides us with an explanation about the foundational principles and the development of public health ethics while also acknowledging the important core challenges of public health ethics. It provides you with many examples of how to recognise, evaluate and communicate ethical issues in public health work and policy. It also concentrates on the application of ethical principles in your public health practice.

Chapter 8 begins by defining, and provides a short introduction to the history of, evidence-based practice. It clearly and succinctly defines the term 'evidence' and discusses the value of public health practice that is based on evidence. In doing this it identifies and appraises the nature of evidence and the sources of public health evidence. The chapter provides examples of the identification of practice based on evidence and discusses the important principles that apply to public health evidence-based practice. It concludes by discussing the way in which evidence can be applied to achieve advances in public health and health policy and the factors that influence success.

5

Public Health Policy

*Elizabeth Parker and Mary Louise Fleming**

LEARNING OBJECTIVES

After reading this chapter, you should be able to:
- Identify and describe the terms "policy", "public policy" and "health policy".
- Critique a range of factors that influence policymaking.
- Describe the financing of Australia's health system and how public health is funded within the system.

- Examine and discuss influences on Australia's health in the last 50 years, and the implications for contemporary policy and professional practice.
- Review and analyse the impact of policy development and public health policy development on practice through case study examples.

INTRODUCTION

We begin by introducing the concept of policy, health and public health policy and the range of factors that influence policymaking. The chapter provides an overview of the multiple health challenges policy is intended to address within a complex system that is described by ecological, economic, social and political impacts (Baum, 2019). Public health researchers (Holsinger & Scutchfield, 2021) talk about how "good" policy and governance can help us achieve equitable, sustainable and healthy societies and that such policies are "health-in-all" policies rather than a singular focus on health policy (Government of South Australia & Global Network for Health in All Policies, 2019). We address contemporary influences on policy, examine current health spending and the reform challenges in health systems and provide national policy development and implications for practice in chronic conditions (or non-communicable diseases, known as NCDs) and infectious diseases, as examples.

WHAT IS "POLICY"?

A policy is a statement of beliefs, goals, objectives and recommendations on a specific subject area (Peters, 2021). Public

policies are policies made by government that affect the whole population.

Policies can refer to past, present or future action, for example:
- A general statement of future intentions or objectives, such as: "It is our policy to support universal healthcare access".
- The past set of actions of government in a particular area, such as economic, refugee or health policies and/or a specific statement of future intentions—for example, "Our policy will allow people to opt out of Medicare in order to take up private health insurance".
- A set of standing rules, such as: "It is our policy not to interfere in those matters that are the responsibilities of the states" (Peters, 2021).

The focus of policy includes establishing priority goals, achieving reform and accomplishing policy objectives. Governments achieve their policy objectives by combining:
- Regulation—restrictions through laws or codes, such as prohibiting tobacco sales to children.
- Taxation or subsidisation—such as making tobacco more expensive or healthcare cheaper.
- Provision—providing healthcare services in government-operated clinics, or contracting with a non-government organisation to provide healthcare on its behalf.

Therefore, policy is often enacted through legislation or regulations, and incentives enabling access to and delivery of services and programs. It examines priorities and the expectations of a variety of groups as its purpose is to build

---

*Anthony Carpenter contributed to this chapter in the previous edition.

consensus and inform people (Nutbeam & Muscat, 2021, p. 1590)

Different governments' political values are reflected in their choices among these alternatives. Think about health policy choices that your government has made. Maybe you could think about the expansion of emergency departments and ambulance services to cope with increased patient presentation. Does policy change when a State Government or Federal Government changes? Can you think of an example of the change that has occurred in a policy setting with a change of government?

We now turn our attention to an examination of the different types of public policy.

TYPES OF PUBLIC POLICY

Distributive Policies

These policies involve providing services or benefits to particular groups in society. Pensions for people living with a disability, and price concessions on healthcare or prescriptions for people with chronic medical conditions, are distributive policies. They are usually implemented without controversy or without noticeable reduction in benefits to other groups (Noll, 2021).

Redistributive Policies

These policies redistribute resources from one group to another group in society, usually to reduce inequity for a disadvantaged group. Redistributive policies reflect government and societal values about social justice for disadvantaged groups. For example, it is well established that people with lower income levels experience poorer health on average. Higher taxation rates for people earning higher income levels are therefore used to redistribute money to pay for social welfare programs for people with lower income levels (Peters, 2021).

Regulatory Policies

Regulatory policies restrict the behaviours of individuals and groups. For example, tobacco control policies place restrictions on smoking in public places and on tobacco sale to minors. Another example is those policies introduced to manage outbreaks of COVID-19. Health professional regulation requires licensing before health professionals may practise their profession. Many industry associations adopt voluntary self-regulation or codes of conduct to avoid potentially more restrictive government regulations (Porche, 2021).

State and territory health departments determine which health service organisations must be assessed against the National Safety and Quality Health Service (NSQHS) Standards. All public and private hospitals, day procedure services and public dental practices are required to be accredited to the NSQHS Standards. The Australian Health Practitioner Regulation Agency (AHPRA) is responsible for the registration and accreditation of various health professions in Australia.

WHAT IS HEALTH POLICY?

Health policy refers to decisions, plans and actions that are undertaken to achieve specific healthcare goals within a society (Nutbeam & Muscat, 2021). Such a policy clearly refers to healthcare and is about a formal statement or procedure, usually within governments, which defines priorities, timing and the range of actions designed to respond to health needs, resources and other political imperatives. In this chapter we will also be thinking about policies that may have an impact on the determinants of health that focus on intersectoral action for health (HiAP).

Health policies arise from a systematic process of building support for public health action that draws upon available evidence and is integrated with community preferences, political realities and resource availability.

Intersectoral action for health means there are actions taken by different sectors of society to achieve health outcomes in ways that are more effective, efficient or sustainable than perhaps the result of one sector working alone. In order to address the determinants of health, an intersectoral approach to health is essential to both enhance health and achieve greater health equity in populations. A focus on health-in-all policies provides a practical framework for supporting intersectoral action for health within government. Intersectoral action for health is usually concentrated in government, but includes actions across other sectors including civil society and the private sector (Nutbeam & Muscat, 2021, pp. 1592–3).

Inquiries into critical healthcare failures in Australia and the UK have found that they arise in part because governments have relied on periodic external accreditation as proof of the safety and quality of hospitals' healthcare (Duckett et al, 2016). These inquiries suggest that, while accreditation against standards is important, it is insufficient by itself to ensure the quality and safety of hospitals (Duckett & Swerissen, 2016).

FACTORS INFLUENCING POLICY

Federation

Australia became a nation in 1901 when six British colonies joined together to become the Commonwealth of Australia. This process is known as Federation (Parliament Education Office, 2022). In Australia, the federal government and the state governments and territories often make their own policy decisions in areas for which they are responsible. Such autonomy allows them to tailor policy to local circumstances and preferences. It can also enable policy experimentation and learning. However, intergovernmental coordination can be beneficial and desirable.

Coordination is often conceptualised as either a process or an outcome. Process and outcome are used in policy analysis to conceptualise policymaking and its effects (Knill & Tosun, 2020). However, intergovernmental coordination is complex. In policy analysis there are steps between process and outcome, called output and impact; that is, to what extent do policy decisions and their implementation actually bring about expected results (Schnabel & Hegele, 2021)? Schnabel and Hegele (2021) examine the complexity of intergovernmental coordination in Australia and three other Federations during the COVID-19 pandemic as a clear example of the complexity of inter-relationships.

Health policies aim to promote and restore the health of populations. Health, and universal access to healthcare, are considered basic human rights (World Health Organization [WHO], 2022). Health policies and priorities exist in dynamic health and political systems, subject to constant political, economic, social and technological change. Health policy is political because of the nature of health itself.

Politics are central to health policy (Baum, 2019). Political parties design policies based on their ideology—a system of beliefs that guide their actions. Health policymaking occurs in every political system, from liberal Western democracies to socialist, communitarian and authoritarian political systems. Scholars argue that the way in which health resources are allocated by policymakers is more important than the type of political system the policymakers represent (Cairney & Goswell, 2022).

Liberal democratic societies, such as the UK, the US and Australia, are characterised by free speech, free and fair elections, the rule of law and a free press. In these societies, the political voice of citizens is aggregated and expressed through the institutions and processes, such as elections, that represent them (Milner, 2021). A range of governments seek to improve the health of their populations, and some seek to reduce health inequalities. Yet, there remains a large gap between their policy statements, practices and outcomes (Cairney & Goswell, 2022).

Complete Activity 5.1 to gain a better understanding of the types of public health policy.

Implementing policy in a democracy often requires making new laws through the parliament. Achieving support for these new policies requires negotiation among individual members and factions of the governing political party, with other political parties in the parliament, and with interested stakeholder groups.

For example, patient and consumer *advocacy* groups, health professional groups, the media and regulatory agencies independent of government, such as medical practitioner registration boards and human rights authorities, may express alternative views about a policy. This situation requires governments to negotiate, modify and compromise proposed health policies in order to achieve their policy objectives. Many *stakeholders*, such as non-government organisations (NGOs), professional groups and community organisations, advocate for particular health policies that are in their interest (Cairney

---

ACTIVITY 5.1   Types of Public Health Policy

Define distributive, redistributive, regulatory and self-regulatory policies, and list their advantages and disadvantages. How do these types of policies impact on health policy? Do you think there are community groups or health professions that are influential in setting and changing public health policy? How are their voices heard?

Reflection

Discuss the themes you have identified as advantages and disadvantages? Is it possible to use a mix of policy types to improve population health? Are physicians and nurses influential in the distribution of resources for public health?

& Boswell, 2022). (See Chapter 11 for a discussion about policy development related to climate change and health.)

The influence of interest groups on policymakers gives rise to the risk of regulatory capture—where the interests of firms or groups are prioritised over the public interest (McKay, 2022). Some scholars argue that regulatory capture is an example of government failure—where governments fail in the efficient or "fair" allocation of scarce resources such as healthcare (Babacan, 2021).

Alternatively, Cairney and Boswell (2022) argue that if health improvement is approached as a policymaking problem it may be possible to identify and mitigate against some of the most obvious problems while working with likely governance dilemmas. There is no straightforward way to take action on health improvement. A focus on clarity, congruity and capacity does not solve these problems, but it encourages health improvement advocates to maximise their chances by being clear on what they seek to achieve and consistent and realistic in how they seek to achieve it (McGowan et al, 2021).

Widespread use of social media and the rise of populism in politics are two more recent influences on health policy.

Social Media

Social media platforms, such as Twitter and Facebook, provide an opportunity for policymakers and healthcare providers to communicate directly with voters and patients, and vice versa (Yeung, 2018). Social media platforms provide direct and constant qualitative and quantitative feedback on contemporary policy issues by individuals and organisations to politicians and governments. This process reduces reliance on political parties, the press and industry groups, reorienting political power towards populist politicians and issues (Lin, 2022).

Complete Activity 5.2 to gain a better understanding of the potential for damage by the media on populist policy.

The use of web-based applications encourages people to create and share a wide range of content that may enable an understanding of the value they place on health and wellbeing for themselves, their friends and family, and the surrounding community (Yeung, 2018).

ACTIVITY 5.2 Populist Policies and Public Health Evidence

With several colleagues, find an example of a populist policy that may be in contradiction to public health evidence. Review how social media has been used to maintain this populist viewpoint.

Reflection

Imagine that you work at an evidence-based public policy institute. How would you use social media to present evidence against populist media messages from policymakers? How would you convince voters and consumers that the evidence-based perspective is credible?

Many patients examine social and popular media before consulting a health professional for advice. What is your role as a health professional in addressing populist beliefs about health issues with evidence?

Populism

Populism is a political philosophy for the preferences and beliefs of "ordinary people" over those with power, such as governments and institutions (Watson & Barnes, 2022). By valuing the voices of "ordinary people", populism inherently discounts "evidence" generated by institutions, such as government health departments and universities. This response represents a gradual shift from evidence-based to evidence-informed decision-making in policy. Further, it stresses the importance of the community where issues can be identified, where evidence is generated and solutions are contextually bound (Kothari & Smith, 2022). Consider Activity 5.2 about links between populism and evidence.

Populist policies and politicians have gained prominence in recent years, as inequality in income and wealth has continued to grow in liberal democratic societies (Head, 2022).

VALUES AND POLICYMAKING

Policies are shaped by the values of groups, societies and policymakers. These values and concepts of "normal" are often not explicit and change over time, both in societies and in political parties. This means that policies developed even 10 years ago may be considered inappropriate or undesirable by political parties and societies today.

Drug and alcohol policy is a contentious policy area where political parties and professional and community groups have strongly held conflicting views. Should use of illicit drugs be treated through the criminal justice system or through drug rehabilitation, or both?

Governments and NGOs use a variety of programs to reduce and prevent alcohol-related harm in the community. These include:

- Regulation—restricting the sale of alcohol to minors.
- Licensing—controlling where and when alcohol may be sold, limiting advertising of alcohol.

- Taxation—levying alcohol sales tax to reduce consumption.
- Subsidisation of medical and public health services, such as alcohol detoxification and health promotion, and education campaigns about alcohol-related harm.

Case Study 5.1 examines the notion of evidence-based policy. The case study has a focus on city planning, global

CASE STUDY 5.1 Evidence-Informed Policy

Read the following article by Giles-Corti et al 2022 What next? Expanding our view of city planning and global health, and implementing and monitoring evidence-informed policy. Available at: https://www.thelancet.com/action/showPdf?pii=S2214-109X%2822%2900066-3 (Accessed 5 June 2022).

The article covers three major issues: initially it summarises key findings; on the basis of this summary it considers what to do next; and then outlines urgent key actions. What evidence do the authors provide in relation to the effects of city planning on sustainable mobility and health? On the basis of that evidence, what do the authors say could support the development of the compact city as they argue that compact cities are necessary for sustainable development?

The authors conclude that cities and their populations are confronted with multiple health challenges as we have identified in Section 1 of the book. These challenges include preventing chronic conditions, dealing with infectious disease pandemics, an ageing population, severe social disparities, biodiversity loss and climate change. Giles-Corti and colleagues (2022) argue for the development and maintenance of evidence-informed city planning policies and standards.

Questions

1. What impact has COVID-19 had on the compact city and why does high density housing underpin compact housing?
2. How do compact cities mitigate and adapt to climate change and why is biodiversity and urban greening fundamental to human health?
3. What are the five actions and sub-actions associated with the transition to healthy and sustainable cities?

Reflection

This article represents the stark reality facing many developed and developing countries around the world. You may want to work together in small groups to examine the article in detail, and to answer the questions that are posed for you in the material above. How do the authors argue that evidence-informed policy, standards and governance can make a difference? Think back to the early part of the article and consider the importance of evidence in developing policies. The following section deals with this issue in further depth.

health and implementing and monitoring evidence-based policy. The authors conclude with the following comment:

> Widespread adoption will enable city planning policy and spatial indicators to be used to benchmark and track progress, unmask spatial inequities in access to health-supportive built environments, inform interventions and investments, accelerate changes that could help solve multiple related problems, and hold governments to account, with co-benefits for human and planetary health
>
> **(Giles-Corti et al, 2022, p. e926)**

EVIDENCE IN POLICY

The idea of using evidence to inform policy, evaluate its outcomes and guide future investment has more recently received greater attention (Partridge et al, 2020). Many governments and NGOs now invest in gathering evidence to inform policy design, implementation and evaluation, although there has been some criticism that Australian governments do not make evidence more available to help guide policy (Australian Government Productivity Commission, 2017). Political and ideological factors often predominate in policy development, and the use of evidence to guide health policy formation in Australia remains sporadic (McConnell et al, 2020). A range of factors have made efficiency, effectiveness and equity core drivers for health system performance and reform. An ageing population, the social determinants of health and inequitable sub-population mortality and morbidity and governments looking to provide more appropriate health services to acute care services are examples of factors that influence system reform.

HEALTH POLICY AND HEALTHCARE SYSTEMS

Healthcare policy is a subset of health policy concerned with healthcare, but, confusingly, the terms are often used interchangeably. Healthcare policy is central in most health systems because healthcare spending consumes most of the health budget. Australia expends an estimated $105.8 billion, representing 16.8% of the Australian Government's total expenditure in 2022–23 (Vines, 2022). It invested $30.1 million in preventive health measures that include implementing the National Preventive Health Strategy 2021–2030 dealing with chronic conditions and a focus on strengthening the infectious diseases response (https://www.health.gov.au/sites/default/files/documents/2022/03/budget-2022-23-national-preventive-health-strategy.pdf).

This distribution of health spending is one measure of health policymakers' priorities (see Figure 5.1). There is "evidence" (from research, evaluation of programs, and economic models) that public health interventions are cost-effective (McGowan et al, 2021). However, the relatively low level of investment in public health suggests that evidence may have a limited role in informing health policy and in shifting funding responses towards public health advancement (Kothari & Smith, 2022). To read more about the federal government's contribution to health promotion and health protection see the following website: https://www.aihw.gov.au/reports/australias-health/health-promotion.

MANAGEMENT AND REFORM OF HEALTHCARE

The challenges to modern-day health systems (an ageing population, access to care, prevention of chronic conditions and infectious diseases [such as COVID-19], quality and safety, cost and fiscal sustainability) have resulted in many reform efforts in health systems. National public health policies have attempted over the years to deal with the most burdensome and prevalent conditions. The National Preventive Health Strategy 2021–2030 sets out the Australian government's current approach to preventing and treating chronic conditions. The Framework articulates values, such as equity and sustainability, as well as policy objectives, which together help us understand the government's health policy priorities. These, of course, may change with the election of political parties.

Health systems evolved in the 19th and 20th centuries to treat episodic conditions, such as injury, infection and surgical conditions. Up until recently, the success of health systems in reducing injuries and communicable disease has resulted in a predominance of non-communicable conditions (see Figure 5.2). The total burden of disease is attributable to the leading five risk factors (Australian Institute of Health and Welfare [AIHW], 2022a).

These chronic conditions tend to affect disadvantaged groups such as Indigenous populations, Culturally and Linguistically Diverse (CALD) communities as well as socioeconomically disadvantaged communities. Further, Australia's universal health insurance, Medicare, does not cover the costs of most dental services. However, Medicare does pay for some essential dental services for some children and adults who are eligible.

Health systems evolved to treat acute illness and injury, not to prevent chronic conditions, which are preceded by the accumulation of risk factors, often without symptoms, over many years (Duckett & Swerissen, 2016). Reorientation of health systems to prevent chronic conditions and to deal with emerging pandemics while simultaneously maintaining acute healthcare access is an ongoing policy challenge in most developed countries.

Multiple policy challenges face the provision of healthcare across the continuum of promotion, prevention and care in Australia into the future.

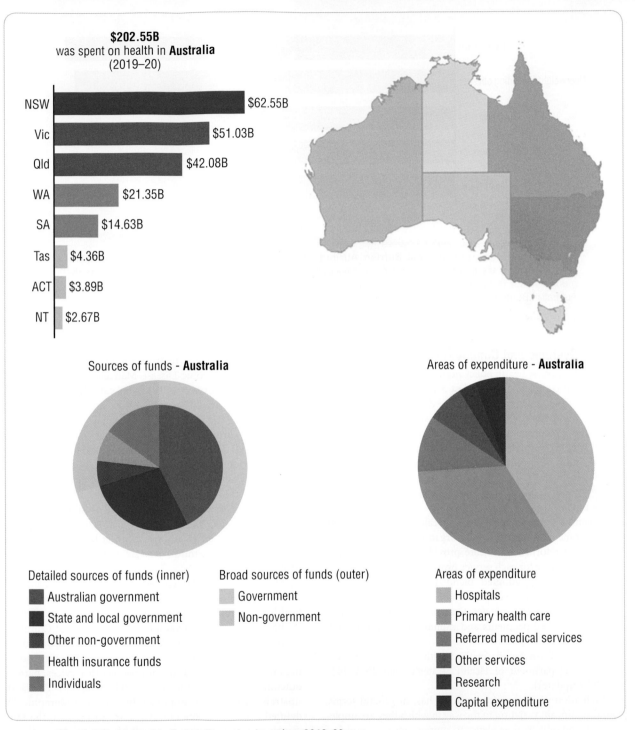

Fig. 5.1 Total Health Expenditure by Location 2019–20.
Total health expenditure in Australia, by state, sources of funding and areas of expenditure. (Source: Australian Institute of Health and Welfare [AIHW] 2021 Health Expenditure Australia 2019–20. AIHW, Australian Government. Accessed 20 July 2022.)

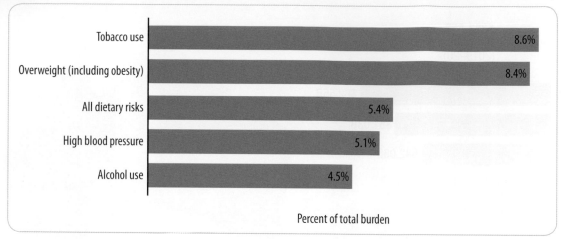

Fig. 5.2 Proportion (%) of Total Burden Attributable to the Leading Five Risk Factors in 2018. In 2018, 38% of the burden of disease could have been prevented by reducing or avoiding exposure to the modifiable risk factors examined in this study. (Source: Australian Institute of Health and Welfare [AIHW] 2021 Australian Burden of Disease Study 2018: key findings. AIHW, Australian Government. Accessed 20 July 2022.)

Health Systems and Complexity

Meeting the diverse health policy needs of the population have always been complex. Over the last 3 years of the COVID-19 pandemic, there was refocused service delivery and additional resources and designated health professionals. Up until this point the predominance of chronic conditions led many health systems to implement policy reforms to improve early identification of chronic disease and their risk factors. These reforms include:

- New models of care—managed care, care coordination, hospital in the home.
- Organisational reform—Primary Health Networks (PHNs), government and not-for-profit organisations.
- Payment reform—healthcare providers have traditionally been paid a fee for each service provided. Healthcare payers have increasingly adopted "blended" payment models that share the risk for healthcare outcomes between the payer and the healthcare provider. Examples include risk adjustment, bundled payments and capitation (see Feldhaus & Mathauer, 2018).
- Broader reform agenda in the health system (see for example, Department of Health Strategic Plan 2021–2025 [2022 update]).

Evaluation of these reform efforts has, in general terms, found significant variation in the way in which they are implemented, and only weak evidence to support any one model of reform over another. There is a need for a focused review of the healthcare system in Australia to gain insights into the areas (e.g. innovation, access, equity, timeliness and costs) where improvements are warranted (Dixit & Sambasivan, 2018).

Other organisational reform examples have included the introduction of Chronic Disease Management (CDM) items for general practitioners (GPs), who can also refer patients to allied health practitioners (Services Australia, 2021). The CDM Medicare items are for GPs to manage the healthcare of people with chronic or terminal medical conditions and/or complex needs. These chronic conditions need to be present for 6 months or longer—for example, asthma, cancer, cardiovascular disease, diabetes, musculoskeletal conditions and stroke. The CDM items are designed for patients who require a structured approach to enable GPs to plan and coordinate their care (Services Australia, 2021). The AIHW (2022b) notes "in 2016 among patients aged 45 and over with at least one long-term health condition, one third (33%; 2.2 million patients) used an MBS CDM item".

Many health systems have established regional "commissioning" organisations to plan, purchase and monitor the health of populations (Silburn & Lewis, 2020) as part of health system reform. Examples include Clinical Commissioning Groups in the UK, Accountable Care Organizations in the US and PHNs in Australia. These health commissioning bodies are intended to improve health services, patient outcomes and value for money. There are 31 PHNs in Australia, each with responsibility for a geographically defined area. Their key objectives are to increase the efficiency and effectiveness of medical services for patients, and to improve coordination of care to ensure that patients receive the right care in the right place at the right time (Australian Government Department of Health and Ageing, 2021).

Each of the PHNs is accountable to the Australian government for health service coordination and improved health outcomes in its geographical area. A review of Australia's healthcare quality demonstrates that the system is of comparatively good quality, but also that funding models, fragmentation of responsibility, lack of quality incentives, inconsistent organisation of care and lack of benchmarking contribute to quality gaps in the Australian system (OECD, 2021).

Health Economics

Health economics evaluations commonly evaluate the cost of a policy in terms of monetary benefit, clinical benefit or benefit for people's health and wellbeing (Hale, 2022). Policymakers use this economic analysis to help allocate resources efficiently, to minimise cost and to maximise the impact of health policies.

Health technology assessments (HTAs) are used to consider whether to fund new medical treatments or devices based on their cost-effectiveness compared with existing treatments (Rejon-Parrilla et al, 2022). For example, manufacturers of medications and medical prostheses (such as artificial hip joints) must submit a health technology assessment when they seek agreement from health funders to subsidise the cost of their treatment for insured patients (Health Technology Assessment, 2022).

Economic analysis of alternative health policies requires modelling or "simulation" about future outcomes. For example, a reduction in the 2015–16 prevalence of smoking in Victoria, to achieve a target of 10% prevalence by 2025, would result in a decline in tangible costs of 14.5%, from $3696.1 million in 2016 to $3161.4 million in 2025 (Greenhalgh et al, 2020). However, policymakers need to be open to the use of simulations and models so that this form of evidence can be incorporated into policymaking.

A FINAL WORD

This chapter has presented definitions and identified types of health and public policy, and stages of policy development. The influence of stakeholders, values and politics on health policy development in liberal democracies has been outlined.

Australia has a tradition of the federal government taking a lead in public health policy developments, and some of the history of this tradition was introduced along with its current public health priorities.

The process of policy development is inherently complex and political, requiring negotiation with many stakeholders and political opponents in order to implement a policy. Health policies are intended to improve the quality and wellbeing of people's lives. Evaluation of health policies is critical in determining which health policies work, and why. Chapter 5 examines social policy and public health and complements the discussions in this Chapter.

REVIEW QUESTIONS

1. What do you understand by the terms "policy", "public policy" and "health policy"?
2. What role do values and politics play in health policymaking?
3. Why is there more policy action on some issues than on others?
4. What are the different types of policy and how do they influence how a policy is developed?
5. What is populism, and how might it affect public health policy?
6. Find and make contact with your local health commissioning organisation, such as a Primary Health Network. Develop five questions that you would ask the manager about the funding of the commissioning organisation and the role of your future profession within these arrangements. Will you be accountable for service standards or clinical quality? How will these be measured?
7. Why do some groups in your society have unequal access to healthcare or health outcomes? What does your government or healthcare organisation do to address this inequality? Are these policies effective?
8. How do terms like access, equity and innovation impact policy development in the health system?

USEFUL WEBSITES

Australian Government Department of Health and Ageing: http://www.health.gov.au (Presents the structure and priorities for attention to improve health and health care for Australians.)

Australian Institute of Health and Welfare (AIHW): http://www.aihw.gov.au (Publishes an annual Health Expenditure Australia series and a profile of the health of Australians in its bi-annual reports.)

Consumers' Health Forum of Australia: http://www.chf.org.au

Australia's Federal Relations Architecture: https://federation.gov.au/

Public Health Association of Australia: http://www.phaa.net.au

REFERENCES

Australian Government Productivity Commission 2017 Data availability and use. Available: https://www.pc.gov.au/inquiries/completed/data-access/report (Accessed 27 July 2022)

Australian Government Department of Health 2021 Primary Health Networks (PHNs). Available: http://www.health.gov.au/primary health networks (PHNs) (Accessed 15 June 2022)

Australian Institute of Health and Welfare (AIHW) 2022a Australia's health 2022. Available: https://www.aihw.gov.au/reports-data/australias-health (Accessed 26 July 2022)

Australian Institute of Health and Welfare (AIHW) 2022b Use of Medicare chronic disease management items by patients with long-term health conditions. Available: https://www.aihw.gov.au/getmedia/4ec4195f-bd1f-40a8-a802-a501cab9d0e0/aihw-phc-7.pdf.aspx?inline=true

Babacan H 2021 Public–Private Partnerships for Global Health: Benefits, Enabling Factors, and Challenges. *Handbook of Global Health*, pp. 2755–88

Baum F 2019 Governing for health: advancing health and equity through policy and advocacy. New York: Oxford University Press

Cairney P, St. Denny E, Boswell J 2022 Why is health improvement policy so difficult to secure? *Open Research Europe* 2:76, 1–16. https://doi.org/10.12688/openreseurope

Dixit SK, Sambasivan M 2018 A review of the Australian healthcare system: A policy perspective. *SAGE Open Med.* 6:2050312118769211. doi:10.1177/2050312118769211 (Accessed 19 July 2022)

Duckett S, Cuddihy M, Newnham H 2016 Targeting zero. Supporting the Victorian Hospital system to eliminate avoidable harm and strengthen quality of care. Melbourne: Victorian Government. Available: https://www2.health.vic.gov.au/hospitals-and-health-services/quality-safety-service/hospital-safety-and-quality-review (Accessed 20 June 2022)

Duckett S, Swerissen H 2016 Chronic failure in primary care. Available: https://grattan.edu.au/wp-content/uploads/2016/03/936-chronic-failure-in-primary-care.pdf (Accessed 3 July 2022)

Feldhaus I, Mathauer I 2018. Effects of mixed provider payment systems and aligned cost sharing practices on expenditure growth management, efficiency, and equity: a structured review of the literature. *BMC Health Services Research* 18(1): 1-14

Giles-Corti B, Vernez Moudon A, Loew M, et al 2022 What next? Expanding our view of city planning and global health, and implementing and monitoring evidence-informed policy. *The Lancet Global Health* 10(6): e919–26. Available: https://www.thelancet.com/action/showPdf?pii=S2214-109X%2822%2900066-3 (Accessed 5 June 2022)

Government of South Australia & Global Network for Health in All Policies 2019 The Global Status Report on Health in All Policies. Adelaide: Government of South Australia

Greenhalgh EM, Hurley S, Lal A 2020 17.4 Economic evaluations of tobacco control interventions. In: Greenhalgh EM, Scollo MM, Winstanley MH, eds. *Tobacco in Australia: facts and issues*. Melbourne: Cancer Council Victoria. Available: https://www.tobaccoinaustralia.org.au/chapter-17-economics/17-4-economic-evaluations-of-tobacco-control-interventions (Accessed 5 August 2022)

Head BW 2022 Policy innovation in turbulent times. In: *Wicked Problems in Public Policy*. Champaign, Illinois: Palgrave Macmillan, pp. 123–139

Health Technology Assessment (HTAs) 2022. Available: https://www.health.gov.au/health-topics/health-technologies-and-digital-health/health-technology-assessments (Accessed 1 August 2022)

Holsinger JWJ, Scutchfield FD (eds) 2021 Contemporary Public Health: Principles, Practice, and Policy, 2nd edn. Lexington: University Press of Kentucky

Knill C, Tosun J 2020 Public policy: a new introduction. London: Bloomsbury Publishing

Kothari A, Smith MJ 2022 Public health policymaking, politics, and evidence. In: Integrating Science and Politics for Public Health. Champaign, Illinois: Palgrave Macmillan, pp. 59–74

Lin Y 2022 Social media for collaborative planning: a typology of support functions and challenges. *Cities* 125: 103641

McConnell A, Grealy L, Lea T 2020 Policy success for whom? A framework for analysis. *Policy Sciences* 53(4): 589–608

McGowan VJ, Buckner S, Mead R, et al 2021 Examining the effectiveness of place-based interventions to improve public health and reduce health inequalities: an umbrella review. *BMC Public Health* 21(1): 1–17

McKay AM 2022 Stealth lobbying: interest group influence and health care reform. Cambridge: Cambridge University Press

Milner HV 2021 Is global capitalism compatible with democracy? Inequality, insecurity, and interdependence. *International Studies Quarterly* 65(4): 1097–10

Noll RG (ed) 2021 Regulatory policy and the social sciences. Berkeley: University of California Press

Nutbeam D, Muscat DM 2021 Health promotion glossary 2021. *Health Promotion International* 36(6): 1578–98

Organization for Economic Cooperation and Development (OECD) 2021 Health at a glance. Available: https://www.oecd-ilibrary.org/social-issues-migration-health/health-at-a-glance-2021_ae3016b9-en (Accessed 13 June 2022)

Parliamentary Education Office 2022 The Federation of Australia. Available: https://peo.gov.au/understand-our-parliament/history-of-parliament/federation/the-federation-of-australia/ (Accessed 10 Mar 2022)

Partridge AC, Mansilla C, Randhawa H, et al 2020 Lessons learned from descriptions and evaluations of knowledge translation platforms supporting evidence-informed policy-making in low- and middle-income countries: a systematic review. *Health Research Policy and Systems* 18(1): 1–22

Peters BG 2021 Advanced introduction to public policy. Cheltenham: Edward Elgar Publishing

Porche DJ 2021 Health policy: application for nurses and other healthcare professionals. Burlington: Jones & Bartlett Learning

Rejon-Parrilla JC, Espin J, Epstein D 2022 How innovation can be defined, evaluated and rewarded in health technology assessment. *Health Economics Review* 12(1): 1–11

Schnabel J, Hegele Y 2021 Explaining intergovernmental coordination during the COVID-19 pandemic: responses in Australia, Canada, Germany, and Switzerland. *Publius: The Journal of Federalism* 51(4): 537–69

Services Australia 2021 Education guide – Chronic disease individual allied health services Medicare items 10950-10970. Available: https://www.health.gov.au/resources/publications/chronic-disease-management-plan-allied-health-checklist (Accessed May 2022)

Silburn K, Lewis V 2020 Commissioning for health and community sector reform: perspectives on change from Victoria. *Australian Journal of Primary Health* 26(4): 332–7

Vines E Budget Review 2022-2023 Index. Health overview. Key figures and trends. Available: https://www.aph.gov.au/About_Parliament/Parliamentary_Departments/Parliamentary_Library/pubs/rp/BudgetReview202223/HealthOverview (Accessed 10 June 2022)

Watson S, Barnes N 2022 Online educational populism and New Right 2.0 in Australia and England. *Globalisation, Societies and Education* 20(2): 208–20

Yeung D 2018 Social media as a catalyst for policy action and social change for health and well-being. *Journal of Medical Internet Research* 20(3): e8508

6

Public Health and Social Policy

Greg Marston

LEARNING OBJECTIVES

After reading this chapter, you should be able to:

- Understand how welfare state trends are impacting on the funding and delivery of public health.
- Briefly describe the history of universal health in Australia, and how this system compares with other countries.
- Understand what is meant by the term 'neo-liberalism', and how it is influencing the design of health services and ideas about risk.

- Understand how other areas of social policy, such as employment, income support and housing policy, impact on population health and wellbeing.
- Differentiate between a health and welfare system that has a high degree of commodification (market-based provision) and one that has a high degree of direct government provision and universal-based health services.
- Discuss the potential benefits of the National Disability Insurance Scheme.

INTRODUCTION

This chapter places public health in the broader context of social policy, and examines how social problems such as growing income inequality, unemployment and insecure housing can impact on health and wellbeing. The term "social policy" is often used to refer to all areas of government, as well as to private and community activity that contributes to health, education, employment and related welfare outcomes. Health policy is somewhat unique compared with other areas of social policy, in that there is a seemingly limitless demand for more and different services, and because issues of life and death are tied up with questions about rationing public resources for healthcare (Lewis, 2014). Health policy analysis, like other fields of social policy, is often concerned with who gets what, when and how in terms of the distribution of public goods and services. Health policy is also about advocating across the policy sectors of housing, urban design, income support and education, not only to improve access to good-quality healthcare, but also to improve community health and create quality of life.

The notion of healthcare as a public good is something that has evolved over time in modern societies. This idea became institutionalised with the advent of the post-war welfare state, following the end of World War II in 1945. The welfare state

has multiple definitions, but central to all of them is a notion of government as either the direct provider or a regulator of private and non-profit provision, of health, education and social welfare services. In Australia, the welfare state includes public schools and hospitals, income support payments (e.g. unemployment benefits, the aged pension), community services, such as counselling and homelessness services, and various forms of occupational welfare, such as superannuation and fringe benefits. The terms 'social policy' and 'welfare state' are sometimes used interchangeably in the academic literature.

This chapter focuses on policy principles and health service delivery, with a particular focus on the relationship between the government and citizens and key social policy principles of access, equity and social justice. It also focuses on the interconnection between social needs and public health outcomes, emphasising that what happens in other fields of social policy, such as housing and unemployment policy, matters a great deal in terms of standard of living and quality of life.

HEALTH POLICY, SOCIAL JUSTICE AND RISK

Discussions of justice within health have often concentrated on questions of how public health priorities should be set, particularly in a fiscal climate of scarcity. Should more resources be spent on infant and prenatal health as opposed to aged care? Should additional resources be directed towards regional and remote areas to help overcome locational disadvantage? Questions of justice are both particular and universal. They are universal in the sense that the principle of redistributing resources towards the groups with the greatest need can form a basis of policymaking irrespective of context; however, the particular requirements for achieving justice will change over time and across different spaces. As Powers and Fadden (2006, p. 5) argue:

> Justice is not a matter of conforming society to an antecedently identifiable set of distributive principles, but rather it is a task requiring vigilance and attentiveness to changing impediments to the achievement of enduring dimensions of well-being that are essential guides to the aspirations of justice.

There are competing discourses about welfare and wellbeing, as Activity 6.1 illustrates, and there are contested representations of health policy problems and solutions in Australian social policy. How we define 'health' and 'illness' shapes the contours of health policy and its legitimate concerns. Moreover, conceptions about health are not 'natural'; they vary from one society to another, and within societies

there are cultural differences about what constitutes health and wellbeing. For social scientists, the terms 'health' and 'illness' are not only defined in terms of anatomy, physiology and genetic makeup, but also in terms of the experience of sickness, disability and pain (Fox & Ward 2006, cited in Pietsch et al., 2010). These experiences are often mediated by class, gender, age and ethnicity, which in turn can affect people's capacity to achieve a level of economic security. In contrast to a biomedical view of the diseased individual body, a social model of health directs the focus from individuals who are ill to social groups with high illness rates; the aim is to find the causes of inequality and, if they include aspects of people's living and working conditions, to use public policy to change them (Burdess, 2011). And in examining public policy, the aim is to see whether the balance is right between funds being directed to biomedical-oriented solutions and public health initiatives that seek to address the social aspects of health, such as occupational health and safety and working conditions. The basic point of a sociological approach is that, in order to understand health, you need to know more than what is going on inside someone's body; you need to know about the social system in which the person lives (Burdess, 2011).

A social perspective on health may look at how the profit motive can affect the delivery of healthcare, or how people from lower socioeconomic groups suffer higher levels of poor health and stress (Pietsch et al, 2010). In Australia, there has been an expanding research and policy agenda around the social determinants of health, which emphasises the social and economic conditions that influence individual and group differences in health status (as discussed in Chapters 1, 2 and 5, and Activity 6.2).

ACTIVITY 6.1 Welfare, Identity and Morality

Answer the following questions:
- How important do you think the work ethic is to shaping attitudes to unemployment and the unemployed in Australia?
- Which groups in society are typically thought to be deserving of government support, and which groups are generally seen as less deserving?
- What are some of the derogatory terms used in Australia to describe someone who is long-term unemployed?

Reflection

Did you find it easy to come up with descriptions of the long-term unemployed? How similar do you think these descriptions are to how citizens and governments in other wealthy countries talk about the problem of unemployment? It is interesting how certain labels for social problems minimise the economic dimensions. Talking about unemployment as the problem of the unemployed individual means less attention is given to systemic factors, such as the shortage of paid jobs in the Australian economy and the role of workplace discrimination in making it more difficult for some groups to get paid work, particularly women, older workers and people from culturally and linguistically diverse backgrounds. An important difference between unemployment benefits and healthcare in Australia is that unemployment benefits are 'targeted' to people who meet certain eligibility requirements, whereas access to healthcare is more universal, which is why it receives wider public and political support.

ACTIVITY 6.2 Health and Society

Answer the following questions:
- How does the World Health Organization's definition of health fit in with Burdess's comments about the importance of the social model?
- As discussed in Chapter 1, can you articulate the definition or perspective of 'health' that you will use in your practice?

Reflection

You may want to consider the WHO definition and then compare and contrast that definition with Burdess's comments relating to a social model of health. In Chapters 1 and 2, and 5 in particular, we discuss a social determinants of health model, and why that is an important model to keep in mind even in a country like Australia, where many people do not have to worry about issues such as equity and access to the healthcare system. You may also want to think back to some of the activities in Chapter 1, where you were asked to think about your definition of health and how other people view a definition of health based on their own experiences.

Health systems are coming under pressure due to increasing demand and the rising costs of health infrastructure and technology. Contemporary media reports in Australia about healthcare and health services often represent the system as being in crisis (Lewis, 2014). Attempts to increase user-charges for primary healthcare to assist with rising budget costs have faced strong opposition from citizens and consumer groups. Demographic and technological changes will be major factors behind increases in health costs in coming decades. Between 2010 and 2050, health spending is expected to increase seven-fold on those aged 65 and over, and twelve-fold on those aged 85 and over; and between 2003 and 2033, health expenditure is set to increase by 189%—from $85 billion to $246 billion (AIHW, 2017). In 2019–20 total health spending in Australia was $202.5 billion, equating to $7,926 per person (AIHW, 2021). As Chapters 2 and 5 indicate, health services constitute one of the largest components of government expenditure.

Health inequalities may intensify as a result of policy measures that seek to reduce government costs for healthcare and individualise risk and responsibility. In recent decades, welfare states have been struggling to meet both old and new lifecycle risks. The old risks are those that the market was generally unable to provide for during the industrial era, such as unemployment, old age, sickness and disability. These risks were a key justification for the 20th-century welfare states. New risks are those generated by post-industrial changes to the labour market, where there has been a decline in full-time work and changing family and household dynamics. New risks include the growth in single-headed households, precarious employment, an ageing population and chronic diseases. Ironically, some of these new risks have been generated by the success of the welfare state in increasing life expectancy and expanding consumption. These risks result in a larger claim being made on governments, which has governments worried about the sustainability of health and welfare measures. To address this challenge, governments are increasingly asking citizens to bear more of the responsibility for life risks, either informally or through

the market. Successive Australian governments, for example, are asking workers to delay retirement and to self-fund their retirement; they are prioritising private rental subsidies rather than building public housing, and encouraging middle- to high-income earners to use private healthcare providers.

The objective of increasing individual and family responsibility for healthcare reflects a body of political thought that less direct government intervention in meeting health and other basic human needs not only reduces government costs, but it also encourages stronger self-reliance among individuals and communities. Critiques of this proposition suggest that the needs of disadvantaged groups in the community will go unmet and that social inequities will widen if markets are seen as the primary mechanism for facilitating access to health and social services.

In practice, the marketisation approach to meeting health and other social needs is patchy and uneven. Some social policy fields, such as employment assistance, have been more or less fully privatised, with a range of for-profit and non-profit providers, such as Salvation Army Employment Plus, providing employment and training services to the unemployed. Other fields, such as education and health, maintain a mixed economy of welfare, although even in these fields of policy and service delivery individuals are encouraged through a range of government-funded rebates and incentives to opt out of the public forms of provision and into private ones. This process of marketised transformation has been legitimated through a neo-liberal economic orthodoxy. While neo-liberalism has many variants, common to all of its manifestations is a belief that market mechanisms of exchange are morally and economically superior to government-provided schemes, which are represented as inefficient and responsible for creating 'welfare-dependent' citizens (Fraser, 1997; Peck, 2010).

While neo-liberalism undoubtedly changed the politics and character of health and welfare provision during the 1990s, it did not lead to an overall decline in social expenditure, as was predicted. Figure 6.1 shows how, even during

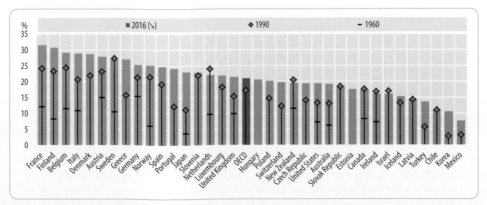

Fig. 6.1 Comparative public social expenditure across Organisation for Economic Co-operation and Development (OECD) countries, 1960, 1990 and 2016. (Source: OECD, 2016.)

periods of fiscal restraint and an espoused ideology of a 'small state', funding for social welfare actually increased. This reinforces the point that neo-liberalism doesn't necessarily mean the end of state regulation and spending; it simply changes the means and ends of government spending and activity.

The demands of neo-liberalism, with its emphasis on market solutions and individual responsibility, can lead to a health and welfare system where people's capacity to pay has a large bearing on whether they receive high-quality healthcare.

What is interesting about comparative health and welfare expenditure is that while Australia is spending about the average on healthcare compared to other countries in the Organisation for Economic Co-operation and Development (OECD), overall social expenditure is towards the lower end of the spectrum. Australia is similar to other English-speaking nations such as the US, the UK, New Zealand and Canada. These countries are referred to as 'liberal welfare states' (Esping-Andersen, 1990), which means they favour market-based solutions to meet social needs (commodification) compared with social democratic countries, such as Sweden and Norway, that give preference to universal health and welfare coverage. The 'social democratic welfare states' are at the high end of expenditure because they have wider coverage, largely funded by higher rates of direct and indirect taxation. The social democratic welfare states have lower rates of income inequality. This kind of welfare state design, and the way it structures social relations, is arguably more conducive to a healthier population.

The landmark study on social inequality and impact on health outcomes by Wilkinson and Pickett (2010) claimed that for different health and social problems, such as physical health, mental health, drug abuse, education, imprisonment, obesity, social mobility, trust and community life, violence and teenage pregnancies, outcomes are significantly worse in more unequal countries. Societies that do best for their citizens are those with the narrowest income differentials, such as Japan and the Nordic countries. The most unequal—the US, the UK and Portugal—do worst. The design of welfare states and their equalising capacity therefore plays a significant role in population health outcomes. If someone has to work three jobs to make ends meet, while constantly living under the threat of eviction from their rental property, then their physical and mental health is likely to be poorer than that of someone who has stable employment and housing. Despite the mantra that 'work is the best form of welfare', precarious paid employment can actually be worse for someone's mental health, compared with no job at all (Butterworth et al., 2011). Thus, what is happening in other fields of social policy has an important bearing on public health outcomes, as Case Study 6.1 illustrates.

Different systems of government and overall policy governance across countries also play an important role in the effectiveness of health systems and outcomes for citizens. The US, for example, spends more on health services per capita than Australia and yet it has poorer outcomes. The costs of drugs, medical technology and a complex profit-oriented, private-sector model of health insurance continue to drive up costs in the US. Sweden, whose healthcare budget is about half that of the US, has a higher life expectancy and an infant

---

CASE STUDY 6.1   Joined-up Problems Need Joined-up Solutions

Joan is a single parent living in a private rental in outer Western Sydney. She has three children, aged 9, 12 and 15. She has her name down on the public housing waiting list, but has been told by the state housing department that it could be 3 years before she gets a place. The two-bedroom flat she is living in has rising damp, and is difficult to keep cool in summer and warm in winter. Her nine-year-old son has asthma, and Joan has noticed that it has been getting worse since they moved into the flat, after she separated from the children's father. Joan wants a permanent part-time job to fit in around school hours, but all she can get is casual work at the local supermarket. The extra income supplements her unemployment benefit, which is less than the single parent's pension, which she had received until her youngest child turned eight. Her casual job makes it difficult for her to predict what her income will be each fortnight, and reporting her income to Centrelink is a challenge. Joan finds that she has very little money left over after paying the rent and bills. She feels ashamed of her situation and guilty that she can't buy her kids the things they need, such as new shoes for school. She manages to put food on the table for them, but sometimes goes without meals herself. She feels stressed and tired a lot of the time and wishes she had both more time and more money.

Questions

1. List the problems Joan faces, and describe how they are interconnected.
2. How does Joan's precarious employment impact on her health?
3. How do you think Joan's feeling of stress might impact on her health and on her children's health?
4. Who should Joan contact to get something done about her poor-quality housing?
5. Can you identify any common themes in the problems Joan is facing? There is a lot of uncertainty in Joan's life, and it is sometimes easy to forget how important it is to have economic security to be able to develop one's full potential in all areas of life, not just in paid work.

mortality rate of around 40% of the US rate (OECD, 2017). Sweden also has a different model of governance compared with the US and Australia. The US, like Australia, has a federal system of government; therefore, different levels of government have different levels of responsibility in terms of the funding, regulation and provision of healthcare. Sweden has a unitary system of government, making it easier to stipulate and implement national standards of healthcare. Joint responsibility for health between levels of government does not necessarily lead to cooperative and effective outcomes. Funding inadequacies and poor services tend to be explained by reciprocal allocation of blame and 'buck passing' in federal systems of government. While different levels of government have different views about the best way forward, industry and health professionals also have competing interests.

HISTORY OF AUSTRALIAN HEALTH POLICY: POLICY DESIGN AND FUNDING ARRANGEMENTS

Compared with most other Western countries, with the exception of the US, Australia was late in developing a national health insurance scheme (Lewis 2014, p. 198). A national health scheme named Medibank was established by the reforming Whitlam Labor Government, which was elected in 1972. Its aim was to provide public insurance for the whole population. At that time, around 20% of the adult population, most of whom were on low incomes, did not have private health insurance.

The original Medibank program proposed a 1.35% levy (with exemptions for low-income earners) to fund the scheme. However, the Senate rejected the Bills, and Medibank was originally funded from general revenue. The Medibank scheme was partially dismantled by the Fraser Government, which came to office in 1975. Medibank was then restored, in a slightly different form, by the Hawke Labor Government in 1983. Renamed Medicare in 1984, it provides a fixed subsidy for different types of medical services and procedures, with patients responsible for paying out of their own pockets any charges levied by providers above this subsidy. The Medicare program is now nominally funded by an income tax surcharge, which is currently set at 1.5%, with a higher levy for high-income earners.

Universal access to primary healthcare has been a political football since it was first introduced in the 1970s. This backwards and forwards policy movement led academic Frank Castles (1985, p. 30) to conclude that Australia has the world's 'most reversible' welfare state. This form of policy development has been particularly acute in relation to the public versus private health insurance debate in Australia. Private health insurance declined significantly following the introduction of Medicare (Colombo & Tapay, 2003). To reverse this decline,

the Howard Government, elected in 1996, introduced various measures, including a substantial subsidy in the form of a non-means-tested 30% rebate to residents on the purchase of private health insurance (Duckett, 2005; Hurley et al., 2002), and a range of financial penalties imposed on those who did not take out private cover (Butler, 2002). As a result of these contested public policy measures, private health insurance membership rose from around 30% in 1998 to 46% in 2001 (AIHW, 2008) and has settled at around 44% ever since (AIHW, 2020).

The expansion of government support for private health insurance was framed in terms of supporting a *universal public health insurance system*. Critics say that the private health insurance rebate is an unfair subsidy to those who can afford health insurance (Lewis, 2014). A key argument is that the money would be better spent on public hospitals where it would benefit everyone. Supporters of the tax subsidy say that people must be encouraged into the private healthcare system, claiming the public system is not universally sustainable for the future. Even after the introduction of the rebate, private health insurance organisations have raised their premiums most years, which negates the rebate somewhat. Roff and Segal (2004) argue that policies to boost private health insurance membership have undermined the efficiency and equity of the Australian healthcare system and have not reduced waiting lists in public hospitals. Walker and colleagues (2006) argued that the boost to private health insurance through the rebate provided substantial public subsidies to the wealthiest quintile of Australians, the group most likely to purchase private health insurance, while the impact of the reforms for the poorest 40% was minimal.

The Australian government's reliance on private health insurance as a tool of public policy is delivering a disproportionate benefit to high-income earners. Some areas of surgery are now performed predominantly in the private sector, and the 55% of Australians without private health insurance must wait, often for months, for elective surgery in the public system. Another example is dental health (discussed in Box 6.1).

The example of dental health illustrates that timely access to healthcare in Australia can still be based on ability to pay, rather than degree of need. It is also worth noting that despite the expansion of the private health subsidy and the continuation of Medicare, the costs of healthcare for individuals continue to rise. In fact, Australia has one of the highest rates of per-capita out-of-pocket health expenditures in the OECD (OECD, 2017). The largest component of non-government funding for healthcare came from out-of-pocket payments by individuals, equating to 20% of total funding in Australia, compared with 10% in the UK, 13% in New Zealand and 14% in Canada (OECD, 2016). When low-income status intersects with disability or ethnicity, it can create an even more

---

BOX 6.1   Dental Health: Australia Falling Behind

Dental health is another area where those who rely on the state-based system must wait longer for basic dental health services than those who can access privately provided dental care. A recent study showed that adults in the highest income quartile were more likely to have visited a dentist in the past 12 months than those in the lowest income quartile (76% compared with 55%), and were nearly twice as likely to have visited for a check-up (55.3% compared with 31.5%). Those in the highest income quartile were also more likely to receive a scaling of their teeth (60.7% compared with 35.6%) and less likely to receive an extraction (3.7% compared with 13.5%) than those in the lowest income quartile (Chrisopoulos et al., 2016).

Dental health is excluded from the Medicare scheme, although universal dental healthcare gained some traction with the Labor Government in office from 2007 to 2013, when the government made a commitment to expand public dental health coverage. The dental profession argued against the inclusion of dentistry in any universal health insurance scheme. This objection was on the basis that universal coverage would potentially act as a price control system within oral healthcare delivery (Matthew, 2007). Despite these objections, new investment in dental care was one of the main conditions on which the Greens political party pledged their support for Labor in forming a minority government in 2010. A proposal debated in the federal parliament in 2012 sought to implement a 6-year package. This would include $2.7 billion for children aged 2–18, $1.3 billion for adults on low incomes, and $225 million to expand services in outer metropolitan, regional and remote areas. The incoming Coalition Government, elected in late 2013, indicated its continuing support for the Child Dental Benefits Scheme, but not whether it would support other components of the 6-year package.

Following the 2016 election, a dental health policy package was announced that would support adults through a National Partnerships Agreement, involving state and federal governments, which would provide targeted support for around 400,000 adults across Australia at a cost of $242 million from July 2017 to June 2019. While this funding was sorely needed, it was insufficient to address overall levels of poor oral health. (Tooth decay remains the most common chronic health condition in Australia.) The most recent Federal Budget, delivered in March 2022 by the then Federal Treasurer, Josh Frydenberg, gave little attention to oral health, with the exception that the National Partnerships Agreement would be extended for another 2 years. The incoming Labor Government elected in May 2022 made an election pledge that it would make more dedicated investments in the dental health system, as part of a package of increased expenditure on health overall. Whether this investment will be sufficient to improve overall oral health in Australia remains to be seen.

---

dramatic profile of health inequalities, as the next section demonstrates.

DISABILITY AND EQUITY CONSIDERATIONS

As discussed earlier, a social model of health is concerned with the health status of different groups in society, in terms of such characteristics as income, ethnicity, place, gender, disability and age. While many fields of social policy, particularly income support and public housing, have been tightening eligibility criteria, disability policy in Australia has been subject to major reforms that seek to increase choice and autonomy and relax eligibility criteria to provide higher levels of support and services for a greater number of Australians with a disability. The National Disability Insurance Scheme (NDIS), which has been rolled out across Australia since 2013, provides support to around 485,000 Australians at a cost of $26 billion per year, which is expected to rise to $40.7 billion per year by 2024–25 (Coorey, 2021). The NDIS was designed as an actuarial system to make short-term investments that reduce long-term costs by increasing an individual's independence and ability to participate in society (Ardill & Jenkins, 2020). The scheme is administered through a national fund, the National Disability Insurance Agency, with money contributed at federal and state levels. The NDIS has been touted as the most significant reform in health in Australia since the introduction of Medicare.

In practice, the NDIS is a national, no-fault insurance scheme that guarantees a level of financial support to people with a disability. Currently, people with similar levels of functionality get access to quite different levels of support, depending on their location, and the timing or the origin of their disability—what some call the 'lottery' of access to services. The NDIS has individualised funding packages based on a client's level of need. The person with the disability, together with their family and carers, are able to choose where they spend their entitlement, meaning that disability and some health service providers no longer receive block funding from the government but will instead compete for a client's funds. Theoretically, the aim is to increase efficiency and give the client choice.

Supports and assistance associated with the implementation of the NDIS aim to increase opportunities for people with disability by tackling such things as inadequate housing, the need for personal care, and assistance in participating in the community. As with all social policy, much depends on the implementation in determining whether this area of social reform meets its intended aims. Individuals and families participating in the scheme are reporting problems with the quality of the care planning process, with people being unable to locate care providers for their approved plans, and there being insufficient flexibility in the budgets (Ardill & Jenkins, 2020). A 2019 government review of the NDIS identified a range of implementation problems from the perspective of partici-pants, including lack of transparency around decision making, difficulty navigating a complex system of assessment and sup-port and some participants feeling like they are not being recognised as the experts on their disability (Department of Social Services, 2019). Despite these implementation issues, there is still a strong push from advocacy groups and partici-pants in the scheme that the original vision for the NDIS to have a person-centred, rights-based approach to disability support can be delivered.

SOCIAL DETERMINANTS OF HEALTH AND ENVIRONMENTAL HEALTH DISCOURSES

This chapter has emphasised the importance of context, cul-ture and other structural factors in making sense of the health inequalities in Australia and in explaining the class, gender and ethnicity differential when it comes to assessing who benefits from quality healthcare. This framework is consistent with the social determinants of health perspective, which can be con-trasted with the biomedical discourse and the way in which this discourse tends to individualise explanations and solu-tions to disease and poor health. It is also evident that environ-mental factors are important, and that the major determinants of health or ill health are inextricably linked to social and economic context (Marmot, 2017). Factors such as housing, income, employment, geography—indeed, many of the issues that dominate political life—are key determinants of popula-tion health and wellbeing. Environmental health impacts, for example, tend to affect disproportionately those population groups that have limited choices about where they live, where they work and what they eat. A shiftworker living alongside a major freeway in poor-quality or overcrowded housing has poorer health outcomes than does the individual who has a good job and lives in appropriate housing located close to public amenities. Yet this analysis is missing when the policy problem is constructed in terms of behavioural explanations, where individuals are positioned as being responsible for mak-ing 'sensible choices' (Habibis & Walter, 2009, p. 232).

The definition of health that has conventionally been operationalised under Western capitalism has two interre-lated aspects: health is considered both as the absence of disease (biomedical definition) and as a commodity (eco-nomic definition). These definitions both focus on individu-als, as opposed to society, as the basis of good health. From this worldview, health is seen predominantly as a product of individual factors such as genetic heritage or lifestyle choices, and as a commodity that individuals can access via either the market or the health system. Health in this sense is an indi-vidualised commodity that is produced and delivered by the market or the health service. Inequalities in the distribution of health are therefore either a result of the failings of indi-viduals through their lifestyle choices or a result of the way

in which healthcare products are produced, distributed and delivered.

Since the beginning of the 20th century, there has been a dramatic decrease in the mortality rates of babies and children in Australia. However, after decades of progress, children's health is under fresh threat from an array of modern condi-tions that impair their life expectancy and quality of life. In what is described as 'modernity's paradox', many Australian children are now not as healthy as were children of earlier generations. Technological advances, new industrial processes, changes in food production and processing, increased mobil-ity, intensified urbanism, global warming, new individualised work practices and the increased consumption of media, pro-cessed foods and drinks, alcohol, personal care products and cosmetics have not only radically changed the quality and patterns of life for children and young people (Wyn, 2009), but have also been linked with a range of 'new childhood mor-bidities' (Baur, 2002). These include low birth weight; rising rates of obesity and diabetes; childhood asthma and increasing allergies; a range of developmental disorders; autism; dental decay; congenital malformations; and mental health problems, including depression, anxiety and behavioural disorders.

Australia could follow the lead of Britain, where there has been a paradigm shift since the early 2000s in terms of linking healthcare reforms with wider public sector reforms to address the determinants of health inequalities (Lewis, 2014). How-ever, cutbacks to public sector expenditure in the UK since 2010, following the Global Financial Crisis, and associated austerity measures are undoing these achievements (Pemberton et al., 2016). Preventative health requires a long-term ap-proach to achieving the policy goals of improving access and equity, and is therefore always vulnerable to budget cuts and short-term electoral cycles. The global health pandemic asso-ciated with COVID-19 further revealed the vulnerabilities in healthcare systems as countries around the world grappled with the overwhelming demand on hospitals and other health-care services. The significant increases in healthcare spending in many OECD countries during the pandemic were seen by many national governments as temporary rather than per-manent. How nations recover from the pandemic has sparked public debate about how much countries should spend on health and what is needed to make nations more resilient in the face of future economic and health shocks (Reed et al, 2021).

A FINAL WORD

Social justice is a matter of life and death. It affects the way people live, their consequent chance of illness and their risk of premature death. We watch in wonder as life expectancy and good health continue to increase in some parts of the world, and in alarm as they fail to improve in others. A girl born in 2012 can expect to live to 82 years if she is born in a high-income country, compared with 63 years in a low-income country (WHO, 2014).

As this chapter has shown, the entitlement to free medical care in Australia is not sufficient to ensure equitable access to timely and good-quality healthcare. Geographical location and demographic factors continue to have an important bearing on access to health services (AIHW, 2013, 2016). Financial barriers to health service could be removed through policies that re-emphasise the universal nature of Medicare, by encouraging bulk-billing for patients and by abolishing the private health insurance rebate (Lewis, 2014, p. 207). Abolishing the rebate would lower health costs overall and reduce the inflationary pressures within the dual insurance system. Health budgets, however, are only part of the picture. Spreading the benefits of quality healthcare and addressing entrenched health inequalities will also require going beyond an individualised discourse of what good health means.

REVIEW QUESTIONS

1. How does the broader context of social policy and the history of the welfare state shape public health policy?
2. How do contemporary notions of risk and responsibility inform social policy decisions?
3. What role do private sector interests, such as health insurers and food-processing manufacturers, play in public health?
4. Why did a public health insurance scheme take longer to develop in Australia compared with the UK?
5. What is the difference between a biomedical and a social model of health?
6. How does the National Disability Insurance Scheme differ from how services to people with a disability have traditionally been provided?

USEFUL WEBSITES

Australian Institute of Health and Welfare: http://www.aihw.gov.au
Australian Policy Online: http://www.apo.org.au
Social Policy Research Centre: http://www.sprc.unsw.edu.au

REFERENCES

Ardill A, Jenkins B, 2020 Navigating the Australian National Disability Insurance Scheme: a scheme of big ideas and big challenges. *Journal of Law and Medicine* (1), 145–64

Australian Institute of Health and Welfare (AIHW) 2008 Australia's health 2008. AIHW Cat. No. AUS 99. Canberra: AIHW

Australian Institute of Health and Welfare (AIHW) 2013 Australia's welfare 2013. AIHW Cat. No. AUS 174. Canberra: AIHW

Australian Institute of Health and Welfare (AIHW) 2016 Australia's health 2016, AIHW Cat. No. AUS 199. Canberra: AIHW

Australian Institute of Health and Welfare (AIHW) 2017 Health expenditure Australia 2015–2016. Available: https://www.aihw.gov.au/getmedia/3a34cf2c-c715-43a8-be44-0cf53349fd9d/20592.pdf.aspx?inline=true

Australian Institute of Health and Welfare (AIHW) 2020 Private health insurance. Available: https://www.aihw.gov.au/getmedia/3a34cf2c-c715-43a8-be44-0cf53349fd9d/20592.pdf.aspx?inline=true

Australia Institute of Health and Welfare (AIHW) 2021 Health Expenditure Australia 2019-20. Available: https://www.aihw.gov.au/reports/health-welfare-expenditure/health-expenditure-australia-2019-20/contents/about

Baur L, 2002 Child and adolescent obesity in the 21st century: an Australian perspective. *Asia Pacific Journal of Clinical Nutrition* 11(3), 5524–5528

Burdess N, 2011 The social basis of health and illness. In: Germov J, Poole M, eds. *Public Sociology: an Introduction to Australian Sociology*. Sydney: Allen & Unwin; pp. 330–48

Butler J, 2002 Policy change and private health insurance. *Australian Health Review* 25(6): 1–12

Butterworth P, Leach L, Strasdins L, et al 2011 The psychosocial quality of work determines whether employment has benefits for mental health: results from a longitudinal national household panel survey. *Occupational and Environmental Medicine* 68(11): 806–12

Castles F, 1985 The Working Class and Welfare. Sydney: Allen & Unwin

Chrisopoulos S, Harford J, Ellershaw A, 2016 Oral health and dental care in Australia: key facts and figures 2015. Cat. No. DEN 229. Canberra: AIHW

Colombo F, Tapay N, 2003 Private health insurance in Australia. Directorate for Employment, Labour and Social Affairs (DELSA). OECD Working Papers No. 8

Coorey P, 2021 NDIS to cost $60b by end of decade without reform: actuary. Available: https://www.afr.com/politics/ndis-to-cost-60b-by-end-of-decade-without-reform-actuary-20210702-p586dv#:~:text=The%20actuarial%20report%20projects%20the,will%20cost%20%2459.9%20billion%20annually

Department of Social Services 2019 Review of the NDIS Act and the NEW NDIS Participant Service Guarantee. Available: https://engage.dss.gov.au/review-of-the-ndis-act-and-the-new-ndis-participant-service-guarantee/

Duckett S, 2005 Private care and public waiting. *Australian Health Review* 29, 87–93

Esping-Andersen G, 1990 Three worlds of welfare capitalism. Princeton, NJ: Princeton University Press

Fraser N, 1997 Justice interruptus: critical reflections on the post-socialist condition. New York: Routledge

Habibis D, Walter M, 2009 Social inequality in Australia: discourses, realities and futures. Melbourne: Oxford University Press

Hurley J, Vaithianathan R, Crossley T, et al 2002 Parallel private health insurance in Australia: a cautionary tale and lessons for Canada. Canberra: Centre for Economic Policy, Australian National University, Discussion Paper No. 448

Lewis J, 2014 Recent changes in health policy: stepping back and looking forward. In: McClelland A, Smyth P, eds. *Social Policy in Action: Understanding for Action*, 3rd ed. Melbourne: Oxford University Press

Marmot M, 2017 Social justice, epidemiology and health inequality. *European Journal of Epidemiology* 32(7): 537–46. Available: https://doi.org/10.1007/s10654-017-0286-3

Matthew J, 2007 EPC scheme developments. *Australian Dental Association News Bulletin* 357, 22–4, 26.

Organisation for Economic Co-operation and Development (OECD) 2016 Social spending stays at historically high levels in many OECD countries. Social Expenditure Update 2016. Available: http://www.oecd.org/els/soc/OECD2016-Social-Expenditure-Update.pdf

Organisation for Economic Co-operation and Development (OECD) 2017 OECD health statistics 2017. Available: https://www.oecd.org/social/health-at-a-glance-19991312.htm

Peck J, 2010 Constructions of neo-liberal reason. Oxford: Oxford University Press

Pemberton S, Fahmy E, Sutton E, et al, 2016 Navigating the stigmatised identities of poverty in austere times: resisting and responding to narratives of personal failure. *Critical Social Policy* 36: 21–37

Pietsch J, Graetz B, McAllister I, 2010 Dimensions of Australian Society, 3rd ed. Melbourne: Palgrave Macmillan

Powers M, Fadden R, 2006 Social Justice: the Moral Foundations of Public Health and Health Policy. Oxford: Oxford University Press

Reed S, Schlepper L, Appleby J, 2021 Health spending during Covid-19: how does the UK compare. Available: https://www.nuffieldtrust.org.uk/news-item/health-spending-during-covid-19-how-does-the-uk-compare#:~:text=In%20many%20countries%2C%20governments%20increased,European%20OECD%20countries%20reporting%20data

Roff M, Segal L, 2004 Why it is time to review the role of private health insurance in Australia. *Australian Health Review* 28(1): 106–7. Available: https://doi.org/10.1071/AH040106 (Accessed 14 Oct, 2014)

Walker A, Percival R, Thurecht L, 2006 Distributional impact of recent changes in private health insurance policies. *Australian Health Review* 29: 467–73

Wilkinson R, Pickett K, 2010 Spirit level: why equality is better for everyone. London: Penguin

World Health Organization (WHO) 2014 World Health Statistics 2014. Available: http://apps.who.int/iris/bitstream/handle/10665/112738/9789240692671_eng.pdf;jsessionid=0CA9AF175D72BDB8B245FE566D986B80?sequence=1

Wyn J, 2009 Young people's wellbeing: managing the healthy self. *Australia Healthy Lifestyle Journal* 56(1): 1–5

7

Ethics and Public Health

Trish Gould and Mary Louise Fleming

LEARNING OBJECTIVES

After reading this chapter, you should be able to:

- Recognise that the term "ethics" is often defined and applied in different ways.
- Explain why ethics are at the very core of public health.
- Describe the foundations and development of public health ethics.
- Understand the core challenges of public health ethics.
- Recognise, evaluate and communicate ethical issues in public health work and policy.
- Apply ethical principles in your public health practice.

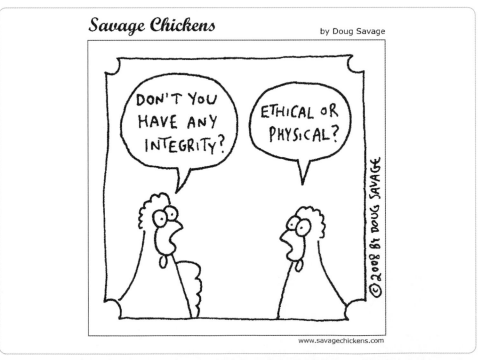

"Integrity". (Source: Savage Chickens cartoon © 2008 Doug Savage.)

INTRODUCTION

Ethics are not only important for health professionals and their client populations, but also for politicians, lawmakers and policymakers, who depend on health professionals for guidance about health-related issues. For example, as human populations increasingly become part of a global monoculture, with the consequent increase in pandemic and epidemic risks, decision-makers need help from health professionals to deal with difficult and controversial decisions arising from those risks.

One of the pivotal challenges in public health ethics is balancing the rights of the individual with the wellbeing of the population as a whole. For example, a person with an infectious disease might have their freedom restricted to protect the rest of the population. Thus, we must decide when it is acceptable to limit the rights of one category of people to ensure the wellbeing of others. Questions of this sort demonstrate the importance of such factors as power, fairness and values in public health ethics. There is already an implicit expectation from the public and health professions that health and wellbeing services are ethical because there is likely to be an outcry if service delivery or policy is perceived to be unfair or corrupt.

Formerly, the bulk of public health ethics tended to concentrate on two main areas: research ethics and responses to infectious diseases. However, public health ethics must also consider such things as: population health, safety and wellbeing; impartiality in service delivery; and the rights of both individuals and groups (Ortmann et al, 2016).

What relevance do ethics have to your own practice? As the considerable expenditure and work hours that go into public health initiatives and policies are, fundamentally, ethically motivated (an intention to "do good"), health professionals are constantly making explicit or implicit ethical decisions.

Public health ethical problems are also thrown up in debates on various cultural, environmental, economic and political issues. For example, with worldwide concerns over dwindling energy resources, must we choose between different types of pollution, such as the toxic chemicals associated with "fracking" versus radioactive waste from nuclear energy production, both of which carry risks to the environment and to people's health? Can public health ethics help with such decisions?

What is your understanding of "ethics"? Is your ethical perspective influenced by other factors, such as your religious, socioeconomic or cultural background? (See Activity 7.1.)

This chapter examines the characteristics of "ethics", the foundations of public health ethics and how we apply ethics to our practice. These themes are illustrated by some ethical challenges in professional health practice. As there is an ethical dimension to everything that is done—or not done—in public health, ethics is a practical field critical to effective health service delivery to consumers, and is of great concern to health professionals, politicians and, not least, the public.

ACTIVITY 7.1 Ethical Practice

Discuss with your classmates how you would define "ethical practice". Imagine and discuss some instances of unethical conduct within your professions.

Reflection

Some of your classmates' ideas may have been very different from your own. Nonetheless, you may find that if you look at the underlying basis for their arguments, many people had similar ideas—for example, "treat others as you would like to be treated". If there were major differences, do you think you can work effectively with those people?

Ethics typically inquires into a variety of concerns—*normative* ethics, *applied* ethics, *descriptive* ethics and *meta-ethics*. This chapter discusses normative and applied ethics in the context of public health.

NORMATIVE ETHICS IN PUBLIC HEALTH

Normative ethics tries to decide what are good and right actions and motives in practice; thus, it is particularly relevant to public health practice. However, as we might expect with such controversial questions, there are differing positions on how to decide what is good or right. The following are five common normative ethical positions:

1. *Consequences:* Consequentialism focuses on the most good for the most people (Greaves, 2020).
2. *Duties and rights:* Deontology maintains that every individual has fundamental duties and rights—and these should underlie ethical decisions (Lazar & Graham, 2021).
3. *Character:* Virtue ethics emphasises an individual's intrinsic qualities (whatever people agree are desirable characteristics, e.g. compassion) in preference to rules or consequences (Löfquist, 2018).
4. *Liberty and human rights:* Liberalism's focus is usually rights, equality, freedom and democracy (Phelan & Dawes, 2018).
5. *Community:* Communitarianism emphasises relationships and shared values; this perspective may require limiting an individual's autonomy for the benefit of the community (Chang, 2022).

Activity 7.2 demonstrates how these different beliefs and theories in normative ethics have real-world impacts. It illustrates how these normative theories offer a range of perspectives on the ethics of any particular public health action, and thus all should be considered when assessing the ethics of any given public health research or intervention. However, we do need to agree on the meanings of these theories and approaches to help us communicate in our efforts to be ethically effective in public health.

ACTIVITY 7.2 Quarantine

Discuss the following with your classmates. The age-old methods of preventing the spread of infection are quarantine and isolation. Imagine a situation where there is an infectious disease with a high mortality rate—for example, COVID-19. The Australian government's response is to order isolation and quarantine for people arriving in the country from places around the world where COVID-19 has high mortality rates.

- What do you think would be an appropriate response to the threat of a virulent virus like this one? Should you isolate sick people, and quarantine people who only *might be* infected?
- Do you think one ethical perspective is better than the others? Or is it more useful to use a range of viewpoints?

Reflection

- A *consequentialist* might argue that it is right to isolate someone with a highly lethal, infectious disease because of the *consequences* of not doing so—a pandemic, and subsequent deaths.
- A *deontologist* might claim that, regardless of the possible outcomes, there is a *duty* to protect people, and everyone has a *right* to be protected from disease.
- A *virtue ethicist* might defend isolation based on the good intentions of those enforcing isolation and quarantine.
- *Liberalists* might argue against enforced isolation and quarantine, and make a case for education in order to persuade infectious people to isolate themselves from others.
- *Communitarians* may argue that it is justifiable to limit individual freedoms—that is, isolating an infected person—if it benefits the whole community.

Clearly, there are many differences between these approaches—for example, the divergence between the "rights" of the individual (liberalism) and the "good" of the community (communitarianism). Nevertheless, they also have things in common; for example, utilitarianism and communitarianism both tend to favour the community over the individual.

THE DEVELOPMENT OF PUBLIC HEALTH ETHICS

Authors have differentiated between medical ethics and bioethics (Kass, 2017). *Medical ethics* refers to a health professional's ethical responsibility towards their (individual) patient. *Bioethics* has tended to concentrate more on the ethics of such issues as research, genomics, stem cell therapies and cloning, rather than medical treatment. The discipline of bioethics developed as a reaction to objectionable research, such as the Tuskegee Syphilis Study (see Case Study 7.1); and the "medical" experiments conducted by the Nazis during the Second World War (Annas & Mariner, 2016).

Although frameworks for public health ethics have partially derived from the bioethical tradition, public health ethics is now a separate discipline (Fairchild et al, 2017). Public health ethics refers to the values that are associated with the practice and institution of public health itself. Ethics in public health is about an analytical understanding and the philosophical or bioethical critique of public health activities and agendas. Essentially, it is about advocacy or activism focused on the promotion of the public's health (Coogan & Costin, 2020). Public health, unlike medicine, focuses more on preventing disease than on treating it. While the core values of public health tend to prioritise the needs and rights of the population (many individuals) over those of specific individuals, public health ethics also has to consider that those populations are made up of specific individuals; thus, individual rights are also important (Smith & Upshur, 2019).

PUBLIC HEALTH LAW AND HUMAN RIGHTS

There is an intricate relationship between public health, law, political philosophy and human rights. Although distinct social institutions, ethics and law are crucial tools for regulating behaviour, and can work in partnership to provide guidance for

CASE STUDY 7.1 The Tuskegee Syphilis Study

Beginning in 1932, a syphilis study took place in Tuskegee, Alabama, in the US. The participants were mainly underprivileged African-Americans. At that time, the accepted treatments for syphilis were not very effective and had toxic side effects. The researchers wanted to establish whether outcomes were better if patients were not treated with these medications. By the mid-1940s, penicillin was the orthodox therapy for syphilis, but the researchers continued with the research, and withheld penicillin and the relevant information. The study finally ended in the 1970s, when details were disclosed through the press. By this time, many of the participants had died from syphilis, and their families had become infected (Centers for Disease Control and Prevention [CDC] Public Health Ethics (https://www.cdc.gov/os/integrity/phethics/).

Imagine you are part of the Tuskegee study research team. In view of the social and ethical environment of today, are the issues any different? Can the researchers' actions be justified, considering

that laws, practices and attitudes were very different at that time?

Reflection

In the 1930s, doctors frequently did not disclose information to patients about their illness, as the doctors thought they "knew best" or did not want to "worry" their patients. Furthermore, the medical ethics of that period did not have the requirements for informed consent that exist today. As a consequence of this and similar studies, many African-Americans have little confidence in medical and public health authorities (CDC Public Health Ethics (https://www.cdc.gov/os/integrity/phethics/), which can have negative consequences for both the individuals and the population as a whole. Despite the differences, there is also a large amount of overlap between medical ethics (the physician's duty towards his or her patient), bioethics (medical research ethics) and public health ethics, as you can utilise all of these approaches together in exploring the above example.

public health. Practitioners must use their judgment to make decisions within the boundaries of the law. Ethics entails evaluating any proposed strategy, together with giving good reasons for any action. Thus, being able to collaborate with others to reflect on all of the potential actions and their ethical implications will enable acceptable decisions to be identified (Abbasi et al, 2018). In addition, if a legal or political controversy arises over a particular public health decision or policy, the fact that an ethical assessment was done as part of that decision-making process or policy analysis may provide reassurance to both the public and the court.

In 1948, the Universal Declaration of Human Rights was adopted by the General Assembly of the United Nations (UN) (UN, 1948), as part of the International Bill of Human Rights (Office of the High Commissioner for Human Rights). Australia has a Human Rights Commission established in 1986 and several States have a Bill of Human Rights.

Jonathan Mann (Mann, 1997), an influential scholar of health and human rights, claimed that a human rights-based paradigm provided a more practical framework for contemporary public health ethics than do frameworks modified from medical, biomedical or earlier public health ethics. Such an approach considers all of the social, economic, political and structural determinants of health, and human rights and public health both promote human wellbeing (Annas & Mariner, 2016; Mann, 1997).

Nay suggests that "legislatures ensure that health surveillance and monitoring policies should be prescribed by law, balanced to public health requirements, done in a clear fashion, controlled by independent regulators, with continual ethical reflection, non-discriminatory, and recognises fundamental rights" (Nay 2020, p. e239).

CODES OF ETHICS

A *code of ethics* is a published collection of standards for practitioners and organisations that dictates certain benchmarks as to their practice and their character while demonstrating their values to the public, as well as the standards of care that the public can expect (Lee et al, 2019).

Many health practitioners will be "covered" by their organisation's codes of ethics. For example, all employees of the Queensland government are covered by the Code of Conduct for the Queensland Public Service (Queensland Government, 2022). In addition, Australia has guidelines for ethical conduct in research with humans. These include the National Health and Medical Research Council's (NHMRC) National Statement on Ethical Conduct in Human Research (NHMRC, 2018), and Ethical Conduct in Research with Aboriginal and Torres Strait Islander Peoples and Communities: Guidelines for Researchers and Stakeholders (NHMRC, 2018). All health researchers in Australia must follow these guidelines.

The NHMRC (2018) research guidelines concerning Aboriginal and Torres Strait Islander peoples emphasise six core values:

1. *Spirit and integrity*—there must be respect for the cultural heritage of past, present and future generations, and credibility of intent when negotiating with Australian Indigenous communities.
2. *Cultural continuity*—the research acknowledges and respects Indigenous people's identities, their bonds with family and community and their relationships with the environment
3. *Equity*—there must be a commitment to fairness and justice.
4. *Reciprocity*—the research recognises the contributions of all partners, and ensures benefits are equitable and of value for communities.
5. *Respect*—there must be respect for, and acceptance of, dignity and diverse values.
6. *Responsibility*—researchers must ensure that they do not harm Aboriginal and Torres Strait Islander peoples or the things they treasure, and must be accountable to the people (NHMRC, 2018).

Similar guidelines are also in place for research with Indigenous peoples in other countries—for example, Canada and New Zealand (Canadian Institutes of Health Research, 2018; Health Research Council of New Zealand, 2022). Example 7.1 concerns the application of the *Values and Ethics* (NHMRC, 2018) guidelines.

EXAMPLE 7.1 Application of Research Ethics to Health Work

The *Values and Ethics* (NHMRC, 2018) guidelines were developed to guide health researchers in their *research* activities with Aboriginal and Torres Strait Islander Australians.

- Do you think they can be applied more generally to any *health-related work* undertaken with Aboriginal and Torres Strait Islander Australians, such as health promotion programs?
- Can these same guidelines be used with non-Indigenous populations?
- Do you understand the principles?
- How can you determine whether you have complied with the guidelines?

Reflection

Although devised for health *research*, the NHMRC guidelines (NHMRC 2018)—with their emphasis on such concepts as respect, reciprocity and responsibility—might also offer a positive model for implementing *public health programs* with Aboriginal and Torres Strait Islander communities. More importantly, however, Aboriginal and Torres Strait Island peoples need to have ownership of, and control over, any research or health initiative for it to be worthwhile and appropriate (Onemda VicHealth Koori Health Unit, 2008). These guidelines might also be suitable for any group with whom you work in partnership, especially different ethnic groups or nations (Parker et al, 2007). However, there may be difficulties reconciling the views of practitioners from different cultural traditions; from the perspective of many non-Indigenous practitioners, the good of the community can often conflict with that of the individual. Conversely, for many Aboriginal and Torres Strait Islander people, an individual would never be considered in isolation from his or her community. (See Chapter 4 for a discussion of Aboriginal and Torres Strait Islander Australians' health issues.)

Elves and Herring (2020) discuss a decision-making framework as one that sets out the general ethical principles that govern individual and societal responses and hence the background against which particular decisions need to be made.

THE APPLICATION OF ETHICS IN PUBLIC HEALTH PRACTICE

The below examples of ethical problems will help you to apply the theories to your profession, and demonstrate the relevance of ethics to your practice.

Public Health Research

When undertaking research projects, you are required to obtain ethical approval from at least one institution (e.g. a university ethical board). In addition to your responsibility to respect confidentiality and the participants' rights to informed consent, there are many other associated issues and risks. These include paying people to participate in a study, and the implications for the notion of voluntary consent, as payment might be considered to coerce people into participating (Jennings et al, 2015); and research funding and the potential conflict of interest—for example, a tobacco company who funds research on whether "vaping" encourages young people to smoke cigarettes (Coggon & Gostin, 2022).

Anthropological Research

In 2007, the UN General Assembly adopted the (non-binding) *Declaration on the Rights of Indigenous Peoples* (UN,

2008). Article 31 acknowledges the rights of Indigenous peoples to:

> . . . maintain, control, protect and develop . . . the manifestations of their sciences, technologies and cultures, including human and genetic resources, seeds, medicines, knowledge of the properties of fauna and flora, oral traditions . . . (UN, 2008)

Example 7.2 demonstrates some of the disadvantages for Indigenous peoples who are "researched".

Screening

Screening is arguably a "good" public health action. For example, in Australia, prostate cancer is the second leading cause of cancer-related mortality in Australian males (Prostate Cancer Foundation of Australia, 2022). If found early, prostate cancer can be treated. However, the treatments have significant side effects, including impotence and incontinence. In addition, some prostate cancers are very slow-growing and unlikely to kill the patient (Crawford et al, 2016). There are other limitations, such as high rates of false positives (Crawford et al, 2016). Activity 7.3 examines some of the issues surrounding screening.

DISEASE CONTROL

Disease control sometimes involves the enforcement of rules and/or control of individuals' behaviour for the good of the population as a whole. While diseases such as Zika virus, Ebola virus disease (EVD), HIV/AIDS, tuberculosis and COVID-19

EXAMPLE 7.2   Ethical Issues Arising from the Genographic Project

A study of genetic anthropology, the Genographic Project aimed to collect 100,000 DNA samples from Indigenous peoples to investigate human migration (Genographic Project website). The project ran into opposition from some Indigenous groups, with Harry (2009 p 10) commenting that it "is a highly invasive continuation of the NGS's [National Geographic Society's] practice of exploiting, objectifying, and capitalising on the lives of Indigenous peoples".

- Why do you think people would protest about this research?
- For the Indigenous peoples of the Pacific region, what are the likely advantages and/or disadvantages of participating?
- Who owns the samples and resources, the research outcomes and the intellectual property rights (Nicholas & Hollowell, 2009; UN, 2008)?

Reflection

Did you consider principles of privacy, autonomy and ownership? Despite the potential benefits, there are many drawbacks with this project. In many societies, the human body is "sacred", and must be kept "whole"; to remove blood or any other body part is inappropriate.

Peoples' own knowledge of their creation, ancestors, oral histories and languages, and their cultural and spiritual beliefs, may be damaged by the (Western) interpretation of any data acquired (Kanehe, 2007; Nicholas & Hollowell, 2009), and this can impact on health. Furthermore, if the results indicate that some Indigenous peoples did not arrive as early as their own histories indicate, the research could have negative consequences for their land and resource rights, and their sovereignty (Kanehe, 2007; Tallbear, 2013), which might negatively impact on their socioeconomic status and, therefore, their wellbeing. In addition, the researchers have not explained whether there are any direct benefits (health or other) for the participants. Therefore, it is likely that a social, spiritual and/or emotional burden is imposed on the people, with no guarantee of receiving any benefits. Do the *means* (collecting samples from Indigenous groups) justify the *ends* (a more comprehensive picture of human migration patterns)? Finally, the importance given to a group's genetic inheritance could result in people being stigmatised as "being somehow inherently flawed", and disregards other factors that impact on health status (Harry, 2009 p 154), such as the social, political and economic environment (see Chapters 2, 5 and 6).

ACTIVITY 7.3   Screening Issues

Discuss these questions with your classmates:

- Is it ethical to screen for any particular condition or disease predisposition if there is not always an effective and acceptable treatment, or if the side effects of treatment are significant and irreversible?
- Conversely, is it ethical not to screen when there is the potential to save lives, whatever the extent of that potential?

Reflection

Did you consider any of the following issues? A false negative may give the person peace of mind when it is unwarranted, while a false positive may lead to unnecessary diagnostic tests and anxiety. Should the participants be advised of the rates of false positives/negatives? Is it ethical to spend limited health funds on screening a subpopulation, where the number of positives identified may be minimal? How would you respond if a screening program had the potential to save one life for every 10,000 people screened? Should we ignore the life of that one individual?

are important public health problems, they also raise critical ethical issues. For example, should we enforce treatment for someone with an infectious disease who refuses to cooperate with the health professional's advice—for example, should they be detained against their will—or can you envision any alternatives?

In Australia, under federal law, a biosecurity officer can direct a person to remain in isolation if they are suspected of having a "listed human disease" (e.g. COVID-19). If the person is non-compliant with such an order, they can be detained and quarantined (Australian Government, 2015). There have been a number of other requirements on individuals or communities, such as "lock downs", travel restrictions or wearing of face masks in a variety of different situations.

While governments do have an obligation—and the legal power—to enforce measures to protect the "common good", they must also ensure they use the "least restrictive alternatives", at the same time choosing the most effective means to achieve the public health objectives (Gostin, 2018).

Do you think the legal powers to isolate/quarantine people adequately balance the rights of the individual against those of the rest of the population? Would it be wrong to let a person with COVID-19 come into contact with the public? The answer to that question initially was "yes", but more recently that question has been now answered "no" or at least we do not know who has COVID as the requirements for testing and reporting have been relaxed.

Another aspect of disease control is contact tracing, which involves finding people who may have had contact with someone who has an infectious disease. However, these people have not in any way sought diagnosis and treatment, nor given their consent to be traced. Conversely, do they have a right to be informed of their possible risk status? Which right, if any, should take precedence? What about protecting the public? Unquestionably, one of the core issues for public health ethics is the necessity to use authority to protect "the people's" health, while also preventing the abuse of such power (Gostin, 2018).

Social Media for Public Health

New technologies offer opportunities for health promotion and education, research and disease control (like contact tracing) (Hunter et al, 2018). A variety of different social networking apps, can be used to educate people about diseases, and for research (Hunter et al, 2018). For instance, the Centers for Disease Control and Prevention uses a range of social media for "health communication campaigns, activities and emergency response efforts" (CDC, 2019). Banerjee and Meena (2021) suggest that public health and social media need to have a more symbiotic and mutually stronger relationship so that social media can become an integrated approach in public health promotion and can help facilitate better psycho-social and global wellbeing. However, using social media can raise ethical problems, including threats to anonymity, confidentiality (Pagoto et al, 2019) and authenticity—for example, the existence of fake accounts (Pulido et al, 2020).

In Activity 7.4 we discuss a case where a person with COVID-19 was seriously ill, and thus unable to tell the health authorities the names of people he had been in contact with. A friend posted the information on the patient's Facebook page to inform possible contacts of their risk. (See Activity 7.4.)

Health Promotion

As discussed in other chapters in this book, health professionals must consider not only individuals' responsibility for their

ACTIVITY 7.4   Privacy Versus the Public Interest

Imagine you are diagnosed with COVID-19. Your family are all treble vaccinated but you know many of your young friends are not vaccinated. The public health authorities contact you advising of the need to isolate for you and your family. They have asked you for a list of your friends that you have been in contact with before the diagnosis.

- Do you feel that this would violate your right to privacy, or would you be relieved that your friends would be informed and tested?
- What if you were very unwell and unable to provide consent?

Reflection

Clearly, there is a conflict between safeguarding your privacy and considering the needs of your friends who may have been infected. Such a case requires a careful balancing of the rights and responsibilities of the relevant authorities, the patient and the public.

EXAMPLE 7.3 Community Perceptions of Their Health Priorities

Imagine you work with a community that has a high rate of type 2 diabetes. You provide information to the community about the role of diet and exercise in controlling diabetes, and you establish an exercise group. However, the results are disappointing—community members seem indifferent. People with diabetes and pre-diabetes do not pay more attention to their diets, nor do they increase the amount of exercise they do.

• What do you think went wrong?
• Do people not care? Do they think that diabetes is "no big deal"?

Reflection

Did you consider the people's own perceptions of their problems? There could be other issues that they consider more urgent. If you identified a health issue and its solution without consulting the community, not only have you ignored the principles of effective health promotion practice (see Chapter 13), but you have also disregarded people's autonomy. Perhaps they did want to address their health problems but could not afford healthy food, or had inadequate exercise facilities (e.g., no safe area to exercise). As well as these more practical issues, it raises problems of meaning—perhaps your idea of "health" or "diabetes" does not accord with theirs. Importantly, there is the possibility that your approach may have been interpreted as coercive and paternalistic.

---

own health, but also the range of other factors that impact on health. In order to prevent unethical (and counterproductive) victim-blaming (Laverack, 2017) they need to recognise that there are numerous, interrelated health determinants (Annas & Mariner, 2016).

Health promotion interventions also have the potential to be patronising and coercive, and the practitioner's definition of "health" may not be congruent with the community's (see Example 7.3).

Advocacy

As described in Chapters 2, 5 and 6, there is ample evidence that social and economic environments impact on a person's health. Does this mean that health professionals have a duty to advocate for equity with regard to the direct determinants of health? What about the broader determinants, such as housing and employment? The Public Health Association (2022) claims that people in the health professions have an obligation to "act as advocates for health at all levels in society". What does this mean? Should health professionals advocate restructuring of a range of elements, such as institutions, policies and laws? For example, a number of organisations advocated for Rapid Antigen Tests (RATs) for the community to check for COVID-19 and to be available to the public at large. They wrote, "A public health crisis requires a public policy response. The current distribution model . . . leaves too many behind and too often the financial means of people will determine whether they have adequate access to RATs. This leaves the whole community vulnerable" (Public Health Association, 2022).

CONTEMPORARY AND FUTURE PUBLIC HEALTH ETHICS

There is a need for more research and discussion on public health ethics. Should health professionals consider more than just public health-related ethical concerns? What about all of the factors that promote or damage health, including social, environmental, political and economic determinants?

A FINAL WORD

In this chapter, we have explored "ethics" and ethical theories relevant to public health ethics. This chapter has endeavoured to unite ethics and public health to demonstrate that good public health practice is intrinsically ethical, and that ethics should be an ordinary part of our day-to-day public health activities. As health professionals, your understanding of ethical practice is a significant aspect of your professional competence. This knowledge and insight will enable you to anticipate and address any potential ethical issues prior to taking action, and to practise in such a way that your motives and values are clearly apparent to others. Anyone working in a public health-related environment needs to understand that there may be more than one ethically correct approach to a given situation, a range of equally unattractive compromises, or none at all. Nevertheless, if you practise systematically, and reflect on your practice, you will be able to justify your actions, both to yourself and to others.

▮ REVIEW QUESTIONS

1. What is the best theoretical approach to public health ethics—for example, consequence—or rule-based? Is there only one best approach, or must all be applied in a balanced way? Justify your response.

2. Think of an example of a conflict between the principles of autonomy and of the good of the community. Why is there a conflict, how would you approach it and is there an outcome where both principles can be respected?

3. Do you think it is possible to ethically practise in, or research with, a culture or community different from your own? Do you see any likely ethical dilemmas?

4. Identify some key contemporary challenges for public health ethics, and outline their significance.

5. After reading some of the chapters in this book, try to identify an ethical dilemma that could potentially arise as a result of a public health action (or lack of action). Explain why it would be a problem, and outline your solution.

6. Why does the Public Health Association of Australia (2021) claim that health professionals have an obligation to "act as advocates for health at all levels in society"?

7. What are some of the challenges with using social media for health research?

USEFUL WEBSITES

Centers for Disease Control and Prevention—Public Health Ethics: https://www.cdc.gov/os/integrity/phethics/
Nuffield Council on Bioethics: http://nuffieldbioethics.org/
World Health Organization, Global Health Ethics: https://apps.who.int/iris/bitstream/handle/10665/164576/9789240694033_eng.pdf

ACKNOWLEDGEMENT

Special thanks to Briin Gould for his perceptive editorial comments in earlier editions of this chapter.

REFERENCES

Abbasi M, Majdzadeh R, Zali A et al 2018 The evolution of public health ethics frameworks: systematic review of moral values and norms in public health policy. *Medicine, Health Care and Philosophy* 21(3): 387–402

Annas GJ, Mariner WK 2016 (Public) health and human rights in practice. *Journal of Health Politics, Policy and Law* 41(1): 129–39

Australian Government 2015 Biosecurity Act, No. 61, 2015 Available: http://legislation.gov.au (Accessed 16 Feb 2018)

Banerjee D, Meena KS 2021 COVID-19 as an "infodemic" in public health: critical role of the social media. *Frontiers in Public Health* 9: 231

BUGA-UP (Billboard Utilising Graffitists Against Unhealthy Promotions) website 2012 Available: http://www.bugaup.org/ (Accessed 18 Feb 2018)

Canadian Institutes of Health Research, Natural Sciences and Engineering Research Council of Canada, Social Sciences and Humanities Research Council of Canada 2018 Tri-Council Policy Statement: Ethical Conduct for Research Involving Humans. Available: https://ethics.gc.ca/eng/tcps2-eptc2_2018_chapter9-chapitre9.html (Accessed 25 March 2022)

Centers for Disease Control and Prevention (CDC) 2019 CDC social media tools, guidelines and best practices. Available: https://www.cdc.gov/socialmedia/tools/guidelines/guideforwriting.html (Accessed 11 May 2022)

Centre for Disease Control and Prevention (CDC) CDC Public Health Ethics. Available: http://www.cdc.gov/os/integrity/phethics/

Chang YL 2022 Communitarianism, properly understood. *Canadian Journal of Law & Jurisprudence* 1–23

Coggon J, Gostin LO 2020 The two most important questions for ethical public health. *Journal of Public Health* 42(1): 198–202

Crawford ED, Rosenberg MT, Partin AW et al 2016 An approach using PSA levels of 1.5 ng/ml as the cutoff for prostate cancer screening in primary care. *Urology* 20: 116–20. Available: https://doi.org/10.1016/j.urology.2016.07.001.

Elves CB, Herring J 2020 Ethical framework for adult social care in COVID-19. *Journal of Medical Ethics* 46(10): 662–7

Fairchild AL, Dawson A, Bayer R et al 2017 The World Health Organization, public health ethics, and surveillance: essential architecture for social well-being. *American Journal of Public Health* 107(10): 1596–8

Gostin LO 2018 Mandatory vaccination: understanding the common good in the midst of the global polio eradication campaign. *Israel Journal of Health Policy Research* 7(4). doi:10.1186/s13584-017-0198-4.

Greaves H 2020 Global consequentialism. In: Portmore DW, ed. *The Oxford Handbook of Consequentialism*. Oxford: Oxford Academic

Health Research Council of New Zealand 2022 Guidelines for researchers on health research involving Māori. Available: https://www.hrc.govt.nz/sites/default/files/2022-02/Ethics%20Committee%20Terms%20of%20Reference.pdf (Accessed April 2022)

Hunter RF, Gough A, O'Kane N et al 2018 Ethical issues in social media research for public health. *American Journal of Public Health* 108: 343–8. doi:10.2105/AJPH.2017.304249

Jennings CG, MacDonald TM, Wei L et al 2015 Does offering an incentive payment improve recruitment to clinical trials and increase the proportion of socially deprived and elderly participants? *Trials* 16, 80. doi:10.1186/s13063-015-0582-8

Kass NE 2017 A journey in public health ethics. *Perspectives in Biology and Medicine* 60(1): 103–6

Laverack G 2017 The role of health promotion in disease outbreaks and health emergencies. *Societies* 7(1): 2. doi:10.3390/soc7010002

Lazar S, Graham PA 2021 Deontological decision theory and lesser-evil options. *Synthese* 198(7): 6889–916

Lee LM, Fairchild AL, Jennings B et al 2019 New Public Health Code of Ethics (organized by APHA & Ethics Section). In: *American Public Health Association (APHA) 2019 Annual Meeting and Expo (Nov 2-Nov 6)*. APHA

Löfquist L 2018 Virtue ethics and disasters. Disasters: core concepts and ethical theories. *Advancing Global Bioethics* 11, 203

Mann JM 1997 Medicine and public health, ethics and human rights. *The Hastings Center Report* 27(3): 6–13

National Health and Medical Research Council (NHMRC) 2018 Ethical Conduct of Research with Aboriginal and Torres Strait Islander Peoples and Communities: Guidelines for Researchers and Stakeholders. Commonwealth of Australia, Canberra. Available: https://nhmrc.gov.au/about-us/publications/ethical-conduct-research-aboriginal-and-torres-strait-islander-peoples-and-communities#block-views-block-file-attachments-content-block- (Accessed 9 Oct 2018)

Nay O 2020 Can a virus undermine human rights? *Lancet Public Health* 5: e238–9. Available: www.thelancet.com/publichealth

Ortmann LW, Barrett DH, Saenz C et al 2016 Public health ethics: global cases, practice, and context. Public health ethics: cases spanning the globe. *Public Health Ethics Analysis* 3: 3–35

Pagoto S, Waring ME, Xu R 2019 A call for a public health agenda for social media research. *Journal of Medical Internet Research* 21(12):e16661. doi:10.2196/16661

Phelan S, Dawes S 2018 Liberalism and neoliberalism. In: *Oxford Research Encyclopedia of Communication*. Oxford: Oxford University Press

Prostate Cancer Foundation of Australia 2022 Prostate cancer in Australia—what do the numbers tell us. Available: https://www.prostate.org.au/news-media/news/prostate-cancer-in-australia-what-do-the-numbers-tell-us/ (Accessed 20 May 2022)

Public Health Association of Australia 2022 ACTU, PHAA and other organisations – Joint statement on the need for free and accessible rapid antigen tests to protect public health and the economic recovery. Available: https://www.phaa.net.au/advocacy-policy/advocacy-letters/letters (Accessed 12 May 2022)

Pulido CM, Ruiz-Eugenio L, Redondo-Sama G et al 2020 A new application of social impact in social media for overcoming fake news in health. *International Journal of Environmental Research and Public Health* 17(7): 2430

Queensland Government 2022 Code of Conduct for the Queensland Public Service. Available: https://www.forgov.qld.gov.au/__data/assets/pdf_file/0024/182292/code-of-conduct.pdf (Accessed 10 April 2022)

Smith M, Upshur R 2019 Pandemic disease, public health, and ethics. *The Oxford Handbook of Public Health Ethics*, 10

Tallbear K 2013 Native American DNA: tribal belonging and the false promise of genetic science. Minneapolis: University of Minnesota Press

United Nations (UN) General Assembly 1948 Universal Declaration of Human Rights. Adopted and proclaimed by General Assembly resolution 217 A (III) of 10 December 1948. Available: http://www.un.org/Overview/rights.html (Accessed 12 Feb 2018)

United Nations (UN) 2008 United Nations Declaration on the Rights of Indigenous Peoples. Available: http://www.un.org/esa/socdev/unpfii/documents/DRIPS_en.pdf (Accessed 12 Feb 2018)

8

Evidence-based Practice

Mary Louise Fleming and Gerry Fitzgerald

LEARNING OBJECTIVES

After reading this chapter, you should be able to:
- Define "evidence" and "evidence-based practice", and describe their value to public health.
- Identify and appraise the nature and sources of evidence.
- Identify and discuss the principles of evidence-based practice as it applies to public health.

- Discuss the way in which evidence can be applied to achieve advances in public health and health policy, and the factors that influence success.

INTRODUCTION

This chapter traces the history and rationale for evidence-based practice (EBP), defines EBP, and differentiates it from "evidence-based medicine". The important skills for EBP, and the processes of attaining the necessary evidence, are considered, and the barriers and facilitators to identifying and implementing "best practice" are examined. The limitations of EBP and other processes to guide practice are discussed and concluding information about the application of evidence to guide policy, organisations and practice is considered.

THE EVOLUTION: EVIDENCE-BASED MEDICINE

In 1972, epidemiologist Dr Archie Cochrane criticised the medical profession for not providing reviews of clinical interventions so that policymakers and organisations could base their practice on empirically proven evidence (Faria et al, 2021). Researchers from McMaster University in Canada first coined the term "evidence-based medicine", which they defined as "the conscientious, explicit, and judicious use of current best evidence in making decisions about the care of individual patients" (Dimitri, 2021). It is about integrating individual clinical expertise and the best external evidence

(Sackett, 1996). Researchers more recently talk of evidence, expertise and patient desire.

The subsequent impact of evidence-based medicine has been to develop the means of accumulating the evidence systematically, analysing it and converting it into guidelines and standards for clinical practice. Thus, enormous quantities of research data are converted into a usable format for clinicians. This emphasis on evidence-based medicine has served to reduce the previous reliance on "opinion" as unqualified "evidence" in its own right.

Evidence-based medicine has an intrinsic clinical focus, but these same principles have been applied to public health, health policy, planning and management. Hence the adoption of the more general term "evidence-based practice" (Egger et al, 2022).

DEFINING "EVIDENCE, EVIDENCE-BASED PRACTICE" AND KEY CONCEPTS

What defines "evidence" and "EBP"? How does EBP inform complex areas such as public policy, public health and healthcare?

We live in an "information age", which means increased accessibility to enormous amounts of information (Egger et al, 2022). Consider Activity 8.1 as a means of beginning to think about what evidence you might use and where you might access it.

ACTIVITY 8.1   Appraising the Evidence

A family member's favourite celebrity is campaigning against mobile phone towers being placed near schools. The family member asks you about the health impact of mobile phone towers, as you are studying for a health degree. Because your studies have taught you to base your decisions on evidence, you research information on the health impact of mobile phone towers. What sources might you consult and trust? What sources do you think would interest your family member the most?

Reflection

There is a range of information sources—journals, textbooks, newspapers, magazines, editorials, online newspapers, telecommunications industry/associations' reports, blogs written by companies or individuals, and government and private health agencies' websites and reports. Some information sources are more trustworthy than others. Information from the internet or in news clips may not be as reliable as that provided by rigorous scientific studies. There has been a significant increase in the number of research studies being conducted, papers being published and journals available. Technological advancements have meant that the quality of research methodologies has improved and research findings are more accessible (Karampela et al, 2019).

This abundance of information justifies EBP. However, we need to know how to interpret information and critically analyse it for its value. Values and beliefs influence how evidence is applied, sometimes at the expense of the research outcomes. Is there a single truth? How is knowledge created? Is it neutral, or is it influenced by social, economic and political factors?

While we are lucky to have so much information at our disposal, it does mean that there is more information to assess to determine what constitutes evidence. Information must be sorted, analysed and then given meaning, or moulded into knowledge by describing its practical application in specific settings (Escoffery et al, 2019).

This process can be very time-consuming, and other factors increase the complexity of identifying and implementing "best practice", including problems with dissemination and communication of the implications of research, and the methods employed to obtain these results (Sahin et al, 2020). Political pressure might influence what research is conducted, published and used to influence practice, and organisational barriers might hinder health professionals who are implementing EBPs within their organisations (Brownson et al, 2018a).

WHAT IS "EVIDENCE-BASED PRACTICE"?

Evidence-based practice (EBP) is the integration of the best research evidence, expertise and population needs that will result in the best health outcomes (Ding et al, 2020). The key elements of the "conscientious, judicious and explicit use of evidence" are critical to an understanding of the approach.

Conscientious implies a systematic and organised approach. *Judicious* implies the wise application of the evidence to particular circumstances, and *explicit* means that it is clear and available. To become an evidence-based practitioner, you need to critique the evidence and be willing to change your practice if doing so is indicated.

KEY CONCEPTS OF EVIDENCE-BASED PRACTICE

EBP originated from concerns to improve healthcare and health outcomes by basing practice on the best available evidence (Brownson et al, 2018a). However, there are risks in using the results of only one study to guide practice. Case Study 8.1 discusses the dangers of reliance on a single study. By contrast Ding and colleagues (2020) suggest a road map for future research in the field of physical activity. In doing so the authors argue for research that provides solutions, and that connects knowledge into translation. They argue that, like many public health issues, physical inactivity is a "wicked problem" that needs a systems-based approach, and that researchers and stakeholders need to work across disciplines and sectors to co-design research and co-create solutions (p. 6).

In practice, what does "evidence based" mean? Is it about using strategies that the research suggests are the best means

CASE STUDY 8.1   Dangers of "Research Utilisation"

Several studies reported that travellers were not at increased risk from deep vein thrombosis compared with the general population. However, other studies suggested that travellers were at increased risk. Reports of a woman who was travelling by air to Australia who had died from a pulmonary embolus might have further persuaded the public of the dangers of long-haul flights.

Several studies conducted over a short period of time reported conflicting data. Consumers who sought advice from their general practitioner on the health risks of long-haul flights may have received an incomplete picture of the risks if healthcare providers relied on only a small number of studies.

Questions

1. Should health professionals only use the results from randomised controlled trials (RCTs) to guide their practice? (Note that not all health issues could ethically be tested using an RCT.)
2. When there are differences of opinion about an issue in the scientific literature, how should health professionals make an informed decision to guide their practice?
3. What type of evidence, and how much evidence, should be collected before making a decision?

for achieving the stated aims? Is it about changing practice? Is it about a systematic appraisal of the best available evidence? The answer to all of these questions is "yes". However, in practice, there is never absolute certainty, as programs that are implemented even in similar circumstances are never quite the same.

The gold standard for research is the randomised controlled trial (RCT). However, there may not be sufficient research on a particular topic, or it may be ethically inappropriate to conduct an RCT. For example, one of the most successful public health interventions of the 20th century led to the recognition that smoking was associated with an increased risk of lung cancer. Despite it being widely accepted by the public and health professionals alike that tobacco use is responsible for many cases of lung cancer, this has not been empirically proven, and it is unlikely that it ever will be. It would be unethical to subject some individuals to tobacco smoke and not others, which is what would be required to conduct definitive research via an RCT.

In addition, research is not always reliable and valid, even if it is available on a particular issue. Evidence evolves over time and this evolution poses challenges, as it requires repositioning of policy and this creates uncertainty and reduces trust in the evidence.

Researchers refer to the approach to EBP being more like a journey towards more effective practice, and along this journey the practitioner must become more open-minded (Brownson et al, 2018a) (see Box 8.1).

Using evidence to make decisions about the most appropriate practice is similar to undertaking primary research, which involves five steps:

1. Identifying the problem.
2. Identifying the evidence that relates to the problem.
3. Finding the evidence.
4. Critically appraising the evidence to determine its suitability.
5. Synthesising the available evidence into a practical application.

Table 8.1 describes these five EBP steps in more detail.

BOX 8.1   What is an Evidence-based Practitioner?

An evidence-based practitioner uses problem-solving skills to determine:

- What they need to know
- The extent to which the intervention is effective, acceptable, equitable, implemented consistently and safely, and is cost-effective
- Whether they have the best available evidence
- Whether the quality of the evidence is good
- Whether the evidence is appropriate for the population and the context in which they will use the evidence

Source: Brownson et al, 2021.

Why is There a Gap Between Research and Practice?

The causes of the evidence–practice gap are multiple, and vary from setting to setting. A number of surveys of health practitioners have been conducted to assess attitudes to EBP and barriers to its implementation. Although data indicate that practitioners welcome EBP, a number of significant barriers to its implementation have been identified:

- Reasons relating to the *evidence base*, such as gaps in the evidence base, or the poor quality of evidence; additionally, the evidence may need to be tested and retested before it is acceptable.
- Personal reasons relating to the *individual practitioner*, such as lack of skills to undertake EBP, or a lack of time.
- Reasons related to the *organisation*, such as inappropriate or inadequate support for EBP, a perceived threat posed by EBP, a lack of understanding of the process, economic constraints, access to evidence, resistance from colleagues, competing agendas, lack of technical support or lack of facilities (Aarons et al, 2018).

Studies suggest that apart from evidence-related reasons and personal barriers, organisational barriers are highly significant in preventing the implementation of EBP (Aarons et al, 2018). Reasons seemingly related to the individual practitioner, such as a lack of time or motivation, can also be influenced by organisational factors.

Organisational Barriers to EBP

Why don't healthcare organisations use EBP? First, healthcare practice has evolved over a long period of time, during which the role, expectations and environment of the health practitioner have changed dramatically. A shift to practice based on evidence rather than based solely on experience and judgment represents a fundamental change (Hailemariam et al, 2019). Healthcare delivery is complex. Policy is developed at the international, national, state and local levels. There are a variety of funding mechanisms and public and private ownership of services, all of which influence decisions (Jacob et al, 2017). Health-related organisations also frequently have multiple (sometimes conflicting) goals, such as improving health, gaining funding, reducing expenditure, fostering staff development and influencing government and community stakeholders. Aspects of organisations themselves also influence the uptake of EBP, as shown in Example 8.1.

The following organisational and environmental supports are suggested for practitioners to apply EBP (Aarons et al, 2018; Brownson et al, 2018a):

- Supportive organisational culture, policies and procedures (e.g. the organisation is open to change, and provides information technology support, opportunities, incentives and funding for EBP)

TABLE 8.1 Evidence-based Practice Steps

Steps	Actions
Identifying the problem	The problem must be adequately and specifically defined to be useful for the search for evidence.
Identifying evidence that relates to the problem	Important considerations include looking, where possible, for sources that rely on primary research, and deciding how to use the evidence to make an informed decision about practice. Consideration should include the effectiveness of the intervention in meeting its goals, the evidence available on the transferability of the intervention to other settings and with other populations, the positive and negative effects of the intervention and the barriers to implementing the intervention (Brownson et al, 2021).
Finding the evidence	The scientific model has gained prominence as a quantitatively objective method for *finding the evidence*; contextual factors, such as environment, socioeconomic factors or education, are considered as *confounding variables*, and study designs often try to eliminate their effects. RCTs are viewed as the "gold standard", but when we are dealing with populations it becomes very difficult, if not impossible, to adopt an RCT methodology (Shelton et al, 2021). Research findings are graded according to an established *hierarchy of evidence* (see Table 8.2), according to how valid and reliable the methodology for the research is considered to be (Shelton et al, 2021). There are a number of ways in which evidence can be sourced. Table 8.3 shows the five characteristics involved in systematic reviews. Searches need to be undertaken systematically, using consistent key words or phrases. They need to be transparent to ensure that others can gauge their suitability and comprehensiveness (Yoo et al, 2021). Numerous sources of evidence can be used to guide practice, such as bibliographical databases (e.g. Medline, Cinahl, Scopus) and the Cochrane (health and medical research) and Campbell collaborations (systematic reviews of the effectiveness of social and behavioural interventions).
Determining the usefulness of the evidence (i.e. critically appraising the evidence to determine its suitability)	*Determining the usefulness of the evidence* is termed *critical appraisal*. It involves a systematic evaluation of the relevance of the study, and the ability to critically appraise a range of study types. An understanding of the epidemiological concepts discussed in Chapter 3 is crucial to understanding the results as they have been presented, as well as having a systematic approach to the appraisal (Brownson et al, 2018a). Standardised checklists for the systematic appraisal of different types of study design can assist in determining the validity of the study findings and their generalisability to other populations. Critical appraisal has to be pragmatic. The focus should be on studies that reach a certain standard of rigour and relevance, while recognising that flaws in published research studies occur, as well as the ways in which the context of the research and one's own practice differ.
Synthesising the available evidence into a practical application	*Putting evidence into practice*. There is still an evidence–practice gap, and research findings frequently cannot be translated into action. Although you might assume that having the research evidence required will lead to rational practices and policies, this is often not the case. Desirable methodological characteristics of research into the effectiveness of interventions include issues such as whether: • The level of detail of an intervention would enable it to be replicated • The participants who are the target of the intervention are fully described • The size and effect of non-respondents are detailed • There are clear outcomes, and these outcomes are compared with baseline measurements taken before the intervention commences.

Adapted from Brownson RC, Baker EA, Deshpande AD et al 2018a Evidence-Based Public Health, 3rd edn. Oxford University Press, New York.

• Supportive external environment to the organisation (e.g. funders, accreditation groups, national/regional/local authorities), which provides opportunities and incentives for EBP
• Organisational procedures to ensure implementation of guidelines and other evidence-based prescriptions for practice

• Methods for systematically evaluating the implementation of EBP and providing feedback to stakeholders on practice effectiveness
• Staff trained as evidence-based practitioners capable of working in evidence-based organisations.

Li (2018) identified six organisational contextual features that are important to EBP implementation across healthcare

TABLE 8.2	**Hierarchy of Evidence**
Type 1 evidence	Systematic reviews and meta-analyses including two or more RCTs
Type 2 evidence	Well-designed RCTs
Type 3 evidence	Well-designed controlled trials without randomisation
Type 4 evidence	Well-designed observational studies
Type 5 evidence	Expert opinion, expert panels, views of service users and carers

RCT = randomised controlled trial.
Source: Dang et al, 2021.

TABLE 8.3	**Systematic Review Process**
THE SYSTEMATIC REVIEW SEARCH SHOULD BE:	
Explicit	Use key terms, record your search, ensure that it is transparent so that others can assess value and it can be replicated
Appropriate	Look where evidence is likely to be
Sensitive	Collect all information that is relevant to your question
Specific	Collect only information that is relevant to the question
Comprehensive	Include all available information

settings that are slightly different to those suggested by Aaron and colleagues (2018) and Brownson and colleagues (2018). These features include organisational culture, leadership, communication and networks, resources, champions and evaluation, monitoring and feedback activities within healthcare organisations.

Organisational structures, such as those that distribute power using centralised and decentralised organisational models, also influence the adoption of EBP. Practitioners require real power to change practices, so EBP may be easier to implement in a decentralised organisation, where individual practitioners make decisions influencing their practice. However, centralised structures may more easily be able to coordinate system-wide support, such as funding. (Consider Activity 8.2 as a means of using evidence to build a case for funding.)

Additionally, we may expect that as individuals with new ideas enter an organisation, these ideas will diffuse through the organisation. However, organisations may display "defensive routines", or resist new ideas as a way of "protecting" the way everything has always been done. Conflict is particularly likely when a proposed change is at odds with existing values and assumptions (Kennedy et al, 2020). To some extent, the existing evidence-based "standards or guidelines" may impede change as they act to prescribe "how things are done here".

The final part of this chapter discusses the role of evidence in policy development.

EXAMPLE 8.1 **Impact of Different Organisational Cultures on EBP Uptake**

Allison

Allison is a recent graduate who works as a dietitian for a public hospital in community A. Allison was taught how to critically appraise research during her university course, and is keen to ensure that her practice is based on current evidence. The organisation Allison works for is very busy, and Allison finds she has little time to review journals and keep up-to-date during her work time. One day when she was reading abstracts online, her supervisor noticed and said, "That's not your job; get back to work". Allison also finds it difficult to follow evidence-based practice (EBP) as her organisation has limited information resources and has not subscribed to many journals electronically. After working at the hospital for a few months, Allison finds that, despite her best intentions, she is largely following the organisational line and basing her practice on what is standard practice in the hospital, even though she suspects that new research regarding dietetic practice is available.

Bianca

Bianca is another recent graduate, and she works as a dietitian for a private hospital in community B. Although understanding of EBP varies among the staff, the rganisation's CEO believes that the ability to adapt to change is crucial for the organisation's future success. Ongoing training is mandatory. Thus, EBP is widely understood and valued. Groups of staff working in various areas also meet monthly to discuss the latest developments in their field and how they could be applied in their practice. Bianca is expected to be familiar with the latest research, and has access to journals online at work. Although her job is very busy, Bianca schedules time in her diary during work hours each week to peruse the evidence and reflect on current practice. She is currently working in conjunction with other hospital staff to identify and overcome potential barriers to changing an aspect of current practice, and feels confident that she will be able to implement this change to improve patient outcomes.

Reflection

Allison's and Bianca's organisations clearly differ in their organisational culture. Some cultural beliefs that operate in organisations that make it difficult to introduce new practices include:
- A reluctance to change historical practices (e.g. "This is how we've always done things").
- A belief that practice is already at a high level.
- A lack of preparedness to ask questions (e.g. "Why do we do things this way?").

You work for a state health department in their population health unit. You are planning to establish a community walking group in some suburban areas, particularly for people who have had cardiac surgery or who are living with coronary heart disease. Partners and family members are also welcome. You need to obtain funding for the program.

Reflection
- How would you go about justifying the program on the basis of evidence?
- How did you define the problem?
- Do you need more information to identify the real issues?
- Try to decide what the focus of your search strategy should be in order to provide the evidence.

EVIDENCE AND POLICY DEVELOPMENT

Although you may not believe that you will be a policymaker, you are likely to be influenced by or to influence policy decisions at some time in your working life. Policy (discussed in Chapters 5 and 6) can be made within legislative, judicial or executive arenas, and within both large and small organisations. Based on what you have read about the barriers to using evidence, do you believe that health policy is likely to be evidence-based?

But why is policy not based on evidence? When you have the skills to find and evaluate evidence, you might expect every decision to be based on a careful consideration of the available data and application to the appropriate context.

However, criticism of policymakers must be tempered by an understanding of the complexity of policymaking (see Chapters 5 and 6). Policymaking is not a linear process, and policymakers may be influenced by information from a variety of sources (not solely scientific evidence), other individuals, personal and political agendas, and longstanding practices (Brownson et al, 2018b; Brownson et al, 2018c). Additionally, there is often conflicting evidence and rarely high levels of evidence (such as RCTs) to inform policy.

The use of implementation science, however, can support progress towards achieving health equity goals as an example. Implementation science seeks to understand and influence how scientific evidence is put into practice for health improvement (Brownson et al, 2021). The challenges of such an approach include the limitations of the evidence base, inadequate measures and methods and the need to pay attention to context (Emmons & Chambers, 2021). Brownson and colleagues (2021) offer a set of steps to address these challenges as follows:
- *Link social determinants with health outcomes*
- *Build equity into all policies*

- *Use equity-relevant metrics*
- *Study what is already happening*
- *Integrate equity into implementation models*
- *Design and tailor implementation strategies*
- *Connect to systems and sectors outside of health*
- *Engage organisations in internal and external equity efforts*
- *Build capacity for equity in implementation science, and*
- *Focus on equity in dissemination efforts.*

Brownson et al, 2021, pp. 4, 9, 10, 11 and 12

Consider the study by Wild and colleagues (2021) that can be found at the following website: https://www.phrp.com.au/wp-content/uploads/2021/03/PHRP3112105.pdf

This study examined the challenges of communicating COVID-19 directives to culturally and linguistically diverse communities in Australia.

Read through this study and then answer the questions that follow:
- What did the study present as evidence-based solutions to influence policy and practice on promoting relevant health behaviours?
- What suggestions did the study support in relation to partnerships and how was this achieved?
- What suggestions do the researchers offer for shifting health behaviours?
- What should be placed at the centre of health communications?
- How might this impact behaviour change strategies?

A FINAL WORD

In summary, the practice of evidence-based public health (EBPH) is influenced by epidemiology, behavioural and policy research, knowing which information is important and how it should be disseminated and an emphasis on practice-based evidence. It is important, however, that we do not ignore the context and the complex processes of decision-making that are central to EBPH (Brownson et al, 2018a). Also, the translation of evidence into practice is inevitably subject to political consideration. Not just considerations at the "political" level of governance but also the interplay of ideas and conflict of special interests within and external to an organisation.

This chapter has introduced you to the reality of evidence–practice gaps, and why policy is not always based on evidence. We have described the influence of organisational and other factors in influencing evidence uptake, and described techniques for identifying barriers to change in your workplace.

REVIEW QUESTIONS

1. What is "evidence-based medicine", and how does this term differ from "evidence-based practice (EBP)"?
2. What are the main elements of EBP, and how might they be useful to you in your day-to-day work?

3. Why do you think evidence is not used consistently to guide practice?
4. One of the issues you may have identified in the previous question was the organisational context in which a person works. What issues might arise in an organisation that might make it difficult to use EBP?
5. What are the steps involved in identifying evidence that should guide practice?
6. Outline a health issue in Australia where technical, social, economic, cultural and political rationalities compete to influence evidence-based implementation.

USEFUL WEBSITES

Cochrane Collaboration: http://www.cochrane.org
Health Evidence: https://www.healthevidence.org/
National Health and Medical Research Council website on contemporary evidence: https://www.nhmrc.gov.au/about-us/news-centre?tid=All&tid_1=All&combine=hierarchy%20of%20evidence

REFERENCES

Aarons G, Moullin J, Ehrhart M 2018 The role of organizational processes in dissemination and implementation research. In: Brownson RC, Colditz GA, Proctor EK (eds) *Dissemination and Implementation Research in Health: Translating Science to Practice*, 2nd edn. New York: Oxford University Press

Brownson RC, Baker EA, Deshpande AD et al 2018a Evidence-Based Public Health, 3rd edn. New York: Oxford University Press

Brownson RC, Colditz GA, Proctor EK 2018b Dissemination and Implementation Research in Health: Translating Science in Practice, 2nd edn. New York: Oxford University Press

Brownson RC, Fielding JE, Green LW 2018c Public health building capacity for evidence-based public health: reconciling the pulls of practice and the push of research. *Annual Review of Public Health* 39: 27–53. Available: https://www.annualreviews.org/doi/pdf/10.1146/annurev-publhealth-040617-014746

Brownson RC, Kumanyika SK, Kreuter MW et al 2021 Implementation science should give higher priority to health equity. *Implementation Science* 16(1): 1–16

Dang D, Dearholt SL, Bissett K et al 2021 Johns Hopkins evidence-based practice for nurses and healthcare professionals: model and guidelines. Indianapolis: Sigma Theta Tau International

Dimitri P 2021 The evolution of evidence based clinical medicine. In: *Practical Pediatric Urology*, pp. 1-15. Champaign, IL: Springer

Ding D, Ramirez Varela A, Bauman AE et al 2020 Towards better evidence-informed global action: lessons learnt from the Lancet series and recent developments in physical activity and public health. *British Journal of Sports Medicine* 54: 462–8

Egger M, Higgins JP, Smith GD 2022 Systematic reviews in health research: an introduction. In: *Systematic Reviews in Health Research: Meta-Analysis in Context*. 1–16. Available: https://onlinelibrary.wiley.com/doi/abs/10.1002/9781119099369.ch1

Emmons KM, Chambers DA 2021 Policy implementation science—an unexplored strategy to address social determinants of health. *Ethnicity & Disease* 31(1): 133–8 Available: https://doi.org/10.18865/ed.31.1.133

Escoffery C, Lebow-Skelley E, Udelson H et al 2021 Evidence-based medicine: a brief historical analysis of conceptual landmarks and practical goals for care. *História, Ciências, Saúde-Manguinhos* 28(1): 59–78

Hailemariam M, Bustos T, Montgomery B et al 2019 Evidence-based intervention sustainability strategies: a systematic review. *Implementation Science* 14(1): 1–12

Karampela M, Isomursu M, Porat T et al 2019 The extent and coverage of current knowledge of connected health: Systematic mapping study. *Journal of Medical Internet Research* 21(9): e14394

Kennedy M, Carbone EG, Siegfried AL et al 2020 Factors affecting implementation of evidence-based practices in public health preparedness and response. *Journal of Public Health Management and Practice* 26(5): 434

Li SA, Jeffs L, Barwick M et al 2018 Organizational contextual features that influence the implementation of evidence-based practices across healthcare settings: a systematic integrative review. *Systematic Reviews* 7: 72. Available https://doi.org/10.1186/s13643-018-0734-5

Sackett DL, Rosenberg WM, Gray JA et al 1996 Evidence based medicine: what it is and what it isn't. *BMJ* 312:371

Sahin O, Salim H, Suprun E et al 2020 Developing a preliminary causal loop diagram for understanding the wicked complexity of the COVID-19 pandemic. *Systems* 8(2), 20

Shelton RC, Adsul P, Oh A et al 2021 Application of an antiracism lens in the field of implementation science (IS): recommendations for reframing implementation research with a focus on justice and racial equity. *Implementation Research and Practice* 2. Available: https://doi.org/10.1177/26334895211049482

Yoo JY, Kim JH, Kim JS et al 2019 Clinical nurses' beliefs, knowledge, organizational readiness and level of implementation of evidence-based practice: the first step to creating an evidence-based practice culture. *PLoS One* 14(12): e0226742

Public Health Strategies

INTRODUCTION

The three chapters that make up this section focus on a continuum of public health activity based on a socioecological model of health that emphasises people through individual and interpersonal strategies, place through organisational and community strategies, and enabling environments for health. We discuss a range of strategies and intervention activities that provide the population or subpopulations with appropriate interventions to meet their diverse needs.

The first of these, Chapter 9, traces individual and interpersonal strategies by providing examples applicable to chronic diseases and infectious diseases. The chapter will enable you to understand a little more about the similarities and differences in definitions of 'non-communicable disease', 'chronic condition' and 'chronic disease'. From a strategies perspective it describes an integrated approach to chronic disease management. Similarly, the section on the broad nature and causes of infectious diseases focuses on identification and examination of the public health principles and strategies to prevent, treat and manage infectious diseases. Highlighting the importance of public health strategies in dealing with infectious diseases across the continuum of care. This chapter concludes with a discussion about the importance of multiple strategies at multiple levels to fully address a range of public health issues.

Chapter 10 focuses on place by contextualising and then examining a range of strategies that can be used in communities and organisations. The chapter begins with an understanding of terminology in the context of public health. In addition to an understanding of organisations and communities as contexts for public health strategies this chapter also explains why the terms 'equity', 'access' and 'participation' are important in influencing health outcomes. The chapter has an emphasis on how you can relate the principles of working with communities, organisations and social institutions to case studies and your own emerging practice.

Chapter 11 addresses environmental impacts on human health. This chapter enables you to consider definitions and comparisons of environmental health and planetary health and includes a discussion about the importance of both perspectives to public health. In the international and national contexts the chapter discusses the major changing environmental exposures and challenges experienced by human populations. This means that mortality and morbidity changes may occur with shifts in types of diseases that dominate our environments now and in the future. Further, we examine the way in which evidence from environmental epidemiology can be applied to health risk and health impact assessment to achieve advances in public health and health policy. Environmental health improvements are discussed in the context of enabling global poverty reduction, facilitating substantial advances in human health. Importantly we investigate the key direct and indirect health and social consequences of climate change and other environmental challenges impacting on our planetary systems.

9

People

Mary Louise Fleming and Gerry Fitzgerald

LEARNING OBJECTIVES

After reading this chapter, you should be able to:
- Understand the similarities and differences in definitions of "non-communicable disease", "chronic condition" and "chronic disease".
- Describe an integrated approach to chronic disease management strategies.
- Identify the public health principles and strategies used to prevent, treat and manage infectious diseases.
- Understand the need for multiple strategies at multiple levels to fully address a range of public health issues.

INTRODUCTION

The aim of this chapter is to introduce the nature and extent of chronic and infectious diseases at the individual level and describe the *public health strategies* used to provide protection and to reduce their burden. It focuses on the importance of implementing multiple strategies at multiple levels to provide a comprehensive overview of the content and strategies that make a difference to the promotion, prevention, rehabilitation and treatment associated with chronic and infectious diseases.

A Brief Overview

At the beginning of the third decade of the 21st century, people across the globe face an infectious disease pandemic arguably not seen since the ravages of Spanish influenza in the early 1900s. As well, there is the continued march of chronic conditions. While infectious diseases have continued to impact heavily on developing countries, COVID-19 has demonstrated vulnerabilities that pay no attention to social and economic determinants of health between developed and developing countries, stretching the resources of health systems across the world. However, as the Global Burden of Disease (GBD) studies suggest, structural inequities in society must be addressed and more liberal approaches to immigration policies adopted, so communities can be better protected from future infectious disease outbreaks (Editorial, *The Lancet*, 2020).

Globally, age-specific mortality has steadily improved over the past 40 years (Global Burden of Disease [GBD], 2020). Despite such improvements, population growth and ageing have led to an increase in most chronic disease causes, putting increased demands on health systems (Wang et al, 2020). The Australian Institute of Health and Welfare (AIHW) regularly reports on chronic conditions that pose significant health problems, have been the focus of ongoing AIHW surveillance efforts and, in many instances, action can be taken to prevent their occurrence (AIHW, 2022; see https://www.aihw.gov.au/reports-data/health-conditions-disability-deaths/chronic-disease/overview). Chronic disease management needs integrated approaches that incorporate interventions targeted at both individuals and populations, alignment of intersectoral policies for health, formation of partnerships and engagement of communities in decision-making with an emphasis on the shared risk factors of different conditions (Australian Government Department of Health and Aged Care, 2022a; 2022b).

Infectious diseases have been a common and significant contributor to ill health throughout the world. In many countries, this impact has been minimised by the combined efforts of preventative health measures and improved treatment methods. However, in low-income countries, infectious diseases remain the dominant cause of death and disability (World Health Organization [WHO], 2021a). In 2021, the WHO produced an evidence brief on the impact of COVID-19 on the social determinants of health and health equity. The following quote from that document is a sober reminder of the complexity facing society.

A sustained, collaborative approach is needed that reaches across health, social and economic actors, across communities and countries, with health and social justice at its core, to manage the current pandemic and build back fairer for the future to ensure future outbreaks do not exact such a heavy and unequal toll on health, wellbeing and economic stability.

WHO, 2021, p. v

DEFINING "CHRONIC CONDITION" AND "CHRONIC DISEASE"

It is useful to define these terms, because "non-communicable disease", "chronic condition" and "chronic disease" are sometimes used interchangeably (https://www.aihw.gov.au/reports/chronic-disease/chronic-condition-multimorbidity/contents/about).

The term *non-communicable disease* is used by the WHO as an overarching definition for chronic disease (https://www.who.int/news-room/fact-sheets/detail/noncommunicable-diseases). *Chronic condition* "encompasses disability and disease conditions that people may 'live with' over extended periods of time, for example more than six months" (WHO, 2021b). *Chronic disease* is a subset of chronic condition. It may be more likely to have a progressively deteriorating path than other chronic conditions (WHO, 2021b). In this chapter, the term "chronic condition" will be used. Chronic conditions are those involving a long course in their development or their symptoms. They account for a high proportion of deaths, disability and illness, and are a major health problem worldwide. Yet many of these conditions are preventable, or their onset can be delayed, by relatively simple measures (AIHW, 2022). You can also refer back to earlier chapters of the book, where the complexity of managing chronic conditions in the health system and in the development and application of health policy are addressed.

Many people with chronic conditions do not have a single condition, they have what is defined as *multimorbidity*. This term refers to people living with two or more chronic conditions at the same time. Multiple chronic conditions can influence quality of life, work and social life and finances (AIHW, 2021).

A number of positive behaviours can prevent or delay the development of many chronic diseases. They include controlling body weight, eating nutritious foods, avoiding tobacco use, controlling alcohol consumption and increasing physical activity (AIHW, 2021).

Table 9.1 and Activity 9.1 examine the relationship between risk factors and chronic diseases in Australia (AIHW, 2022; WHO, 2022).

The success of public health initiatives, in part, means that people are living longer, and this increased life span allows more time for chronic illness to develop and a longer period of life living with chronic disease (Centers for Disease Control and Prevention [CDC], 2022). Chronic diseases place an extra burden on healthcare systems. Chronic diseases continue to be the leading cause of disability in the world (GBD, 2020), with over 70% of the global burden of illness mainly attributable to cardiovascular disease (which covers all diseases and conditions of the heart and blood vessels), cancer, diabetes and chronic respiratory diseases, as well as mental health problems, injuries and violence (WHO, 2022). Similar to the WHO, Australia continues to acknowledge chronic disease as a major health challenge (AIHW, 2022).

INTEGRATED APPROACH TO CHRONIC DISEASE CARE

Australia has a National Strategic Framework for Chronic Conditions (2019), accompanied by a National Strategic Framework for Chronic Conditions, reporting framework and an indicator results report (2022).

Earlier, Wilcox (2015) proposed a preventive action strategy for chronic disease that includes seven core underpinning principles and three strategic priorities, as presented in Figure 9.1.

Using these underpinning principles as a guide to action, it is possible to tackle chronic disease along a continuum of care from promotion and prevention to early detection and early intervention, self-management, comprehensive management in the community and, for those with advanced chronic illnesses, coordinated care, high-quality palliative care and dying with dignity. This process will ensure evidence-based and coordinated care that embraces multidisciplinary programs with a focus on the complete chronic condition pathway.

CHRONIC DISEASE STRATEGIES ACROSS THE CONTINUUM OF CARE

Table 9.2 provides an overview of a range of public health strategies for chronic illness across the continuum of care. Examples of such strategies are provided below.

Promotion and Prevention

It is essential that a major focus of public health is on the prevention of chronic disease. Evidence suggests that chronic disease is related to a variety of risk factors and determinants and, importantly, to a life-course perspective (Australian Institute of Health and Welfare [AIHW], 2022). Interventions introduced early to keep people healthy for longer will reduce the burden of disease and the costs to the health system in treating people with chronic illness. For example, obesity is a chronic disease that is an international health priority that contributes to a range of

TABLE 9.1 Selected Chronic Diseases, Risk Factors and Determinants

Disease/Condition[1]	RISK FACTOR AND DETERMINANTS: HEALTH BEHAVIOURS; BIOMEDICAL FACTORS; SOCIOENVIRONMENTAL FACTORS						Biomedical Factors	Socio-Environmental Factors		
	Health Behaviours									
	Poor Diet	Physical Inactivity	Tobacco Use	Alcohol Misuse	High Cholesterol	Excess Weight	High Blood Pressure	Social Support	Early Life	Low Socio-economic Status
Cardiovascular disease (heart attack and stroke)	✓	✓	✓	✓	✓	✓	✓		✓	✓
Cancers	✓	✓	✓	✓		✓				✓
Depression		✓		✓	✓	✓		✓	✓	✓
Diabetes type 2	✓	✓	✓			✓			✓	✓
Respiratory/asthma			✓						✓	✓
Chronic kidney disease	✓	✓	✓			✓	✓		✓	
Oral diseases	✓		✓		✓				✓	✓
Musculoskeletal disorders	✓	✓	✓	✓		✓				

✓ = established link.

[1]Diseases/conditions' risk factors and determinants are based on "Determinants of Health" in *Australia's health* (AIHW, 2020) and "Evidence for chronic disease risk factors" (AIHW, 2022).
Source: Modified from Wilcox, 2015; AIHW, 2022; WHO, 2022.

comorbidities, including diabetes, kidney disease and 'several types of cancer' (to eliminate ambiguity). The complex interplay of individual and societal drivers of obesity is a key challenge for prevention, and calls to engage with this complexity are a key part of obesity prevention (Maitland, 2021).

Early Detection and Early Intervention

Early detection and treatment can reduce complications, comorbidities and mortality. Approaches to early detection and early intervention include population-based screening, and opportunistic screening by health workers for risk factors and/or early signs and symptoms. Examples of the former include mammography for women and bowel cancer screening.

Comprehensive Management in the Community

While the presence of a single risk factor can lead to illness, there is an increasing risk of developing chronic conditions when more than one risk factor is present. There is a need to focus on collaborative efforts between the public health and healthcare sectors. Also, the healthcare system needs to focus on better use of prevention and early detection services, and improved and sustained population health is achieved by improved collaborations between communities and healthcare providers. Self-management is an important strategy to foster cooperation between the person and his or her family, health service providers and the healthcare system. We need approaches that will improve health equity by building communities that promote health rather than disease, have more accessible and direct care and focus the healthcare system on improving population health (Kwan et al, 2022).

The Australian National Strategic Framework for Chronic Conditions has a focus on five priority strategies to support people with a chronic condition, which include the engagement of people with a chronic illness, their families and carers. This engagement should occur in a context of continuity of care that is consistent, holistic and coordinated, and where

ACTIVITY 9.1 Sorting Risk Factors and Determinants

Consider Table 9.1, which is divided into health behaviours, biomedical factors and socioenvironmental factors. Why are the risk factors and determinants for cardiovascular disease (CVD) spread across the full Table when compared with musculoskeletal disorders, and why might depression be influenced by many biomedical and socioenvironmental factors? Read on if you are having trouble with the answers, and see the following websites (AIHW, 2021; Australian Burden of Disease Study 2018 – Key findings. https://www.aihw.gov.au/reports/burden-of-disease/burden-of-disease-study-2018-key-findings/contents/key-findings. Also, AIHW, 2022: Australia's Health 2022 in brief. https://www.aihw.gov.au/getmedia/c6c5dda9-4020-43b0-8ed6-a567cd660eaa/aihw-aus-421.pdf.aspx).

Reflection

Most chronic diseases have multiple risk factors, and the situations that lead to their initiation often begin early in life, or even in the womb. Therefore, a life-course perspective of chronic diseases and their risk factors is important, as it recognises the interactive and cumulative impact of social and biological influences throughout life (AIHW, 2022).

there is collaborative sharing of secure, consistent and relevant health information. Most importantly, people with chronic conditions need equitable and accessible health services and supportable systems that work together to meet the needs of community members (McGill et al, 2021).

Complex and Advanced Chronic Disease Management

Integration and continuity of prevention and care includes care planning and coordination through a range of providers and settings. An example is the chronic disease management items available for patients with chronic conditions and complex care needs; these include diabetes, heart disease and other chronic conditions (AIHW, 2022). Describing integration refers to strengthening patient-centred health systems by:

1. Promoting comprehensive delivery of quality services across the life-course.
2. Designing such programs for the multidimensional needs of the population and the individual.
3. Delivering by coordinated healthcare providers working across settings and levels of care.
4. Tackling upstream causes of ill health, and promoting wellbeing through intersectoral and multisectoral actions (Goniewicz, 2021).

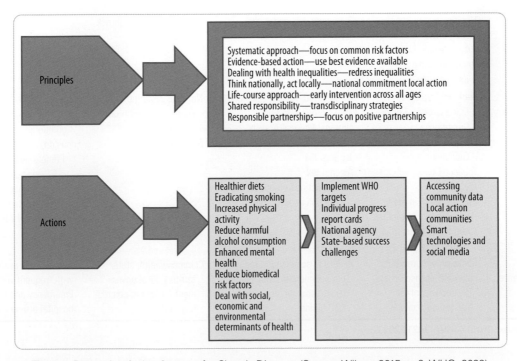

Fig. 9.1 Prevention Action Strategy for Chronic Disease. (Source: Wilcox, 2015, p, 2; WHO, 2022).

TABLE 9.2   Public Health Strategies for Chronic Illness Across the Continuum of Care

Settings	Promotion/ Prevention	Screening and Early Intervention	Management in the Community	Complex Advanced Care
Individual and intrapersonal	Active travel options Healthy environments Targeted exercise programs Life-course *perspective*	Access and equity for all Australians to a range of screening, e.g. breast, bowel, prostate, cholesterol Nicotine patches Quit Smoking programs	Rehabilitation programs Effective care that is coordinated Primary care for Aboriginal and Torres Strait Islander populations	Effective primary care GP-led In-home support Culturally appropriate primary, secondary and tertiary care for Aboriginal and Torres Strait Islander populations
Schools	Active travel options Healthy tuck-shops Urban design Physical education in all school curricula No advertising of unhealthy foods to children Plain packaging of tobacco products	Active screening programs for at-risk child and adolescent populations		
Communities	Active travel Urban design Targeting sporting clubs and food outlets Positive media	Emphasis on rural and remote communities and provision of services to enable access and equity Access for Aboriginal and Torres Strait Islander populations Focus on at-risk groups for early screening	Community-based and sub-population interventions Reduction of risk factors for people with chronic conditions Media for chronic condition management	Home healthcare Appropriate treatment Integration of care Culturally appropriate care
Workplaces	Healthy food options Active travel Urban design Range of workplace interventions	Screening provided in the workplace	Interventions for high-risk groups	
Whole-of-government policy and strategic intent	National Strategic Framework for Chronic Conditions National Physical Activity Guidelines Tobacco tax Alcohol tax Salt reduction in foods and sugar in beverages Avoid policy focus from vested interests	National Strategic Framework for Chronic Conditions National Physical Activity Guidelines Tobacco tax Alcohol tax Salt reduction in foods and sugar reduction in beverages	National Strategic Framework for Chronic Conditions Build local action commitment	National Strategic Framework for Chronic Conditions Focus on Primary Health Networks, GP and community care, in-home care and hospice care Coordination of care
Economic circumstances	Reducing or eliminating chronic disease boosts productivity of the Australian economy	Access to screening to reduce the prevalence of risk factors could boost the economy by $2.3 billion	Commonwealth, state/territory, local government funding at community level	Reduced costs associated with frequent visits to Emergency and long-stay hospital attendance

Source: Wilcox, 2015; AIHW, 2021; 2022.

Furthermore, a large proportion of funding for chronic disease management is directed at programs that target comparatively restricted categories of populations, diseases or risk factors; therefore, managers of comprehensive chronic disease programs need to ensure that programs are integrated to reduce unnecessary duplication (CDC, 2022).

Clearly, it is essential to coordinate realistic and comprehensive strategies to advance the Australian health system's ability to provide comprehensive chronic disease prevention and management (AIHW, 2020). Table 9.2 describes the range of stages along the chronic disease continuum, the differing settings and the public health strategies that can be put in place. Activity 9.2 uses this table and asks you to consider "where to begin" for the selection of strategies.

In summary, chronic conditions have many related determinants and risk factors that should be considered through a broader approach to chronic condition management that spans the life-course, uses multiple settings and focuses on multiple levels of intervention from promotion to care and treatment.

DEFINING "INFECTIOUS DISEASE"

Infectious diseases are a common and significant contributor to ill health throughout the world, particularly in developing countries. There are a diversity of terms and definitions used to describe infectious diseases and their impact.

Communicable diseases are those that can be communicated from one person to another. The overwhelming majority of these are infections disease.

Infectious diseases are caused by pathogenic microorganisms (also known as pathogens), such as various species of bacteria, viruses, parasites or fungi. More specifically, *zoonotic diseases* are infectious diseases of animals that can cause disease when transmitted to humans (Adams & Butterly, 2015).

Most infectious diseases are spread directly from one individual to another, but some can only be transmitted by an inert life stage (e.g. tetanus spores) or via a vector (e.g. malaria transmitted by mosquitoes). Others can be acquired from another source, such as contaminated water or spoilt food.

Infectious diseases are still very common, even in developed countries, and include relatively common diseases such as the common cold, dental caries and acne vulgaris. They may have highly significant economic and social impacts, but do not have significant morbidity or mortality. However, infectious diseases continue to be a major cause of death and disability in developing countries. Such countries often lack the economic capacity to provide the community with the public health infrastructure required to prevent or manage infectious diseases. Consequently, infectious diseases still account for a number of the top 10 causes of death in low-income countries (WHO, 2018). Infectious diseases may be endemic in communities at various levels, but also subject to outbreaks or epidemics.

MODELS OF INFECTIOUS DISEASE

The concept of human infectious disease is multidimensional, and includes our interaction with the pathogen, the impact within our body of contact with the pathogen and the interaction between our body and the various environments in which we live. For any infectious disease to occur, there are always three elements (Abubaker et al, 2016):

1. A person or host who is the target of the disease, and who may be susceptible to it.
2. An agent, which is either the direct cause of disease or a contributing or predisposing factor to its onset.
3. The environment, which may influence the existence of the agent, the exposure of the host to the agent or the susceptibility of the host.

These interactions are commonly described in terms of two models of infectious diseases: the *agent–host–environment triangle*, which is also known as the *epidemiological triad*, and the *chain of infection* model.

For both models of infectious diseases, the following elements may apply:

- *Susceptible host*—despite living in a sea of microbes, people are generally healthy due to intrinsic and specific host defences. Susceptibility includes the host being immunocompromised, there being other defects in the host's normal defences.
- *Infectious agent*—an agent must be present and capable of causing infection (e.g. virus, bacteria, fungi, protozoa).
- *Reservoir*—the agent may have a reservoir where it can propagate—that is, live, reproduce and die in the natural state. This includes humans, animals and the environment.

- *Portal of exit* from reservoir and *portal of entry* into a susceptible host—examples include the respiratory tract, the gastrointestinal (GI) tract, skin and mucous membranes.
- *Transmission*—the agent needs to be transmitted, directly or indirectly, from one place to another.

INFECTIOUS DISEASE MANAGEMENT

Managing infectious diseases in society is reliant on a range of complementary strategies, which together aim to prevent, monitor and treat disease. These strategies include those targeted at disease prevention, those involved with surveillance and early detection and those aimed at managing disease when it occurs.

This text focuses on the public health aspects of disease prevention along three key aspects of managing infectious diseases: (1) disease prevention, through societal and environmental structures, immunisation, vector control and personal protection; (2) surveillance, early recognition and early intervention; and (3) infection control (see Case Study 9.1).

CASE STUDY 9.1   COVID-19

In December 2019, the health authorities in Wuhan in China advised the World Health Organization of the emergence of a novel Coronavirus that was causing severe respiratory disease. By the middle of 2022, despite the availability of multiple vaccines, the pandemic continues to spread around the world. More than 6 million people have been identified to have died from the disease, although estimates of excess mortality suggest a figure closer to 20 million (COVID-19 Excess Mortality Collaborators, 2022). The pandemic has had widespread social, economic and health impacts.

Endeavours to control the spread of the disease have featured enhanced population-based hygiene measures and social isolation, including community wide lockdowns. The extent to which this has been applied and successful has depended on a variety of social, economic and health system influences. Australia's broad approach was to eliminate domestic transmission and control entry until such time as vaccines were available. As a result, the mortality rates are much less than those in countries that experienced considerable transmission in an unvaccinated population.

While it is too early to evaluate the international response, the pandemic has demonstrated challenging peculiarities that have resulted in added complexity.

- Vaccines have proven less effective than hoped for in preventing transmission although there is evidence that they reduce severity and mortality
- New viral variants and sub-variants have eluded the acquired immunity from vaccines and prior infection
- Moderate levels of social cohesion and social compliance have resulted in control of the spread but were not sustainable.

DISEASE PREVENTION

Societal and Environmental Structures

Our societal and environmental systems and structures are designed to minimise the risks of disease transmission. We have laws and regulations to provide access to safe drinking water, clean, safe food and hygienic waste disposal. A long-established, but now rarely used, social prevention measure is that of quarantine (i.e. the compulsory isolation of individuals). In many countries, we value our personal space; in addition, we have rules and standards of social conduct that help to limit disease transmission. We expect people to cover their noses and mouths when sneezing, not to spit in public and to wash their hands after toileting. All of these approaches contribute to the reduction of infectious diseases.

Immunisation

The primary aim of immunisation is to protect the individual who receives the vaccine. Additionally, vaccinated individuals are less likely to be a source of infection for others, thus also reducing the risk to unvaccinated individuals. This concept is known as *population immunity* or *herd immunity*. When vaccination coverage is high enough to produce high levels of population immunity, infections can be eliminated from a community. However, if vaccination coverage is not maintained, it is possible for these diseases to return. Consequently, health authorities are vigilant about vaccine coverage levels in their community, and encourage the widespread uptake of immunisation through public and professional awareness campaigns and free access to vaccines.

Immunisation is credited with dramatically reducing morbidity and mortality from infectious diseases during the 20th century. There has been significant public health success from immunisation activity in Australia (National Centre for Immunisation Research and Surveillance [NCIRS], 2022). For example, consider the following information, from the NCIRS website, about human papillomavirus (HPV) and the benefits of the new 9vHPV, Gardasil9 (https://ncirs.org.au/ncirs-fact-sheets-faqs-and-other-resources/human-papillomavirus). The vaccine has had a major impact on young people and young adults.

Immunity is the ability of the human body to protect itself from infectious disease. Humans can *acquire* immunity by natural or artificial means. The most common natural means of acquiring immunity is through exposure to the disease, either by contracting it personally or by coming into contact with someone who has the disease. In response, the body produces *antibodies* to the *antigens* that are contained in the organisms that produce the disease. Vaccination programs aim to replicate this naturally acquired immunity through artificial means that avoid the risks of the disease itself. Unfortunately, no vaccine offers complete coverage. In addition, a vaccine may cause an adverse event. Even though most vaccines cause minor adverse

CASE STUDY 9.2   Vaccine Hesitancy

The COVID-19 pandemic has highlighted what was already a growing concern in the population at large about a reluctance to receive safe and recommended available vaccines, described as "vaccine hesitancy" (Machingaidze & Wiysonge, 2021). Achieving high COVID-19 vaccine coverage has been a significant challenge given Australia's supply, access and hesitancy challenges (Leask et al, 2021). For example, shipment delays, issues coordinating delivery across jurisdictions and other challenges meant it took 45 days to deliver Australia's first million doses. Vaccine hesitancy also impacted vaccine uptake, particularly after the clotting syndrome (TTS) vaccine safety signal was identified (Kaufman et al, 2022). It is fair to say that throughout the pandemic issues with communication, shifts in recommendations and fluctuations in cases have all impacted on government trust (Seale et al, 2021). Dettori and colleagues (2022) suggest that promoting vaccine uptake must be linked to well-structured information and communication campaigns, implemented through all available channels, including ICTs, if they are to prevent negative changes in behaviour. It must also be remembered that the complexity of communication processes are important to achieve vaccination compliance, and that listening forms the basis for clear and effective communication with users.

Further, vaccine hesitancy will still need to be addressed in parents and other socioeconomically disadvantaged groups. This means by providing effective vaccine campaigns in languages other than English for migrants and refugees.

Read the article by Machingaidze and Wiysonge 2021 Understanding COVID-19 vaccine hesitancy. Nature Medicine 27(8), 1338–9. Available: https://www.nature.com/articles/s41591-021-01459-7.pdf.

Questions

Vaccine hesitancy has been shown to be a reluctance to receive safe and recommended vaccines. After you have read the article cited above, consider the range of positive and negative factors that influence people to be vaccinated. COVID-19 is a good example of this issue that is contemporary. Write up your information in a decision-making matrix that could include the following information.

DECISION-MAKING MATRIX

Immunisation	Immunisation facts	Social Commentary	Political/ Economic Commentary	Evidence Summary and Conclusion
For		+	+	+
		−	−	−
Against		+	+	+
		−	−	−

In your final evidence and summary comments, you must use evidence that you have collected. If you are not sure what evidence is, review Chapter 8 on evidence-based practice and consider the appropriate use of evidence in this context.

---

events, such as fever, pain or redness at the site of injection (NHMRC, 2022), there could be more substantial adverse events for a small number of individuals, particularly from live virus vaccines. However, misinformation campaigns about immunisation (see Case Study 9.2), often propagated on the internet, present an inaccurate view of the reality (see Box 9.1).

Vector Control

Vector-borne transmission of an infectious agent is generally caused by an arthropod (i.e. an insect), either by simple mechanical transfer of microorganisms from the external parts of the vector (e.g. on its legs), or through the vector ingesting and later expelling the agent, often through penetration of the skin of a susceptible host, as is the case for mosquitoes (Abubaker et al, 2016).

In 2019, expenditure on the control and elimination of the most deadly vector-borne disease, malaria, was estimated at US$4.3 billion (Haakenstad et al, 2019). Dengue is of particular concern for northern areas of Australia, which regularly have outbreaks due to the presence of the dengue mosquito, *Aedes aegypti*. In other parts of Australia, diseases such as Ross River virus infection and Barmah Forest virus infection are commonly associated with mosquito vectors. The

environmental health links with vector-borne diseases include poorly designed irrigation and water systems, inadequate housing, poor waste disposal and water storage, deforestation and loss of biodiversity.

Even though well-planned vector control measures can significantly contribute to reducing the burden of vector-borne diseases, the preventative power of vector control is grossly under-utilised in public health (WHO, 2022). Rather than relying on a single method of vector control, the WHO recommends implementing integrated vector management (IVM), which stresses the importance of first understanding the local vector ecology and local patterns of disease transmission, then choosing the appropriate vector control tools from the range of options available (WHO, 2022). In Australia, most of the vector control activities are carried out by local governments in consultation with state health and environmental agencies.

Personal Protection

Actions can also be taken to protect individuals on a personal level. These include:

- Encouraging behaviours that ensure safe practices, such as handwashing and covering your mouth when coughing.

BOX 9.1   **The Internet and Immunisation**

With more than 90% of young people in developed countries being regular internet users, and the worldwide web being an important source of health information for laypeople, the potential for the internet to play an important role in providing accurate and up-to-date information on immunisation issues is clear. One public health concern is the potential for the internet to be used to spread incorrect and potentially dangerous information on immunisation. An example is the use of the internet and other social media platforms by the anti-vaccination movement to portray highly emotional messages that counter the messages inherent in public health campaigns. In order to help laypeople judge the quality of immunisation information on social media platforms, the WHO has developed criteria for assessing website quality in terms of credibility, content, accessibility and design. These criteria are available at the WHO's Vaccine Safety Net website: https://vaccinesafetynet.org/.

Adapted from Amicizia D, Domnich A, Gasparini R et al 2013 An overview of current and potential use of information and communication technologies for immunization promotion among adolescents. Human Vaccines and Immunotherapeutics 9 (12): 2634–42.

- Encouraging "safe sex" to reduce disease transmission, particularly sexually transmitted diseases, including HIV/AIDS.
- Encouraging the safe use of clean needles for drug addicts to reduce the risks associated with cross-infection from dirty needles.
- Encouraging the use of personal protective barriers—for example, condoms for safe sex, and mosquito netting.
- Encouraging and supporting the use of prophylactic medication in circumstances where exposure is possible—for example, malaria prophylaxis for travellers to malaria-prone areas.
- Actively managing secondary (post-exposure) prophylaxis—for example, in the event of needlestick injuries to health workers.

SURVEILLANCE, EARLY RECOGNITION AND EARLY INTERVENTION

In Australia, systems and structures are in place to screen for the presence of disease and to investigate and manage outbreaks. Early warning functions are fundamental for national, regional and global health security. Outbreaks such as the severe acute respiratory syndrome (SARS) and avian influenza, and potential threats from biological and chemical agents, demonstrate the importance of effective national surveillance and response systems (CDC, 2021).

Public health surveillance includes vital statistics (e.g. birth and death certificates), sentinel surveillance/early warning systems for key health indicators and registries such as those maintained for cancer and birth defects (UNSW, 2022). Public health officials also maintain a system of compulsory reporting of particular infectious diseases to facilitate early recognition and intervention. In Australia, surveillance of infectious disease is through the National Notifiable Diseases Surveillance System (NNDSS) (NNDSS, 2022). Diseases are reported by diagnostic laboratories or by clinicians to state health agencies, who then forward the information to the NNDSS. The reports are made to state health agencies so that immediate outbreak investigation, contact tracing and public health interventions can occur. Part of this response is analysing the incoming data. The basic analytic approaches used in surveillance systems involve describing and analysing data in terms of:

- *Time*—patterns of disease incidence, which may generate hypotheses, or may reflect patterns in reporting
- *Place*—geographical distribution of disease or of its causative exposures or risk-associated behaviours
- *Person*—characteristics of people or groups who develop disease or sustain injury, which helps in understanding the risk factors for disease or injury, and targeting interventions. (Refer to Chapter 3 for further details on the use of epidemiological methods for disease surveillance and control.)

INFECTION CONTROL

Tertiary prevention is the third level of management, and involves attention to infection control in a range of environments and the appropriate management of infected patients. "Infection control" describes the systems, behaviours and structures that are designed to break the transmission of microorganisms from infected patients to unaffected people.

Infection control practice involves a multitiered approach that consists primarily of standard precautions and *transmission-based precautions*.

Standard precautions include handwashing, wearing clothing to reduce cross-infection, wearing gloves where necessary, and wearing masks to reduce respiratory transmission. Transmission-based precautions are recommended for patients known or suspected to be infected with a pathogen, and include the highest standard of respiratory protection, isolation and barrier nursing and care in a positive-pressure environment with closed-circuit air control. The outbreak of COVID-19 has demonstrated the benefit of disease control strategies, including population-level social isolation and enhanced personal hygiene measures.

Outbreak Investigation and Contact Tracing

The public health strategies implemented to investigate a disease outbreak are an essential part of infectious disease management. The strategies are as follows:

- *Identifying the disease and the causative agent*—this requires specimens from the infected patient(s) and the collection and testing of specimens for any possible or likely causes; for example, during an outbreak of a food-borne illness, specimens from food sources, food-handlers and environmental contaminants may assist with tracking the cause.

- *Investigating the circumstances of the infection*—this may involve taking a detailed history of exposure and contacts.
- *Identifying and testing others who may have been the source of the infection.*
- *Identifying others who may be at risk* from similar exposure, and who may knowingly or unwittingly be a source of further transmission.
- *Timely implementation of appropriate control measures* to minimise further illness.

The choice and type of control measure should be guided by the results of the epidemiological and environmental investigations. However, to protect the public, controls are sometimes implemented based on limited information. Control measures for food-related outbreaks, for example, include food recalls, restaurant closures, excluding food-handlers, decommissioning food-processing equipment and revising maintenance and operating procedures.

Barriers to Effectively Managing Infectious Diseases

Despite the wide range of control measures available, there are many barriers to effective disease control. These generally relate to the failure of systems and structures that are often related to general societal problems—for example, poverty and its associated failure of infrastructure, education and awareness and resources; community ignorance associated with poor education standards; and ideological views. Sometimes individuals or communities hold ideological views that are contrary to known infectious disease management strategies; for example, some individuals believe on religious or personal grounds that vaccination is "unnatural", whereas others believe that vaccines sourced from Western countries are an attempt to subjugate the people of developing nations.

A FINAL WORD

This chapter has covered a wide range of issues related to the development, prevention, management and care of chronic conditions and infectious diseases. It is important to understand the health issue being considered, as well as the range of public health strategies that can be used across the continuum of care. We have defined both chronic conditions and infectious diseases, and briefly discussed models and mechanisms for disease development. We have then focused on various approaches for managing and preventing disease, as well as outlining the importance of public health strategies throughout the continuum of care for both chronic conditions and infectious diseases.

REVIEW QUESTIONS

1. How would you define a "chronic disease"?
2. What is an "infectious disease"? How is an infectious disease different from a communicable disease?
3. How are chronic conditions managed at the state/territory and federal government levels?
4. The Australian Government's National Chronic Disease Strategy concentrates on four key areas for improving outcomes. In a table, identify these four key areas, and describe the contribution of each to the prevention and management of chronic disease.
5. How can microorganisms cause disease?
6. What protective mechanisms does the body use to prevent infection?
7. How might we prevent and/or manage infectious diseases?
8. Discuss the major strategies you would use to manage a disease outbreak.

USEFUL WEBSITES

Australian Government Department of Health and Ageing, updated 2022 Tobacco control: https://www.health.gov.au/topics/smoking-and-tobacco/tobacco-control

Australian Institute of Health and Welfare 2022. Chronic disease: https://www.aihw.gov.au/reports/chronic-disease/nsf-for-chronic-condition-reporting-framework/summary

Australian Government Department of Health and Aged Care 2022 COVID-19: https://www.health.gov.au/funnelback/search?query=covid19

Centers for Disease Control and Prevention: http://www.cdc.gov

Immunise Australia Program: https://www.health.gov.au/our-work/national-immunisation-program

Queensland Government, Queensland Health: https://www.health.qld.gov.au/public-health

NHMRC 2022 Health Advice: https://www.nhmrc.gov.au/health-advice

REFERENCES

Abubakar I, Stagg HR, Chioen T et al 2016 Infectious Disease Epidemiology. Oxford: Oxford University Press

Abubakar I 2020 The future of migration, human populations, and global health in the Anthropocene. *The Lancet* 396: 1133–4

Adams LV, Butterly JR, EBSCOhost 2015 Diseases of poverty: epidemiology, infectious diseases, and modern plagues. Hanover, NH: Dartmouth College Press

Amicizia D, Domnich A, Gasparini R et al 2013 An overview of current and potential use of information and communication technologies for immunization promotion among adolescents. *Human Vaccines and Immunotherapeutics* 9(12), 2634–42. doi:10.4161/hv.26010

Australian Government Department of Health and Aged Care 2022a Reporting nationally notifiable diseases. Available: https://www.health.gov.au/topics/communicable-diseases/nationally-notifiable-diseases/reporting?language=en

Australian Government Department of Health and Aged Care 2022b National Notifiable Diseases Surveillance System (NDSS). Available: https://www.health.gov.au/initiatives-and-programs/nndss#:~:text=The%20National%20Notifiable%20Diseases%20Surveillance,the%20impact%20of%20these%20diseases

Australian Institute of Health and Welfare (AIHW) 2021 Chronic condition multimorbidity, AIHW. Available: https://www.aihw.gov.au/reports/chronic-disease/chronic-condition-multimorbidity/contents/about. (Accessed 16 May 2022)

Australian Institute of Health and Welfare (AIHW) 2021 Chronic disease. Available: https://www.aihw.gov.au/reports-data/health-conditions-disability-deaths/chronic-disease/overview. (Accessed 20 Jul 2022)

Centers for Disease Control and Prevention (CDC) 2022 National Center for Chronic Disease Prevention and Health Promotion (NCCDPHP). Atlanta, GA: Department of Health and Human Services. Available: https://www.cdc.gov/chronicdisease/about/. (Accessed 1 June 2022)

Centers for Disease Control and Prevention (CDC) 2021 Global Health Security Agenda. Available: https://www.cdc.gov/global-health/security/index.htm

COVID-19 Excess Mortality Collaborators 2022 Estimating excess mortality due to the COVID-19 pandemic: a systematic analysis of COVID-19-related mortality, 2020-21. *The Lancet* 399(10334), 1513–36. Erratum in: The Lancet 2022 Apr 16;399(10334), 1468

Dettori M, Castiglia P 2022 COVID-19 and digital health: evolution, perspectives and opportunities. *International Journal of Environmental Research and Public Health* 19(14), 8519. https://doi.org/10.3390/ijerph19148519

Editorial 2020 Global health: time for radical change? *The Lancet* 396: 1129

Global Burden of Disease (GBD) 2020 Viewpoint Collaborators. Five insights from the Global Burden of Disease Study 2019. *The Lancet* 396(10258), 1135–59

Goniewicz K, Carlström E, Hertelendy AJ et al 2021 Integrated healthcare and the dilemma of public health emergencies. *Sustainability* 13(8), 4517

Haakenstad A, Harle AC, Tsakalos G et al 2019 Tracking spending on malaria by source in 106 countries, 2000–16: an economic modelling study. *The Lancet Infectious Diseases* 19(703), 16. Available: http://dx.doi.org/10.1016/S1473-3099(19)30165-3

National Centre for Immunisation Research and Surveillance (NCIRS) 2022. Available: http://www.ncirs.edu.au/ (Accessed 2 Jun 2022)

Kaufman J, Tuckerman J, Danchin M 2022 Overcoming COVID-19 vaccine hesitancy: can Australia reach the last 20 percent? *Expert Review of Vaccines* 21(2), 159–61

Kwan BM, Brownson RC, Glasgow R et al 2022 Designing for dissemination and sustainability to promote equitable impacts on health. *Annual Review of Public Health* 43: 331

Leask J, Carlson SJ, Attwell K et al 2021 Communicating with patients and the public about COVID-19 vaccine safety: recommendations from the Collaboration on Social Science and Immunisation. *Med J Aust* 215(1), 9–12

Machingaidze S, Wiysonge CS 2021 Understanding COVID-19 vaccine hesitancy. *Nature Medicine* 27, 1338–9. https://doi.org/10.1038/s41591-021-01459-7

Maitland N, Wardle K, Whelan J et al 2021 Tracking implementation within a community-led whole of system approach to address childhood overweight and obesity in south west Sydney, Australia. *BMC Public Health* 21, 1233. https://doi.org/10.1186/s12889-021-11288-5

McGill E, Er V, Penney T et al 2021 Evaluation of public health interventions from a complex systems perspective: a research methods review. *Social Science and Medicine* 272, 113697

National Centre for Immunisation Research and Surveillance (NCIRS) 2022. Available: https://ncirs.org.au/

National Health and Medical Research Council (NHMRC) The Australian Immunisation Handbook. Updated 2022. Available: https://immunisationhandbook.health.gov.au/contents/about-the-handbook

National Health and Medical Research Council (NHMRC) 2022 Infection prevention and control. Available: https://www.nhmrc.gov.au/health-advice/public-health/preventing-infection

National Notifiable Diseases Surveillance System (NNDSS) 2023. Introduction to the National Notifiable Diseases Surveillance System. Available: https://www.health.gov.au/initiatives-and-programs/nndss?utm_source=health.gov.au&utm_medium=callout-auto-custom&utm_campaign=digital_transformation. (Accessed 26 May 2022)

Seale H, Heywood AE, Leask J et al 2021 Examining Australian public perceptions and behaviors towards a future COVID-19 vaccine. *BMC Infectious Diseases* 21, 120. https://doi.org/10.1186/s12879-021-05833-1

UNSW. The Kirby Institute 2022 Surveillance. Available: https://kirby.unsw.edu.au/research/surveillance

Wang B, Nolan R, Marshall H 2021 COVID-19 immunisation, willingness to be vaccinated and vaccination strategies to improve vaccine uptake in Australia. *Vaccines* 9(12), 1467

Wang H, Abbas KM, Abbasifard M et al 2020 Global age-sex-specific fertility, mortality, healthy life expectancy (HALE), and population estimates in 204 countries and territories, 1950–2019: a comprehensive demographic analysis for the Global Burden of Disease Study 2019. *The Lancet* 396(10258), 1160–203

Wilcox S 2015 Chronic diseases in Australia: blueprint for preventive action. Australian Health Policy Collaboration Paper No. 2015-01. Melbourne: Australian Health Policy Collaboration

World Health Organization (WHO) 2018 The top 10 causes of death. Available: http://www.who.int/mediacentre/factsheets/fs310/en/ (Accessed 21 Apr 2018)

World Health Organization (WHO) 2021a COVID-19 and the social determinants of health and health equity: evidence brief. Geneva: WHO

World Health Organization (WHO) 2021b Noncommunicable diseases. Available: https://www.who.int/news-room/fact-sheets/detail/noncommunicable-diseases. (Accessed 10 May 2022)

World Health Organization (WHO) 2022 Toolkit for developing a multisectoral action plan for noncommunicable diseases. Overview. Geneva: WHO

World Health Organization (WHO) 2022 Genuine intersectoral collaboration is needed to achieve better progress in vector control. Geneva: WHO. Available: https://www.who.int/news/item/11-04-2022-genuine-intersectoral-collaboration-is-needed-to-achieve-better-progress-in-vector-control

10

Place

Louise Baldwin and Mary Louise Fleming

LEARNING OBJECTIVES

After reading this chapter, you should be able to:

- Understand what place means in the context of terms like "community", "organisation" and "social institution" in public health interventions.
- Identify how the determinants of health relate to these terms.

- Explain why the terms "equity", "access" and "participation" are important in improving health outcomes.
- Understand the interrelationship between participation, engagement and empowerment in the context of place.
- Relate the principles of working in a variety of places through case studies and your own emerging practice.

INTRODUCTION

Public health engages with people in places like communities, organisations and social contexts where they live, work and play. In this chapter, our attention turns to working with population groups in a variety of settings. In this section of the book we use an adaptation of the socioecological model of health. Remember in the first chapter we focused on personal and interpersonal strategies. In this chapter we consider "organisations" and "communities" as aspects of place and discuss the use of strategies that encourage engagement, participation and empowerment. We further explore capacity building and the social determinants of health, including key principles for working in these contexts in public health practice.

Organisations and Other Societal Contexts

The idea of an organisation can be viewed in a number of ways. In this chapter we discuss how an organisation is defined in our society and how public health strategies can occur in that context. An organisation is made up of groups of people who act together in pursuit of common goals or objectives. People are impacted by social movements, markets and hierarchies, and influenced by culture (Hatch, 2011). Social institutions or organisations are a core part of the community. People are reliant on these structures because they enable the fulfilment of expected roles and behaviours (Brown, 2018). For example, we know that society needs a way to keep people

healthy, so we have a community healthcare facility or a large tertiary hospital in our community. Sociologists, when they hear the word "institution", would think of social structures such as governments, families, schools, workplaces and healthcare facilities. Anthony Giddens calls institutions "the more enduring features of social life" (Giddens, 1984, p. 24). They are complex social forms that reproduce themselves.

COMMUNITIES

Community settings are described as various organisations or places in communities such as schools, a range of not-for-profit organisations, social services or public health agencies, or worksites, as examples (Escoffery et al, 2018). Working with communities is core to public health. After all, communities are the intersection between working at the interpersonal level (Chapter 9) and the enabling environments level, where we take a broader, holistic approach focusing on environments, policies and social issues (see Chapter 11).

Community participation was the focus of the 1978 Alma Ata declaration, which framed the community as central to the planning, organising, operation and control of primary healthcare.

A focus for the new SDGs is the provision of people-centred health services and participatory approaches (UN, 2019). Also, intersectoral approaches encompassing community participation and engagement are key to implementing strategies in public health. Engaging communities effectively will have a positive impact on social capital, enhancing community empowerment, improving health status and reducing health inequalities (Haldane et al, 2019).

The term "community" is widely used in many contexts to identify groups of people who may share a geographical area, interests, needs, locality and other collective dynamics (Reynolds & Sariola, 2018). Tembo and colleagues (2021) note that communities can be defined in terms of geography and relationships. In our lives, we are part of many communities, often at the same time. We can be part of the community where we live, contribute to a workplace, attend or work in a school community and participate in a sporting community or one that brings together people with common interests or cultures (see Activity 10.1). Online communities can play an influential role in our lives and expose us to being part of multiple global communities.

Communities can also be defined as a group of people with a common set of circumstances or having common interests. Living in a common area or neighbourhood can indicate a community; however, we should not assume that people who live in close proximity to one another share common beliefs, interests or needs. Many of the programs, initiatives and services provided to us are based on our neighbourhood or local government area, yet not everyone is connected to their local community by postcode or suburb or town boundaries (Tembo et al, 2021).

ACTIVITY 10.1 My Community?

What is your definition of a community? Think about the life you are leading now. How many communities are you a part of? In the table provided below, on the left-hand side list the communities you think you belong to. In the middle column, note down what role you play in each of these communities. In the right-hand column, suggest how public health might relate to each of these communities. Then select two of these communities and discuss the public health activities that you know are or could be a part of each community.

My Community	My Role in this Community	How Can Public Health Play a Role?

Reflection

Have you thought about a broad range of communities that you are a part of? Look again at the definition of community to help you with this activity. What role do you play in a community you have selected? Are you a member of the local hockey club and a player? Are you a volunteer telephone counsellor for Lifeline? Finally, think about how your community, and what you do in that community, might make a contribution to the health of that community.

It is important that the role of social, physical, economic and cultural environments and their impact on health is acknowledged. These determinants of wellbeing need to be taken into account as they influence communities, and impact on people and local environments. For example, think of a rural area where people living a considerable distance apart come together during the week for sporting activities. The sporting environment provides a good example of a community forming around common interests. The environment in which they gather, such as the clubhouse or sports field, makes up a part of that community. Public health relates to this community in many ways. For example, there are physical issues such as clean water and hygiene, opportunities to support healthy behaviours such as physical activity, smoke-free areas, healthy food choices and awareness of important issues such as mental health promotion and sun protection. The diverse perceptions, cultural values and needs of individuals within communities, as well as the relevant environmental surroundings, must be acknowledged in public health practice to ensure optimal health outcomes for the population.

WHY WORK WITH COMMUNITIES, SOCIAL STRUCTURES AND ORGANISATIONS?

Historically, health professionals may have been tempted to work "on" communities, a workplace or a school (a "downstream" approach), rather than "with" them (an "up-stream" approach). Earlier approaches to public health often claimed to have the answers, and so health workers worked on communities to "fix" problems. Today, health workers recognise the importance of supporting local community or organisations to find solutions, and of understanding the social determinants of health and the life circumstances of people where they live, such as their social environments, their workplace, financial circumstances, health literacy and education (Marmot, 2017; Ramanadhan et al, 2018; Reynolds & Sariola, 2018).

COMMUNITY CAPACITY BUILDING

Building the capacity of communities has become the focus of much attention in health. It relates to the physical and social resources, structures and systems within the community to enable cohesiveness and resilience. In the cycle of working with communities, community capacity building must address the social determinants of health (see below) and equip community members and partners with skills and resources for future health challenges (Ramanadhan et al, 2018). In rural communities, as an example, community capacity building is crucial for the development of an appropriate and responsive health service that meets community needs. It draws on social capital to create empowered communities to choose local solutions (Markantoni et al, 2019).

SOCIAL DETERMINANTS OF HEALTH

Many chapters in this book discuss the social determinants of health (see Sections 1 and 2). This issue is pertinent to working with communities. Recognition of the social determinants of health is crucial to improving health outcomes. Social determinants such as housing, transport, crime, safety and employment all affect the health of a community, regardless of how it is defined.

The issues that determine social health also relate to health equity, such as having accessible and locally relevant health services and programs for all. To address the social determinants of health, the engagement of the community, participation and empowerment are integral considerations in needs assessment and the formulation of initial evidence, decision-making processes for the delivery of services, ongoing evaluation and evidence translation. Further, as Paremoer and colleagues (2021) suggest, governments and the international community must take responsibility for "rebuilding social protection and solidarity to protect populations from future health challenges, while civil society and social movements also have a role in holding decision makers to account" (p. 3).

Working across the public health spectrum builds on strengths within communities and empowers processes and people to address social inequity. It can address both traditional (physical, mental and social) wellbeing as well as the environmental factors affecting the broader social determinants of health, such as housing and transport. Further, community ownership of the health issue and the means to improve health outcomes are crucial, whether it is primary prevention strategies to reduce risk factors and improve healthy lifestyles, or the utilisation of local health services. Community ownership leads to empowered communities, and situates health as an integrated and consistent theme in the way the community functions (Paremoer et al, 2021).

WHAT IS COMMUNITY ENGAGEMENT, PARTICIPATION AND EMPOWERMENT?

Community engagement, participation and empowerment are important elements of working with communities to improve health. As early as 1978, the *Declaration of Alma-Ata* recognised community participation, social justice and equity as key foci for health planning and the delivery of locally relevant programs and services (see Activity 10.2).

Community participation plays an important role in achieving social justice and equity. There is consensus that approaches such as community engagement, participation and empowerment in public health are crucial for effective public health practice (Reynolds & Sariola, 2018).

Thought needs to be put into how stakeholders might collaborate to focus on issues that are wicked problems that are contested, and that it is far better to focus on

---

ACTIVITY 10.2 *Alma-Ata* and Community Participation

Search the internet for the *Declaration of Alma-Ata*. List the comments that are made about community participation in the document. Now consider the *Declaration of Alma-Ata* itself. Why do you think this document is considered a "cornerstone" of public health in practice, even today?

Reflection

From the Declaration you will see that the term "primary health care" is used to describe community participation. Why are these comments about primary health care still so important today, 40 years after the Declaration was launched?

---

interdependencies, uncertainty, controversy and complexity (Head, 2022).

Community Engagement

Community engagement is multifaceted. It has a focus on adapting comprehensive local approaches that give communities a voice, and the necessary resources to put ideas into action. Such community-led strategies can ensure diverse local voices are heard, map local concerns and alliances, and the codesign of programs (Burgess et al, 2021).

The process seeks feedback from communities on perceived needs that are health-related, or on broader social issues such as transport or community representation on health committees. Other examples include coming together to shape agendas for action (Reynolds & Sariola, 2018). Community engagement needs to involve people within communities, from the development of ideas and thoughts through to the implementation and ongoing evaluation of programs or services (Eder et al, 2021).

Community Participation

Community participation has a strong focus on "collective action that connects sociocultural affiliations, beliefs, values and customs that use social interactions to encourage and focus outcomes" (Carmen et al, 2022). Collective action involves community participation in all aspects of the planning process, from needs assessment to implementation and ongoing evaluation. The effectiveness of this approach is having deep participation from the community and others as equal partners in the process (Ramanadhan et al, 2018).

Community Empowerment

Empowerment is a concept that describes "feeling in control" of situations. In health, it is important for individuals, groups and communities to feel empowered or in control of their own health, whether it be primary prevention, clinical decision-making, survivorship or end-of-life care decisions.

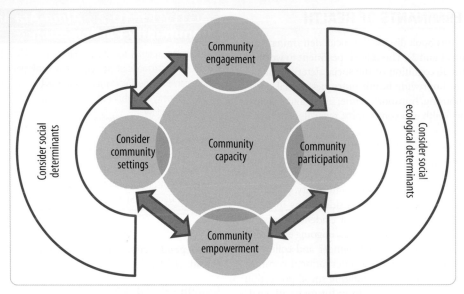

Fig. 10.1 The Working with Communities Cycle.

Empowerment suggests having the knowledge to make informed decisions. It results from "social, cultural, psychological or political processes through which individuals and social groups are enabled to express their needs, present their concerns, devise strategies for involvement in decision-making, and achieve political, social and cultural action to meet those needs" (Nutbeam & Muscat, 2021, p. 1586). Empowerment has the potential to reframe choices about community living and therefore social structures. Community empowerment begins to form along the cycle from participation and engagement (see Fig. 10.1); and, as the community develops, its capacity strengthens so empowerment grows (Smart, 2017).

We have discussed the three integrated strategies of community engagement, participation and empowerment. Note the distinctions between these strategies, but also note why one cannot occur without the other, and why there is no "end" point nor is it a linear process and that working with communities is never "finished". For example, if we ask a community what their health needs are, we are engaging that community in discussion about individual or collective local health issues. By working with communities in collaborative planning, implementation and evaluation (such as identifying needs, appraising the evidence and then creating solutions), the process can lead to community participation. Empowerment can be a subsequent phase of this process, where the community feels empowered and in control of solutions and positive health outcomes. Ongoing collaboration, however, is essential to ensure that communities are a part of public health, and that engagement, participation and empowerment are continually being developed and enhanced (see Activity 10.3).

ACTIVITY 10.3 Notions of Community Empowerment

Remember in Section 1 of the book we discussed the World Health Organization's definition of health. In that definition, a sense of "feeling in control" was included. Go back to our earlier chapters and consider this definition of health. Think about what the term "control" means and identify how the notion of community empowerment relates to being in control of health. Discuss this notion of "feeling in control" in relation to primary prevention (e.g. healthy eating) and in the context of the provision of a health service (e.g. a youth mental health service). What difference would "feeling in control" make to you or to a rural community or to an Aboriginal or Torres Strait Islander person in their community?

Reflection

"Feeling in control" can mean different things to different people. Have you considered what it means to be "in control" in the health context? Does it mean that you make the final decision about what you eat? Or are you influenced by the advertising of food products that you enjoy eating? Do you often consider the food that you eat in terms of kilojoules? In terms of protein, fat or carbohydrate content? How does the notion of "feeling in control" relate to your choices or the influencers that impact on your choices?

COMMUNITY AND ORGANISATIONAL STRATEGIES

In this chapter, we think about settings not just as places, but as opportunities to involve communities through participation, engagement and empowerment across the spectrum of public health activity.

One of the most prominent examples of community empowerment through a settings approach has been the Healthy Cities movement, largely stemming from Europe and the United Kingdom (de Leeuw & Simos, 2021). This means a different way of working with communities. It is described by de Leeuw and Simos (2021) as "the alignment of the conceptual 'software' of a Healthy City with the local government 'hardware' and its strategy and mobilizing power across sectors and civil society" (p. v). What is now an international initiative has provided the opportunity, the legitimacy and the space to experiment with and learn from what are both challenging concepts and ideas of modern public health.

WORKING WITH COMMUNITIES

Engaging with a community requires understanding the way the community works and the underlying social and physical structures, relationships, systems and services. Public health programs can be unsuccessful when they attempt to be "added" onto the community, rather than developed with and for the community. It is important to recognise the role of community and social structures, so as to enable public health to be integrated into the way the community functions.

Access and equity are important aspects of participation in risk factor prevention and participation in healthy lifestyle behaviours. The Heart Foundation Walking program is an Australia-wide initiative that encourages local community groups to form under volunteer leaders who are supported by Heart Foundation staff in each state and territory. The program is based on the need to increase physical activity levels through walking. It is a low-cost, low-risk activity with overarching benefits for cardiovascular health and social wellbeing (Ball et al, 2017). Communities are engaged through local health centres and local governments. Promotion and recruitment are low in cost and utilise community channels such as social media, community noticeboards and access to local organisations. The program includes a recognition system for walkers, such as "milestones" achieved and celebrated with certificates and small rewards such as water bottles. These milestones and achievements are highly valued by participants. Evaluations indicate that the program has achieved 70–80% of participants (walkers and organisers) meeting physical activity recommendations (Ball et al, 2017). An important outcome of community participation in health is that it not only keeps people healthy for longer, it also keeps them in their community and away from hospital engagement for as long as possible.

Williams and colleagues studied the role of playgroups in creating family support for Aboriginal and Torres Strait Islander families (Williams et al, 2016). This work showed that participation in playgroup environments can have positive benefits for home-learning environments, with opportunities to engage families, especially in isolated areas (Williams et al, 2016).

Digital platforms are powerful yet underused tools for engaging the public. Merchant and colleagues (2021) discuss four strategies to advance public health messaging during the COVID-19 pandemic that included deploying countermeasures for misinformation, surveillance of digital data to inform messaging, partnering with trusted messengers and promoting equity through messaging.

Read Case Study 10.1, and then consider the principles for integrated approaches to working with communities in Box 10.1. Think about how they might apply to these communities. How do you think a public health practitioner could facilitate these communities to empower them to work towards their own solutions? What strategies might be used?

CASE STUDY 10.1 Community Engagement in Rural and Regional Communities

Rural and regional areas present different opportunities to engage communities who may share very large geographical areas, and to join together as a community in a number of different ways. In two studies designed to identify the health needs of regional Queensland areas, community workshops, semi-structured group interview and individual in-depth interviews and consultations with other not-for-profit organisations were used to collectively identify the local health issues and concerns of the two communities. This process saw community leaders identified through channels such as local government, the local CWA and representatives from not-for-profits and other health facilities in each region were invited to participate. The consultation identified a range of issues, including mental health, health service access and delivery and mental health service constraints, physical activity and healthy eating and managing alcohol and drug use. These issues were prioritised by each community in order of importance to them for future action. Plans were then developed with key community leaders and health professionals to address these local needs. These detailed interactions with the two communities and attention to the notions of community development through the cycle of working with communities realised a set of foundations for future action through ongoing engagement, building empowerment and capacity (WMR, 2016).

Questions

1. Identify the steps along the cycle of working with communities.
2. How do these steps set the foundation for future action?
3. What do the terms "ongoing engagement", "building empowerment" and "capacity" mean in a rural community?
4. Why do you think community engagement is important for successful community action in rural and remote communities?
5. Does this mean telling communities what the needs assessment identified and what their focus should be? Or does it mean something else?

BOX 10.1 Principles for Working With Communities in an Integrated Approach

Recent literature (Schiavo, 2021) addresses the important principles of community engagement and why they make a difference:

- Local communities are the main beneficiaries of community engagement.
- Communities should be empowered to strengthen local health and social systems, and improve local conditions by owning and leading the decision-making process that would result in community-driven data, solutions and policies, and ultimately in community transformation and well-being.
- True community engagement should create new power dynamics, and serve as a mechanism for changing policies, programs and practices.
- True community engagement is "a key public health, healthcare, communication and international/community development area that seeks to empower communities to achieve behavioural and social results in support of improved health or development outcomes".
- It uses strategies that collaborate with and empower communities.
- It is about listening to local communities and recognising the expert in every community member, and every leader representing the community.
- It works towards and celebrates community ownership of interventions, and research design, implementation and evaluation.
- It builds trust, long-term relationships and willingness for participation among communities and their leaders.
- It is a process that works from the grassroots to change existing systems of power and privilege (Schiavo, 2021, p. 91).

Can you think of other recent examples of communities trying to pursue a community-led recovery after a natural disaster? You could look at some of the episodes of the ABC program: *The People's Republic of Mallacoota*, as an example (https://iview.abc.net.au/show/people-s-republic-of-mallacoota; accessed 20 July 2022). This example demonstrates the possibilities and the barriers to community-led recovery.

A FINAL WORD

Working with communities and organisations in social settings is crucial for public health. Communities and organisations are defined in many different ways in a variety of disciplines. This chapter addresses them in the context of public health. The concept of communities can be diverse. As a student or practitioner, it is important to recognise this fact, and its impact on how public health is contextualised. Working with organisations or social institutions through a settings approach enables a range of comprehensive and complementary public health strategies to be developed in communities by community-led approaches. Of course, this is a complex process and is often fraught with internal and external challenges. Overall, improving health outcomes for the public relies on working effectively in partnership with communities in a manner that is based on respect and equal status, along the cycle from initial engagement to ongoing empowerment and capacity building, underpinned by strong evaluation and integration of contemporary evidence. In the following Chapter and Chapters 12 and 13 in the final section we continue to focus on theory into practice in public health.

REVIEW QUESTIONS

1. How do communities differ in type, and why is this important for public health?
2. How are "organisation" and "social institution" defined as they relate to settings for public health?
3. What role do social determinants of health play in communities?
4. Why is community engagement that has no, or little, community involvement seen as "tokenistic"?
5. Suggest ways in which a public health practitioner can work with communities for more effective outcomes.
6. Why are concepts of equity and access important when working with communities?
7. What is community empowerment, and why is it important?

USEFUL WEBSITES

Australian Government. Head to Health: https://headtohealth.gov.au/meaningful-life/connectedness/community

Australian Institute of Health and Welfare. Healthy Community Indicators: https://www.aihw.gov.au/reports-data/indicators/healthy-community-indicators

World Health Organization. Healthy Settings: https://www.who.int/teams/health-promotion/enhanced-wellbeing/healthy-settings

World Health Organization Western Pacific Region. Building healthy communities and populations: https://www.who.int/westernpacific/about/how-we-work/pacific-support

REFERENCES

Ball K, Abbott G Wilson M et al 2017 How to get a nation walking: reach, retention, participant characteristics and program implications of heart foundation walking, a nationwide Australian community-based walking program. *International Journal of Behavioral Nutrition and Physical Activity* 14, 161

Brown S 2018 Social Institutions. Khan Academy. Available: https://www.khanacademy.org/test-prep/mcat/society-and-culture/social-structures/v/institutions (Accessed 7 Jun 2018)

Burgess RA, Osborne RH, Yongabi KA et al 2021 The COVID-19 vaccines rush: participatory community engagement matters more than ever. *The Lancet* 397(10268), 8–10

Carmen E, Fazey I, Ross H et al 2022 Building community resilience in a context of climate change: the role of social capital. *Ambio* 51, 1371–87

de Leeuw E, Simos J 2021 Healthy cities. In: *The Palgrave Encyclopedia of Urban and Regional Futures* (pp 1–6). Cham: Springer International Publishing

Eder MM, Millay TA, Cottler LB, PACER Group 2021 A compendium of community engagement responses to the COVID-19 pandemic. *Journal of Clinical and Translational Science*, 5(1), e133

Escoffery C, Lebow-Skelley E, Haardoerfer R et al 2018 A systematic review of adaptations of evidence-based public health interventions globally. *Implementation Science* 13(1), 1–21

Giddens A 1984 The Constitution of Society: Outline of the Theory of Structuration. Cambridge: Polity Press

Haldane V, Chuah FL, Srivastava A et al 2019 Community participation in health services development, implementation, and evaluation: A systematic review of empowerment, health, community, and process outcomes. *PloS One* 14(5), e0216112

Hatch MJ 2011 Organizations: A Very Short Introduction. Oxford, UK; Oxford University Press. Online. Available: http://www.veryshortintroductions.com/browse?t1=VSIO_SUBJECTS%3ASOC00450

Head BW 2022 Wicked problems in public policy: understanding and responding to complex challenges. Palgrave Macmillan. Cham: Springer International, p. 176.

Markantoni M, Steiner AA, Meador JE 2019 Can community interventions change resilience? Fostering perceptions of individual and community resilience in rural places. *Community Development* 50(2), 238–55

Marmot M 2017 Social justice, epidemiology and health inequality. *European Journal of Epidemiology* 32(7), 537–46. Available: https://doi.org/10.1007/s10654-017-0286-3

Merchant RM, South EC, Lurie N 2021 Public health messaging in an era of social media. *JAMA* 325(3), 223–4

Nutbeam D, Muscat DM 2021 Health promotion glossary 2021. *Health Promotion International* 36(6), 1578–98

Paremoer L, Nandi S, Serag H et al 2021 Covid-19 pandemic and the social determinants of health. *BMJ* 372, n129

Ramanadhan S, Davis MM, Armstrong R et al 2018 Participatory implementation science to increase the impact of evidence-based cancer prevention and control. *Cancer Causes and Control* 29, 363–9

Reynolds L, Sariola S 2018 The ethics and politics of community engagement in global health research. *Critical Public Health* 28(3), 257–68

Schiavo R 2021 What is true community engagement and why it matters (now more than ever). *Journal of Communication in Healthcare* 14(2), 91–2

Smart J 2017 What is Community Development? Melbourne: Australian Institute of Family Studies.

Tembo D, Hickey G, Montenegro C et al 2021 Effective engagement and involvement with community stakeholders in the co-production of global health research. *BMJ* 372, n178

United Nations, Global Sustainable Development Report 2019 The future is now: science for achieving sustainable development. Department of Economic and Social Affairs

Wesley Medical Research (WMR) 2016 Improving health and wellbeing in regional Queensland —assessing health needs and identifying evidence-based responses: a population health approach. Final Report. Brisbane: WMR

Williams KE, Berthelsen D, Viviani M et al 2016 Participation of Australian Aboriginal and Torres Strait Islander families in a parent support programme: longitudinal associations between playgroup attendance and child, parent and community outcomes. *Child: Care, Health and Development* 43(3), 441–50

11

Enabling Environments for Health

Melissa Haswell and Hilary Bambrick

LEARNING OBJECTIVES

After reading this chapter, you should be able to:

- Compare and contrast Indigenous Peoples' understandings of the environment with Western concepts of environmental health and planetary health, and discuss the importance of all three perspectives to public health.
- Discuss the major changing environmental exposures and challenges experienced by human populations in Australia and abroad, which underlie the shifts in types of diseases that now, or may in the future, dominate morbidity and mortality.
- Appraise the ways in which environmental health improvements enabling global poverty reduction

have led to substantial advances in human health, from reduced infant mortality to increased life expectancy.

- Identify and discuss the key direct and indirect health and social consequences of climate change and other environmental challenges we face as a result of human pressure on our planetary systems and what changes are urgently needed.
- Understand and discuss the way in which evidence from environmental epidemiology can be applied in health risk and health impact assessment to achieve advances in public health and health policy.

INTRODUCTION

Whatever your background or career goals, you will benefit from gaining an appreciation of the inextricable link between the health of the environment and the health of people. This chapter will expose you to the complexity and urgency of issues encompassed by environmental health, which is necessarily interdisciplinary and rapidly evolving. Well-informed ideas, decision making, planning and action in environmental health often provide simultaneous protection for the population from infectious, toxicological, physical and psychosocial risks. Furthermore, maintaining the positive, health-promoting features of the environment is essential for enabling mental health and social and emotional wellbeing, which in turn promote healthy lifestyles and chronic disease prevention.

We have reached a critical point in history where unprecedented human pressure is overreaching the capacity of the Earth's environmental systems to deliver basic needs for good health. This situation and how we respond will have vast implications for public health in coming decades. Public and environmental health professionals are increasingly working together to ensure awareness of the need to act now to

protect and promote ecologically sustainable, health-enabling environments—but much more urgent action is needed.

This chapter aims to 'open the door' for public health students, educators and professionals to gain knowledge and skills to advocate for proactive protection of both public health **and** the environment, in Australia and globally. The chapter seeks to increase your readiness to respond to environmental conditions that threaten multiple aspects of human health today, in the coming decades, as well as for future generations. It discusses how 'thinking global and acting local'— that is, returning to fundamental public health processes by galvanising community action to address these challenges—is needed now to build empowerment, resilience and progress towards sustainability and environmental restoration.

DEVELOPMENT AND DEFINITIONS OF ENVIRONMENTAL HEALTH

Before considering mainstream public health perspectives on the environment, we must first acknowledge and appreciate at least 65,000 years of ecological custodianship of the Australian continent by Aboriginal Peoples, who demonstrated that people can flourish even in the harshest of living conditions as caretakers invested in the protection of our planet's vast biological and geological diversity. Torres Strait Islander Australians have derived great strength and cultural identity through their intimate connection with the waters of the sea, their islands, reefs, the stars and winds for thousands of years (Sharp, 1993). A deep connection with the natural world, a sense of being part of and responsible for guarding and protecting the balance of nature, also lies at the centre of traditional Māori culture in Aotearoa New Zealand and is expressed in the concept of Kaitiakitanga (Royal, 2007). Profoundly embedded across hundreds of diverse Indigenous cultures and languages that make up First Nations Australasia (Australia, New Zealand, Papua New Guinea and some Pacific Islands) is a spiritual connection and an unwavering sense of responsibility to pass on healthy Lands and ecosystems to future generations (Salmon et al, 2019; Cresswell et al, 2021).

There is much to be learned from this timeless knowledge about relationships between the physical and human and non-human living worlds (Woodward et al, 2020). The consequences of European disregard for traditional knowledges have been extremely heavy for the Australasian environment, but there are growing efforts to return environmental management to traditional custodians in some areas, such as through Indigenous rangers, Indigenous Protected Areas (Williamson, 2022), Australian native title legislation, research partnerships (Woodward et al, 2020) and through negotiation between Iwi (Māori tribes) and the New Zealand government.

Complete Activity 11.1 to reflect on influences in your life that impact on your relationship with the environment.

In the Western tradition, the discipline of environmental health has blended environmental science, toxicology and communicable disease with the practice of environmental law, state and federal regulatory agencies, and public health practice. The field has relied heavily on evidence from environmental epidemiology—that is, research measuring associations between potential hazards in the environment, human exposures to those hazards and resulting disease and mortality.

These associations have been informally observed and documented throughout human history. For example, in 1775, London surgeon Sir Percival Pott recognised a high frequency of scrotal cancer among chimney sweeps, postulating a link with excessive exposure to soot (Friis, 2012). In the mid-1800s, anaesthesiologist Dr John Snow demonstrated the spatial connection between supply networks of contaminated water from the Thames River and cholera cases in London (Friis, 2012).

This and other seminal work spawned the fields of occupational and environmental epidemiology—as well as demands for protection, via legislation and regulation, of public and worker health from harmful environmental exposures. Today, Australia and New Zealand have advanced systems in place at national, state and local government levels, most of which adhere to international standards and guidelines. Human Health Risk Assessment is frequently used in Australia to combine evidence on individual hazards and their potential health impacts at expected levels of exposure, to support decision making in general and specific circumstances (enHealth, 2012).

Definitions of environmental health vary widely, particularly in the ways that they have included, or excluded, interactions between the environment and sociobehavioural factors affecting health, as well as consideration of ecological sustainability to ensure the health of future generations. For example, the Australian Government Department of Health (2014) and the current Environmental Health Standing Committee Strategic Plan 2020–2023 (enHealth Council, 2020) adopts the longstanding World Health Organization definition as:

> Environmental health addresses all the physical, chemical and biological factors external to a person, and all the related factors impacting behaviours. It encompasses the assessment and control of those environmental factors that can potentially affect health. It is targeted towards preventing disease and creating health-supportive environment.

Importantly, in Australian states and territories, environmental health is considered a core discipline within public health that is essential to health protection. Adopting a wider terminology, the concept of "environmental public health" offers a greater scope and includes not only potentially harmful "factors" (i.e. hazards), but also of environmental determinants of health, such as "the circumstances, and conditions in the environment or surroundings of humans that can exert an influence on health and well-being" (enHealth Council, 2020).

Figure 11.1 provides a diagrammatic representation of the ecological model of health, reminding us of the interactions between the many different components of the environment

---

ACTIVITY 11.1 Indigenous Worldviews and Environmental Sustainability

Consider as you read through this chapter how the application of Indigenous worldviews is important in addressing today's pressing environmental challenges.

Reflection

What challenges do you face in your own life in reducing your impact on the environment? Which ones are personal choices; which ones are determined by your place of work and/or study? Which ones are determined by your society? Do you think that connecting people with a deeper appreciation of Nature could help address these environmental challenges? How?

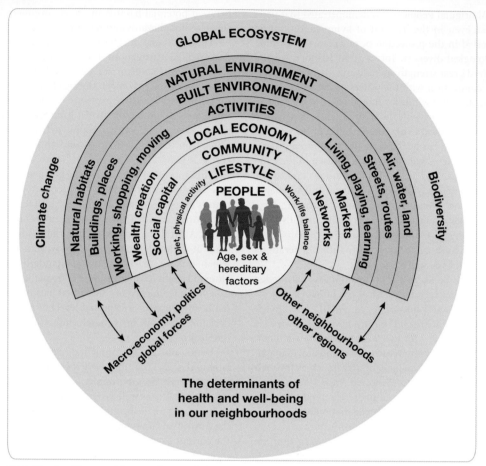

Fig. 11.1 The health map. (Source: Barton & Grant 2006, based on a public health concept by Dahlgren & Whitehead 1991)

and sociopolitical systems that influence people's health (Dahlgren & Whitehead, 1991; Barton & Grant, 2006).

Humans have long altered the environment in order to meet their wants and needs with materials and services, with varying levels of attention to losses to health and the environment. Today, there are many examples of large-scale activities, such as coal and unconventional gas and oil mining, and urban developments that pose multiple chemical, psychosocial, physical, climate and environmental health risks. These complex developments are best examined using Health Impact Assessment (HIA) (enHealth, 2017). HIA uses a range of tools, both qualitative and quantitative, and engages with representatives and stakeholders from affected communities to produce a more comprehensive understanding of potential outcomes. HIA is more consistent with broader public health principles, practice and mixed methods of inquiry. For further information, and to browse through some examples of HIAs, go to https://www.who.int/health-topics/health-impact-assessment#tab=tab_1.

BURDEN OF ENVIRONMENTAL DISEASE: OPPORTUNITIES FOR IMPROVEMENT

Since the mid-1900s, remarkable progress in human health and wellbeing globally has been achieved via improvement of environmental health conditions. The major global efforts launched through the Millennium Development Goals (MDGs) of the United Nations (UN) in 2000 reduced the number of people living in poverty by 50% (UN, 2015). This was enabled by widespread improvement of water supplies, sanitation facilities, vector control measures and housing. It also resulted in reduced infant mortality and increased life expectancy—contributing to unabated population growth in developing countries.

Despite these improvements, however, unhealthy environmental conditions have continued to cause an estimated 22.7% of global mortality (12.8 million deaths annually) and 21.8% of the global burden of disease (combining morbidity

CASE STUDY 11.1 Environmental Health Disparities Experienced by First Australians

Australia's Aboriginal and Torres Strait Islander communities have been sharply impacted by conditions promoting the rising prevalence of obesity and diabetes on top of continuing basic environmental health challenges (Macniven et al, 2016). Children in many remote communities experience higher rates of infectious diseases of the skin, upper and lower respiratory tract, ears and gastrointestinal tract as a result of overcrowded and poorly constructed houses and "health hardware", inadequate waste management systems increasing vector breeding and sanitation and water supply breakdowns (Pholeros et al, 1993; Bailie et al, 2010; 2011). They also face higher risk of nutritional problems linked to poor supply and/or excessive costs of fresh fruits and vegetables compared with highly processed, energy dense foods (Thurber et al, 2017).

Aboriginal and Torres Strait Islander communities are also more vulnerable to the impacts of climate change, including sea level rise, excessive temperatures at home and schools, extreme weather events and grief and loss from environmental degradation (Green et al, 2009; Rigby et al, 2011).

Reflection

Reflect on and discuss the ethical aspects of Australia's failure to address the enormous environmental health gap sufficiently and sustainably between Aboriginal and Torres Strait Islander and non-Indigenous Australians. How does climate change compound these injustices? What steps are taking place to move forward towards equity?

---

in All Policies approach provides a promising framework for boosting these partnerships, but greater focus is needed to promote equity in access and to build climate change resilience into our environments (van Eyk et al, 2017). See Case Study 11.1 examining health disparities for first nations people in Australia and the impact of climate change.

SHIFTING THE LENS BEYOND THE CURRENT BURDEN OF DISEASE TO FUTURE CHALLENGES

While the achievements of the MDGs were considerable, the 15 years of poverty reduction occurred through economic development that was tied directly to environmental degradation (United Nations, 2015). Population growth in the developing world, consumption of goods accessed through processes that have depleted environmental resilience and reliance on greenhouse gas-emitting fossil fuels—coal, oil and gas—continued unabated (Intergovernmental Panel on Climate Change, 2022).

Thus, looking only at the current global and Australian environmental disease burden leaves us with a limited view of the true public health challenges we face today and which will intensify in the near future. As public health has been grappling with these major current health transitions in the last 20 years, prospects for ensuring future health through environmental protection have worsened, particularly regarding climate change. Recent reports have warned that the window for preventative and adaptation actions to protect health is closing, particularly regarding climate change (Intergovernmental Panel on Climate Change, 2022), biodiversity loss (Murphy & van Leeuwen, 2021) and extreme weather events such as the 2019–2020 "Black Summer" bushfires (Australian Institute of Health and Welfare, 2021) and the extreme floods in southeast Queensland and Northern NSW in 2022 (Rice et al, 2022).

As the symptoms of a warming planet have become increasingly obvious, broader recognition has occurred within public health of the many urgent and interrelated issues that tie the health of our planet to the health and wellbeing of current and future generations, but this recognition is yet to translate into widespread political action to adequately address the problem (Horton et al, 2014; Watts et al, 2018).

THINK GLOBAL, ACT LOCAL

The concept underlying 'think global, act local' is credited to one of the Western world's great forward-thinkers, Scottish town planner, biologist and social activist, Sir Patrick Geddes (Thomson & Geddes, 1931; Groom, 2012). In the early 1900s he recognised the need for development to work with both people and the environment to collectively promote broader ecological sustainability in line with human wellbeing. These ecological "think global, act local" concepts also underpinned a *socioecological* approach to health within the Ottawa Charter for Health Promotion (WHO, 1986), which stated:

> . . . the inextricable links between people and their environment constitutes the basis for a socio-ecological approach to health . . . the conservation of natural resources throughout the world should be emphasised as a global responsibility . . . the protection of the natural and the built environments and the conservation of natural resources must be addressed in any health promotion strategy.

Today's recognition of the need to work together across human disciplines and nations to reconstruct a sense of responsibility to replenish natural systems has led to major global efforts towards the implementation of the United Nations' Sustainable Development Goals (Fig. 11.2) and the 2015 *Paris Agreement* (UN, 2015; United Nations Climate Change, 2018). This Agreement encompasses emission reduction pledges from 197 nations who participated in the 21st Conference of Parties of the United Nations Framework Convention on Climate Change (UNFCCC); a majority of which have been ratified by national governments and are becoming embedded into policy.

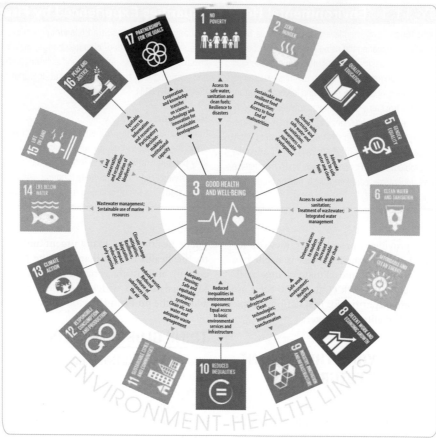

Fig. 11.2 Diagrammatic representation of the Sustainable Development Goals and their links to environmental health (Prüss-Ustün et al, 2016b, p. 96). (Source: http://www.who.int/quantifying_ehimpacts/publications/preventing-disease/en/)

Although highly encouraging, prioritising these essential goals within nations has proved challenging, including in Australia where our *policies* on climate change are highly impacted by the *politics* of climate change. Once a leader on carbon pricing, recent Australian policies have prioritised short-term economic interests, through export income earned through its fossil fuels, above the consequences of climate inaction. In sharp contrast, the New Zealand government and, so far, the new Australian government elected in 2022 are pressing ahead with plans for higher emission-reduction targets and global leadership in renewable energy transitions and clean energy exports. The contrasting policies are explored in Activity 11.2.

The urgency of the public health voice in these arguments is clear. For over two decades, the late Professor Tony McMichael spearheaded global recognition of the gravity of both direct and indirect impacts of climate change and other urgent environmental challenges on public health (McMichael, 2017). Climate change is increasingly contributing to morbidity and mortality across most health conditions, including infectious diseases, non-communicable chronic diseases, nutritional deficiencies, mental health disorders and injuries and death from extreme weather events in Australia and abroad (McMichael et al, 2015; Watts et al, 2018; Hanna & McIver, 2018; Burke et al, 2018; Romanello et al, 2021).

In 2009, *The Lancet* (2009) identified climate change as the "greatest health threat of the 21st century" and established the UCL Commission on Health and Climate Change. In 2014, the Commission reframed the challenge as a call to public health action on the "greatest health opportunity of our time" (Watts et al, 2018). This not only emphasised the urgent threat to health resulting from climate change, but also called attention to the multiple health and environmental co-benefits of reducing carbon emissions via transitioning to cleaner renewable energies, moderating consumption of meat and reducing "food miles"and increasing public and active transport. A significant example of leadership being undertaken through

ACTIVITY 11.2 Examining and Comparing Australia's and New Zealand's Recent and Current Climate Change Policies

The previous Australian government (2018–2022) published its 2017 Review of Climate Change Policies (http://www.environment.gov.au/climate-change/review-climate-change-policies), which drove its methods and targets. Many argue that for a nation with one of the world's largest per capita greenhouse gas emissions (European Commission Science Hub, 2022), failing to stay on track towards its Paris Agreement commitments (NDEVR Environmental, 2022) and contributing substantially to the global supply of coal and gas through exports, Australia's plans were not sufficiently aligned to the magnitude of this global—or even local—imperative (Doherty, 2018). Read through the 2017 Review's executive summary (pp. 5–7) and browse through the main body of text.

Now read how the New Zealand government is currently seeking world leadership on climate change action with a Zero Carbon Bill introduced in 2018 to reduce carbon emissions to net zero by 2050 (https://environment.govt.nz/acts-and-regulations/acts/climate-change-response-amendment-act-2019/). The plan includes an emissions trading scheme, embracing renewable energy opportunities and vigorous engagement with agriculture and forestry. Finally, listen to the speech by then New Zealand Prime Minister Jacinda Ardern to the UN General Assembly on 25 September 2021 (https://www.youtube.com/watch?v=32bn8mhlX40).

Reflection

Answer the following questions:

- To what extent did the last Australian government appear committed to domestic and global leadership on climate action in 2018?
- How well has New Zealand done in putting plans into action for reducing emissions and leading change domestically and internationally?
- Has the Australian Labor government elected in 2022 managed to steer the nation into more committed, effective and ethical decarbonisation policies?
- Can you identify some similarities and differences between the attitudes, priorities and values expressed by the two most recent governments in Australia and currently in New Zealand?

ACTIVITY 11.3 Acting Local: Cities Power Partnership

In attempts to accelerate government action, or to progress forward without it, exciting initiatives are growing around the world. One example is the Cities Power Partnership (http://citiespowerpartnership.org.au/), which is galvanising community action on climate change mitigation, regardless of any emission-reduction requirements at state and federal level. Hosted by Australia's Climate Council, the Cities Power Partnership is a free, non-profit support and networking initiative to facilitate renewable energy projects at local council level, and thereby accelerate Australia's emissions reduction. This opt-in partnership provides opportunities for local governments to share ideas, support each other and showcase their renewable energy activities. Currently, 170 councils around Australia (32% of all councils) have signed up to the partnership, and many more are pursuing renewable energy activities outside the partnership. Some of the activities occurring under the partnership include bulk-buying solar panels to provide a lower-cost option for residents, promoting active and public transport and increasing energy efficiency in council buildings.

Reflection

Discuss the strengths and limitation of local government pressing forward on renewable energy transitions in the absence of strong national policy on climate change. How do you think different levels of government should respond to the health threats and impacts associated with climate change?

supportive partnerships and city councils to drive renewable energy transition is discussed in Activity 11.3.

A FINAL WORD

As economically developed, and still prosperous, nations with very high innovative capacity, Australia and New Zealand are extremely well placed to take a leadership role in promoting health-enabling environments today and in the future. The knowledge, ideas and voice of all health professionals are absolutely essential to achieve this goal, as Horton and colleagues (2014, p. 847) eloquently concluded in their manifesto "From public to planetary health":

> The voice of public health and medicine as the independent conscience of planetary health has a special part to play in achieving this vision. Together with empowered communities, we can confront entrenched interests and forces that jeopardise our future. A powerful social movement based on collective action at every level of society will deliver planetary health and, at the same time, support sustainable human development.

REVIEW QUESTIONS

1. Why do we need to use knowledge from many sources and disciplines—for example, Indigenous knowledges, social and physical science, ecology, medicine and public health—in

order to address the challenges faced in creating and protecting health-enabling environments?

2. How do the tools of Human Health Risk Assessment and Health Impact Assessment help guide decision making on developments that impact on the environment?

3. What early observations of environmentally mediated disease led to the development of the field of environmental epidemiology?

4. What proportion of the global burden of disease can be attributed to unhealthy environmental conditions? Which types of environmentally associated diseases have decreased, and which types have increased, in recent years?

5. What environmental factors contribute to obesity? How are these linked to socioeconomic status?

6. Why is climate change considered the greatest health challenge and the greatest health opportunity of our time?

7. What are the main human activities contributing to climate change, and what actions can be taken to reduce greenhouse gas emissions?

8. How are cities, communities and health leaders leading change and pushing governments to take stronger action to address the challenge of climate change?

9. What actions can you take in your daily life and career to

USEFUL WEBSITES

Australian Government, Department of Health 2014 Overview of environmental health: https://www.health.gov.au/topics/environmental-health

enHealth Council 2020 Environmental Health Standing Committee (enHealth) Strategic Plan 2020 to 2023. Australian Department of Health, Canberra https://www.health.gov.au/resources/publications/environmental-health-standing-committee-enhealth-strategic-plan-2020-2023?language=en

Health Impact Assessment examples: https://www.who.int/health-topics/health-impact-assessment#tab=tab_1

Australia State of the Environment 2021, Australian Government Department of Agriculture, Water and the Environment, Canberra: https://soe.dcceew.gov.au/overview/introduction

New Zealand Prime Minister Jacinda Ardern, speech to the UN General Assembly, 25 September 2021: https://www.youtube.com/watch?v=32bn8mhIX40

Defining the Indefinable: Descriptors of Aboriginal and Torres Strait Islander Peoples' Cultures and Their Links to Health and Wellbeing: https://www.lowitja.org.au/page/services/resources/Cultural-and-social-determinants/culture-for-health-and-wellbeing/defining-the-indefinable-descriptors-of-aboriginal-and-torres-strait-islander-peoples'-cultures-and-their-links-to-health-and-wellbeing

REFERENCES

Australian Government Department of Health 2014 Overview of environmental health. Available: http://www.health.gov.au/internet/main/publishing.nsf/Content/health-pubhlth-strateg-envhlth-index.htm (Accessed 5 Mar 2018)

Australian Institute of Health and Welfare (AIHW) 2016 Healthy Communities: Overweight and obesity rates across Australia, 2014–15 (In Focus). Cat. no. HPF 2. Canberra: AIHW

Australian Institute of Health and Welfare (AIHW) 2021 Data update: Short-term health impacts of the 2019–20 Australian bushfires, AIHW, Australian Government. Available: https://www.aihw.gov.au/reports/environment-and-health/data-update-health-impacts-2019-20-bushfires/contents/introduction (Accessed 20 Jul 2022)

Bailie RS, McDonald EL, Stevens M et al 2011 Evaluation of an Australian Indigenous housing programme: community level impact on crowding, infrastructure function and hygiene. *Journal of Epidemiology and Community Health* 65(5), 432–7

Bailie R, Stevens M, McDonald E et al 2010 Exploring cross-sectional associations between common childhood illness, housing and social conditions in remote Australian Aboriginal communities. *BMC Public Health* 10. doi:10.1186/1471-2458-10-147

Barton H, Grant M 2006 A health map for the local human habitat. *The Journal for the Royal Society for the Promotion of Health* 126(6), 252–61

Bowe B, Artimovich E, Xie Y et al 2020 The global and national burden of chronic kidney disease attributable to ambient fine particulate matter air pollution: a modelling study. *BMJ Global Health* 5, e002063

Bowie C, Beere P, Griffin E et al 2013 Variation in health and social equity in the spaces where we live: a review of previous literature from the GeoHealth laboratory. *New Zealand Sociology* 28(3), 164–91

Burke SEL, Sanson AV, Van Hoorn J 2018 The psychological effects of climate change on children. *Current Psychiatry Reports* 20(5), 35. doi:10.1007/s11920-018-0896-9

Crawford B, Byun R, Mitchell E et al 2017 Socioeconomic differences in the cost, availability and quality of healthy food in Sydney. *Australian and New Zealand Journal of Public Health* 41(6), 567–71

Cresswell ID, Janke T, Johnston EL 2021 Overview: Outlook and impacts. In: *Australia State of the environment 2021, Australian Government Department of Agriculture, Water and the Environment*. Canberra. Available: https://soe.dcceew.gov.au/overview/outlook-and-impacts. doi:10.26194/f1rh-7r05 (Accessed 1 Aug 2022)

Dahlgren G, Whitehead M 1991 Policies and strategies to promote social equity in health. Stockholm: Institute for Future Studies

Dendup T, Feng X, Clingan S et al 2018 Environmental risk factors for developing type 2 diabetes mellitus: a systematic review. *International Journal of Environmental Research and Public Health* 15(1), 78

Diez Roux AV, Mujahid MS, Hirsch JA et al 2016 The impact of neighborhoods on CV Risk. *Global Heart* 11(3), 353–63

Doherty P 2018 Climate change is a fiendish problem for governments – time for an independent authority with real powers. The Conversation

(Australia). Available: https://theconversation.com/climate-policy-is-a-fiendish-problem-for-governments-time-for-an-independent-authority-with-real-powers-93853 (Accessed 15 Jul 2022)

enHealth Council 2012 Environmental Health Risk Assessment: Guidelines for Assessing Human Health Risks from Environmental Hazards. Canberra: Australian Department of Health. Available: https://www.health.gov.au/resources/publications/enhealth-guidance-guidelines-for-assessing-human-health-risks-from-environmental-hazards

enHealth Council 2017 Health Impact Assessment Guidelines. Canberra: Australian Department of Health. Available: http://www.health.gov.au/internet/main/publishing.nsf/content/A12B57E41EC9F326CA257BF0001F9E7D/$File/Health-Impact-Assessment-Guidelines.pdf (Accessed 5 Mar 2018)

enHealth Council 2020 Environmental Health Standing Committee (enHealth) Strategic Plan 2020 to 2023. Canberra: Australian Department of Health. Available: https://www.health.gov.au/committees-and-groups/enhealth

European Commission Science Hub 2022 Emissions Database for Global Atmospheric Research (EDGAR) Fossil CO2 emissions of all world countries. Available: http://edgar.jrc.ec.europa.eu/overview.php?v=CO2andGHG1970-2016&dst=CO2pc&sort=des9 (Accessed 1 Aug 2022)

Friis RH 2012 Environmental epidemiology. In: *Essentials of environmental health*, (2nd ed., pp. 27–48) Burlington: Jones & Bartlett, Ch 2.

Fuentes Pacheco A, Carrillo Balam G, Archibald D et al, 2018 Exploring the relationship between local food environments and obesity in UK, Ireland, Australia and New Zealand: a systematic review protocol. *BMJ Open* 8, e01870

GBD 2019 Diabetes and Air Pollution Collaborators 2022 Estimates, trends, and drivers of the global burden of type 2 diabetes attributable to PM2·5 air pollution, 1990–2019: an analysis of data from the Global Burden of Disease Study 2019. *Lancet Planet Health* 6, e586–600

Green D, King U, Morrison J 2009 Disproportionate burdens: the multidimensional impacts of climate change on the health of Indigenous Australians. *Medical Journal of Australia* 190(1), 4–5

Groom RC 2012 Think Global and Act Local. *Journal of ExtraCorporeal Technology* 44(4), 177

Hann EG, McIver LJ 2018 Climate change: a brief overview of the science and health impacts for Australia. *Medical Journal of Australia* 208(7), 311–15

Horton R, Beaglehole R, Bonita R et al 2014 From public to planetary health: a manifesto. *The Lancet* 383(9920), 847

Intergovernmental Panel on Climate Change 2022 Summary for Policymakers [Pörtner H-O, Roberts DC, Poloczanska ES et al (eds]. In: Climate Change 2022: Impacts, Adaptation, and Vulnerability. Contribution of Working Group II to the Sixth Assessment Report of the Intergovernmental Panel on Climate Change [Pörtner H-O, Roberts DC, Tignor M, et al (eds)]. Cambridge: Cambridge University Press. Available: https://www.ipcc.ch/report/sixth-assessment-report-working-group-ii/

McMichael A 2017 Climate change and the health of nations: famines, fevers and the fate of populations. Oxford: Oxford University Press

McMichael AJ, Butler CD, Dixon J 2015 Climate change, food systems and population health risks in their eco-social context. *Public Health* 129(10), 1361–8

Macniven R, Richards J, Gubhaju L et al 2016 Physical activity, healthy lifestyle behaviors, neighborhood environment characteristics and social support among Australian Aboriginal and non-Aboriginal adults. *Preventive Medicine Reports* 3, 203–10

Murphy HT, van Leeuwen S 2021 Biodiversity: Key findings. In: *Australia State of the Environment 2021, Australian Government Department of Agriculture, Water and the Environment.* Canberra. Available: https://soe.dcceew.gov.au/biodiversity/key-findings (Accessed 1 Aug 2022)

NDEVR Environmental 2022 Tracking Two Degrees. Quarterly Report December 2021. Q2/ FY2022. Melbourne, Australia. Available: https://ndevrenvironmental.com.au/wp-content/uploads/2022/04/T2D-Report-FY2022-Q2-VA.0-1.pdf (Accessed 15 Jul 2022)

Pholeros P, Rainow S, Torzillo P 1993 Housing for health: towards a healthy living environment for Aboriginal Australia. Newport Beach, NSW: HealthHabitat

Prüss-Ustün A, Wolf J, Corvalán C et al 2016a Preventing disease through healthy environments: A global assessment of the environmental burden of disease from environmental risks. Geneva: World Health Organization. Available: https://apps.who.int/iris/bitstream/handle/10665/204585/9789241565196_eng.pdf?sequence=1&isAllowed=y (Accessed 30 Jul 2022)

Prüss-Ustün A, Wolf J, Corvalán C et al 2016b Diseases due to unhealthy environments: an updated estimate of the global burden of disease attributable to environmental determinants of health. *Journal of Public Health* 39(3), 464–75

Rice M, Hughes L, Steffen W et al 2022 A super-charged climate: rain bombs, flash flooding and destruction. Climate Council of Australia Ltd. Available: https://www.climatecouncil.org.au/wp-content/uploads/2022/03/Final_Embargoed-Copy_Flooding-A-Supercharged-Climate_Climate-Council_ILedit_220310.pdf (Accessed 15 Jul 2022)

Rigby CW, Rosen A, Berry HL et al 2011 If the Land's sick, we're sick: the impact of prolonged drought on the social and emotional well-being of Aboriginal communities in rural New South Wales. *Australian Journal of Rural Health* 19(5), 249–54

Romanello M, McGushin A, Di Napoli C et al 2021 The 2021 report of the Lancet Countdown on health and climate change: code red for a healthy future. *The Lancet* 398(10311), 1619–62

Royal, TAC 2007 'Kaitiakitanga – guardianship and conservation – Understanding kaitiakitanga', Te Ara – the Encyclopedia of New Zealand. Ministry for Culture and Heritage, Government of New Zealand. Available: http://www.TeAra.govt.nz/en/kaitiakitanga-guardianship-and-conservation/page-1 (Accessed 16 April 2018)

Salmon M, Doery K, Dance P et al 2019 Defining the indefinable: descriptors of Aboriginal and Torres Strait Islander Peoples' cultures and their links to health and wellbeing. Aboriginal and Torres Strait Islander Health Team, Research School of Population Health. Canberra: The Australian National University. Available: https://www.lowitja.org.au/page/services/resources/Cultural-and-social-determinants/culture-for-health-and-wellbeing/defining-the-indefinable-descriptors-of-aboriginal-and-torres-strait-islander-peoples'-cultures-and-their-links-to-health-and-wellbeing (Accessed 18 July 2022)

Sharp N 1993 Stars of Taigai. The Torres Strait Islanders. Canberra: Aboriginal Studies Press

The Lancet 2009 A commission on climate change. *The Lancet* 373(9676), 1659

Thomson JA, Geddes P 1931 Life: outlines of general biology. London: Williams and Norgate

Thurber KA, Banwell C, Neeman T et al 2017 Understanding barriers to fruit and vegetable intake in the Australian longitudinal study of Indigenous children: a mixed-methods approach. *Public Health Nutrition* 20(5), 832–47

United Nations Climate Change 2018 The Paris Agreement. Available: https://unfccc.int/process/the-paris-agreement/the-paris-agreement (Accessed 15 Mar 2018)

United Nations (UN) 2015 Transforming Our World: The 2030 Agenda for Sustainable Development. New York: UN Publishing. Available: https://sdgs.un.org/goals

Warin B, Exeter DJ, Zhao J et al 2016 Geography matters: the prevalence of diabetes in the Auckland region by age, gender and ethnicity. *New Zealand Medical Journal* 129(1436), 25–37

Watts N, Adger WN, Ayeb-Karlsson S et al 2018 The Lancet Countdown: tracking progress on health and climate change. *The Lancet* 389, 1151–64

Williamson B 2022 Caring for Country means tackling the climate crisis with Indigenous leadership: 3 things the new government must do. The Conversation; 1 June 2022. Available: https://theconversation.com/caring-for-country-means-tackling-the-climate-crisis-with-indigenous-leadership-3-things-the-new-government-must-do-183987 (Accessed 10 Jul 2022)

Woodward E, Hill R, Harkness P, Archer R (eds) 2020 Our knowledge our way in Caring for Country: Indigenous-led approaches to strengthening and sharing our knowledge for land and sea management. Best practice guidelines from Australian experiences. Northern Australia Indigenous Land and Sea Management. Alliance and Commonwealth Science and Industry Research Organisation. Available: https://www.csiro.au/en/research/indigenous-science/indigenous-knowledge/our-knowledge-our-way (Accessed 31 Jul 2022)

World Health Organization 1986 Ottawa Charter for Health Promotion. Geneva; WHO. Available: https://www.who.int/publications/i/item/ottawa-charter-for-health-promotion. (Accessed 6 Jul 2018)

Contemporary Issues

INTRODUCTION

Chapters in the final section of the book follow on from Section 3 in that they build on our conversations about strategies using a socioecological model. They also provide us with the opportunity to explore the role of health promotion to enhance the future wellbeing of the Australian population and to make some relevant comments about the importance of planning and evaluation. We explore the impact of globalisation, and how disaster, emergencies and terrorism are dealt with in a public health context.

Chapter 12 discusses refocusing public health with an emphasis on promotion and protection. It begins by defining a range of definitions to enable us to understand their histories and place in public health. While examining levels of prevention, and how health promotion works across these levels we also have the opportunity to introduce health promotion in a global context, its strategies and applications in various settings and populations. We have a conversation about the opportunities for the health promotion workforce. Concluding this chapter is an analysis of the success of health promotion and its future challenges.

Chapter 13 examines contemporary practice and the importance of planning and evaluation in public health practice. It is important when considering planning and evaluation to understand the integration between the two terms. When setting out an agenda for planning it is important to consider the types of needs assessments available to public health and the range of resources that are available to help you select and use appropriate approaches. Planning is about 'praxis' and the importance of understanding a theory-into-practice approach by examining a range of planning and evaluation models and their strengths and weaknesses. In particular, we discuss the importance of the evaluation cycle, evaluation designs and an evaluation plan. We use case studies in this chapter to explore these concepts and principles.

In our focus on global health in Chapter 14 we discuss the concept of global health and its key characteristics. We identify key aspects of globalisation and how these aspects impact on the health of populations worldwide. In particular, we cover the importance of the Global Burden of Disease Study in informing a global health approach. We deal with issues of migration in Australia and how migration has played an important role in the history of Australia and New Zealand, and the nature and extent of the impacts of migration on the health of individuals and communities. This also enable us to critically evaluate the factors that impact on the health of refugees and asylum seekers, including immigration detention as an example. Importantly, we discuss some of the challenges of a human rights approach to the promotion of global health.

In Chapter 15 we examine issues that impact on public health, such as disasters, emergencies and terrorism. It is timely for us to examine the impact on population health of emergency planning and response, given the number of local and global disasters in recent years. We begin this chapter by defining 'disaster' and the causes and impacts of disaster. We have an opportunity to focus on identifying trends in disasters and the factors influencing those trends as well as discussing the principles of disaster management in the modern context. The key public health implications of disasters are presented and we identify and discuss the role of public health practitioners in disaster management. We introduce you to the impact of terrorism on population health, and we discuss the social, emotional, environmental and political implications.

In our final chapter of the book, **Chapter 16,** we provide you with some concluding remarks about the impact of megatrends on the population and the changing nature of the world in which we live. Initially, we return to our socioecological model as a final statement about the range of factors that impact on public health and the health of the population. We help you to consolidate your learning in this text through an analysis of the future of public health and the broad impact of globalisation on population health processes and outcomes. We consider the range of megatrends globally and locally and how they might impact on public health and population outcomes.

12

Refocusing Public Health with a Health Promotion and Prevention Lens

Louise Baldwin

LEARNING OBJECTIVES

After reading this chapter, you should be able to:
- Understand the role of health promotion and prevention in the broader public health context.
- Introduce health promotion in a global context—its strategies and applications in various settings and populations.
- Identify levels of prevention, and how health promotion works across these levels.
- Discuss different practices and opportunities in health promotion for health professionals.
- Share the successes of health promotion and its future challenges.

INTRODUCTION

Keeping the population healthy and safe may seem like common sense to reduce the incidence of otherwise preventable health issues. When we talk about health promotion and prevention, this largely refers to adapting known risks to reduce a person's or population's likelihood of developing a disease, injury or other health issue. Prevention is not possible for all health issues; however, research has discovered several factors which increase the risk of developing health issues. These issues can be biological (that is, inherited genetically or part of a person's biological make-up) or they can be lifestyle related, which means a behaviour that is participated in that increases the risk of developing a certain health issue or injury. Prevention approaches bring multiple benefits to the health of the public, which is why a prevention lens is important for all public health practitioners. This includes reducing risk of preventable mortality and morbidity; creating healthier, happier lifestyles; reduced burden on the health systems and, potentially, the creation of healthier, connected and productive communities (DoH, 2021). Health promotion takes a community centred, equitable, socioecological approach, in combination with a range of strategies and policies and is at the core of helping to shape the health of populations.

EVOLUTION OF, AND EVIDENCE FOR, HEALTH PROMOTION

The concept of health promotion emerged with the *Declaration of Alma-Ata* in 1978 (World Health Organization [WHO], 1978), and its Health for All strategy. Health promotion was seen as an approach that assumed that people's health was determined not only by their own behaviour, but also by the contexts in which they lived and worked. To improve health within a population, a "new public health" was needed to tackle these determinants, as research revealed that multiple strategies across many sectors—government, non-government and industry—were needed to ensure health opportunities for all. Globally, there were, and are, population challenges: war and the consequent displacement of millions of people as refugees; the globalisation of the workplace; increasing disparities in the standards of living between and within countries; planetary health; and the increase in ageing populations. Public health practitioners need the skills to identify and analyse the impact of these factors on health and the broader determinants, and to advocate for healthy public policies that support individual, organisational and population-wide health changes.

Public health generally takes a population focus as opposed to an individual focus. An easy way to distinguish these approaches is by using practical examples. A medical practitioner treating a patient for signs of heart disease may undertake specific tests on that person, consider genetic risk factors, prescribe medicine and suggest lifestyle changes such as physical activity, healthy eating and quitting smoking. A population approach, however, considers the adaptable risk factors across the whole population and also looks at contributing factors such as where people live, economic issues and other social factors. The definition by Buck and colleagues summarises this well:

> *An approach aimed at improving the health of an entire population. It is about improving the physical and mental health outcomes and wellbeing of people within and across a defined local, regional or national population, while reducing health inequalities. It includes action to reduce the occurrence of ill health, action to deliver appropriate health and care services and action on the wider determinants of health. It requires working with communities and partner agencies.*
>
> *Buck et al, 2018*

There is mounting evidence for the cost–benefit of health promotion, and thus for the need to devote more resources to prevention to improve the health of populations (Australian Health Promotion Association and Public Health Association of Australia, 2021). In a review of available evidence for national expenditure on preventive health, Jackson and colleagues (2017) identified that many preventive health interventions are cost-effective. This is due to interventions either promoting health and reducing the need to treat expensive diseases, or enabling populations to live longer with improved quality of life (WHO, 2021; Vos et al, 2010). In a landmark study Vos and colleagues (2010) identified that policies, including taxation on tobacco, alcohol and unhealthy foods, a mandatory limit on salt in three basic foods (breads, cereals and margarine) and an intensive SunSmart campaign, among others, could achieve a large impact on population health through cost-effective interventions. Complete Activity 12.1 to better understand health education, health promotion and health protection. This work has since been supported by various studies including the World Health Organization through their "Choosing Interventions that are Cost Effective (CHOICE)" program and global position statements such as the International Union for Health promotion and Education's 10 systems requirements for non-communicable diseases (International Union for Health Promotion and Education (IUHPE), 2018; WHO, 2021).

LEVELS OF PREVENTION IN PUBLIC HEALTH AND HEALTH PROMOTION

There are three defined levels of prevention—primary, secondary and tertiary. Some recent health advancements mean that a fourth element of survivorship can be incorporated into these considerations. *Primary prevention* focuses on whole

---

ACTIVITY 12.1 Health Education and Promotion and Protection

Discuss the following questions with other students:

- Discuss the difference between individual behaviour change and population-level public health.
- In a small group, define prevention. Comment on whether you believe there is a lot of attention being paid in the community to prevention. Does this include complementary medicine?
- Search for the IUHPE's 10 systems requirements for prevention of non-communicable diseases (NCDs). Write a short summary of the case for financial investment in preventing premature mortality in Australia.

Reflection

What did you consider when discussing individual versus population approaches for public health? How do you think systems and governments can be shifted to focus on greater prevention programs rather than treatment for otherwise preventable diseases?

---

populations, including healthy individuals, and targets reducing known disease risk factors while promoting factors that are protective of health. These factors include physical activity, healthy eating, sun protection and immunisation. Strategies reflect the *Ottawa Charter*, such as banning cigarette advertising in all media, and implementing legislation or public policies and creating supportive environments to assist people to make healthy choices. These strategies are sometimes called 'upstream strategies'. They work by addressing the causes of poor health, and focus on the promotion of health and wellbeing. *Secondary prevention* aims at detecting and curing the disease before it causes symptoms—for example, cervical cancer screening, the early detection of skin cancer, mammography screening and addressing early warning signs of mental ill health. *Tertiary prevention* focuses on the diagnosis of a disease and minimising its consequences, such as cardiac rehabilitation programs for heart disease.

Survivorship is a fourth element added to this trio of levels of prevention, as we see such vast improvements in secondary and tertiary prevention leading to greater survivorship. For example, cancer or cardiovascular disease survivorship also means opportunities to minimise risk of a secondary diagnosis by embracing health promotion. This includes the need for sun protection and regular skin surveillance following a melanoma diagnosis, or improving physical activity and healthy eating following a cardiovascular diagnosis to improve overall heart health.

These levels of prevention are reflected in the continuum of care and are demonstrated in Figure 12.1. Activity 12.2 aims to develop a deeper understanding of these levels of prevention.

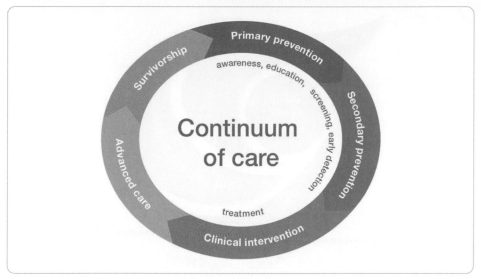

Fig. 12.1 Continuum of care. (Source: Wesley Medical Research, 2016, p. 15)

PRINCIPLES OF HEALTH PROMOTION

In 1986, the WHO declared a set of principles that underpinned health promotion: "'health' as the extent to which an individual or group is able to realise aspirations and satisfy needs; and to change or cope with the environment" (WHO, 2022). The principles are as follows:

- Health promotion involves the population as a whole in the context of their everyday life, rather than focusing on people at risk for specific diseases.
- It is directed towards action on the determinants or causes of health.
- It combines diverse, but complementary, methods or approaches, including communication, education, legislation, fiscal measures, organisational change, community development and contemporary, locally relevant, local activities against health hazards.
- It aims particularly at effective and concrete public participation.
- Health professionals, particularly in primary healthcare, have an important role in nurturing and enabling health promotion.

Health was seen as a "resource for everyday life, not the object of living". This definition represents a positive concept of health, instead of it merely being the absence of disease. The definition of health promotion was to "enable people to take control over their health". The concept of empowerment was implicit in health promotion, and was described as "a process through which people gain greater control over decisions and actions affecting their health" while the role of health professionals in health promotion is to work *with* people, not *on* them.

The *Ottawa Charter* has five essential actions (see Figure 12.2). Examples of these actions are given below.

1. *Build public policies that support health:* Health promotion goes beyond healthcare (e.g. hospitals that treat the sick), and makes health an agenda item for policymakers in all areas of governmental and organisational action. The aim must be to make healthier choices easier. Example: government smoke-free policies in schools, workplaces and transport.

2. *Create supportive environments:* Health promotion recognises that, at both the global and the local levels, environments can be supportive of health actions. Examples: walking and bike paths connecting services within communities encourage active travel; shaded environments encourage active lifestyles and minimise ultraviolet exposure and skin cancer risk.

3. *Strengthen community action:* Health promotion works through effective community action. Communities need to have control of their own initiatives and activities. Health professionals must learn new ways of working with individuals and communities—working *for* and *with*, rather than *on*, them. Example: collaborate with refugee communities to prioritise health needs.

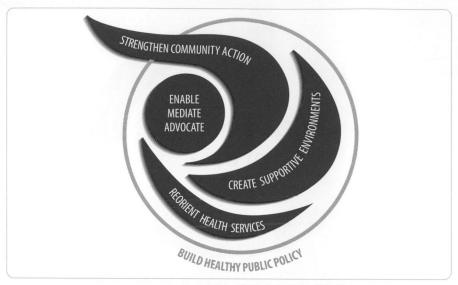

Fig. 12.2 Ottawa Charter for Health Promotion. (Source: WHO, 1986)

TABLE 12.1	**WHO Global Health Promotion Conferences**	
Year	**Place**	**Theme/Scope**
1986	Ottawa, Canada	Action to achieve health for all by the year 2000 and beyond (WHO, 1986)
1988	Adelaide, Australia	Healthy public policy (WHO, 1988)
1991	Sundsvall, Sweden	Creating supportive environments for health (WHO, 1991)
1997	Jakarta, Indonesia	Partnerships and settings (WHO, 1997)
2000	Mexico City, Mexico	Bridging the equity gap, with a focus on the determinants of health (WHO, 2000)
2005	Bangkok, Thailand	". . . identifies actions, commitments and pledges required to address the determinants of health in a globalised world through health promotion" (WHO, 2005)
2009	Nairobi, Kenya	"Promoting health and development: closing the implementation gap" (WHO, 2009)
2013	Helsinki, Finland	"Health in All Policies" (HiAP) and how to implement them (WHO, 2013)
2016	Shanghai, China	Promoting health, promoting sustainable development: health for all, and all for health (WHO, 2016)
2021	Geneva, Switzerland	Health promotion for wellbeing, equity and sustainable development (WHO, 2021b)

4. *Develop personal skills:* Health promotion supports personal and social development through providing information and education for health, and by helping people to develop the skills they need to make healthy choices. Example: educate patients about diabetes self-care.

5. *Reorient health services:* Responsibility for health promotion in health services is shared among individuals, community groups, health professionals, medical care workers, bureaucracies and governments.

Since 1986, the WHO has hosted regular global conferences that focus on and explore specific aspects of health promotion (see Table 12.1). These conferences, actions and frameworks propel continued action for advancing health. They embed the principles of health promotion as an integral part of public health. Complete Activity 12.3 to understand how the five action steps of the *Ottawa Charter* can be applied to reduce alcohol- or drug-related violence.

HEALTH PROMOTION IN PRACTICE: WHOLE-OF-SYSTEM, COLLABORATIVE APPROACHES

Intersectoral collaboration has long been integral to health promotion. It is built on the premise that "health is everybody's business" and that the actions of many sectors can impact on public health. Such sectors may include transport, housing, water services, electricity, education and environmental controls. For example, lack of transport access to health facilities, schools and shopping centres can affect the health of communities, potentially those on lower incomes, such as the aged and unemployed.

ACTIVITY 12.3 Australian National Preventive Health Strategy

Search for the Australian National Preventive Health Strategy 2021–2030. What themes can you identify in the Strategy? What focus can you see on population versus individual level approaches? What do you think this means for public health practice in Australia?

A *whole-of-system health promotion* is the integration of health promotion action within the whole system—across all sectors, including education, workplaces, housing, employment and so on. A good way to think of it is where communities interact—where they live, work, play and learn. The Geneva Declaration from the WHO calls for the creation of Wellbeing Societies—to demonstrate the need for all parts of a society to embrace health (WHO, 2021a).

Settings for Health Promotion

Given that health promotion is everybody's business, and recognising the need to make the "healthy choice the easy choice", the concept of health promotion "settings" became embedded as a core function of health promotion globally. Settings are places or social contexts in which people engage in daily activities, and where environmental, organisational, interpersonal and personal factors interact to affect health and wellbeing. They are places where people, communities, organisations and groups live, work, play and learn. This could include early childhood services, schools, workplaces, sporting clubs, community spaces (often managed through local governments), islands, villages, hospitals, universities and whole cities and towns. They may also be virtual settings, such as websites or online services. Settings provide systems and structures for health promotion actions: creating healthy policies, supportive environments, community action, personal skills and a focus on prevention to make healthier choices, environments, services and systems. Below we discuss three common settings.

Schools

Health promotion in schools includes planning and coordination of prevention actions; cross-sector partnerships and actions across and within school communities; political and financial support and evaluation (Gugglberger, 2021). The *Health Promoting Schools* (HPS) framework provides an effective guide for integrating health promotion throughout the school. The framework includes six key areas:

1. Healthy school policies
2. The school's physical environment
3. The school's social environment
4. Individual health skills and action competencies
5. Community links
6. Health services (Gugglberger, 2021).

The IUHPE outlines a series of tools and resources useful for achieving effective health promotion in schools. Pulimeno and colleagues (2020) note that some settings are multidimensional, such as schools, as they can also be workplaces. Therefore, such settings can model effective health promotion approaches for students, staff and the whole school community.

Communities

A community can be a geographical place—a city, town, neighbourhood—or groups of people who share common bonds—such as age or cultural identity—or who are linked through a common interest or cause (such as protecting the environment) or are coping with the same health condition (e.g. cancer patients). Communities can also include online communities. Community needs assessments are collected by government and non-government agencies and universities. Such needs assessments can be used in your public health practice. (See Chapter 13 for a list of needs assessment tools.)

Communities can be partners in health promotion and should be engaged from the beginning to co-design and collaborate in the development, implementation and ongoing evaluation of public health approaches (WHO, 2020). Local knowledge, expertise and resources are community "assets"; as such, they can form the basis of collaborative ventures to improve local health outcomes

Workplaces

Workplaces are dynamic enterprises with increasing numbers of staff working remotely, and often part-time. A healthy workplace is one where there is collaboration and a continual improvement process to protect and promote workers' health and safety and considerations for sustainability. Workplace health promotion considers the whole environment of the workplace and provides supported approaches to enhancing the health of employees and the extended community within a workplace. In terms of very practical examples, this may include a mentally healthy workplace, support for flexible working and family friendly arrangements, support for physical activity and reducing sedentary behaviour in offices, all aspects of workplace health and safety legislation (see Activity 12.4).

ACTIVITY 12.4 Settings for Health Promotion

With a group of students, choose one of the settings (schools, workplaces or communities) and a health issue of interest. Research and critique two articles on health promotion programs in that setting. What were the strengths of the chosen programs? The limitations? Would you have used alternative strategies? How were the programs to be sustained? What did you learn about the process of engagement in using a settings approach in health promotion?

Search for the Geneva Charter for Well-being published by the WHO in 2021. What are wellbeing societies? How could we consider wellbeing societies in Australia?

HEALTH PROMOTION IN ACTION: PUBLIC HEALTH SUCCESSES

CASE STUDY 12.1　Public Health Success in Australia

The Public Health Association of Australia (PHAA) is the leading professional association for public health in Australia. The PHAA reviewed public health success stories and released a seminal report outlining the top 10 public health successes over the past 20 years to 2018.

The report notes:

> Currently amounting to less than 2% of national health expenditure, public health investments are among our most efficient health buys. They save expenditure through avoided sickness, hospitalisation and lost working productivity. Resourcing public health measures generally saves far more than it costs.
>
> New resourcing of public health initiatives is essential if we are to reduce future national health expenditure (or even merely stem current rates of increase).
>
> Public health is also about equity, and is concerned with achieving fair health and wellbeing for everyone, not just those with better resources.
>
> (PHAA, 2018, p. 4)

The report outlines the 10 successes:

1. A reduction in neural tube defects: severe birth defects with high mortality and lifelong morbidity. Mandatory fortification of folate in wheat flour used for bread was introduced.
2. A world leader in immunisation: The National Immunisation Program provides free vaccination to eligible people and has significantly increased immunisation coverage.
3. Eliminating cervical cancer: through screening, the human papilloma test and the HPV vaccine.
4. Oral health—preventing dental decay through the introduction of water fluoridation.
5. Reduced the incidence of skin cancer in young adults with comprehensive SunSmart programs.
6. Reduced deaths from tobacco-related disease through some of the most advanced and toughest tobacco control laws in the world.
7. Reduced road deaths and injuries with comprehensive road safety strategies.
8. Reduced gun deaths in Australia with legislation.
9. Sustained low prevalence of HIV and AIDS through multiple policies and strategies.
10. Prevented deaths from breast cancer and bowel cancer through dedicated population-level screening programs.

Questions:

1. What trends do you see in the approaches used for these effective public health gains?
2. In small groups, search for the PHAA document on *Top Ten Public Health Successes over the last 20 Years*. Choose two of the successes—what population-level strategies did these public health programs use?
3. Review the Ottawa Charter discussed earlier in this chapter. Which of the public health successes embraced healthy public policy and supportive environments? How was this achieved?

EMERGING CHALLENGES FOR HEALTH PROMOTIONS

The United Nations Sustainable Development Goals (SDGs) are a lever to recognise the inextricable link between the environment, people and other determinants of health such as employment, housing, transport and income. The SDGs also recognise the need for action to enhance and promote health with a prevention lens, rather than focus on treatment of otherwise preventable health issues (UN, 2022). Barry (2021) considers this and outlines key enablers and system requirements for comprehensive approaches to health promotion and prevention. These include effective advocacy for the concept and practice of health promotion—that includes greater capacity of workforces to implement and evaluate prevention efforts across communities. Secondly, the need for enabling policy structures for universal health promotion actions across sectors—this recognises that health issues do not sit in the health promotion—and finally, greater investment in innovative research methods and knowledge transformation. These recommendations are at the core of enabling the broader public health system to shift a lens from treatment to focus on prevention where evidence shows the opportunity to reduce unnecessary diseases and deaths and enhance the health and vitality of communities.

A FINAL WORD

Public health professionals make a positive difference to the health of individuals, communities and populations. Public health globally faces multiple challenges, with a distinct role for promotion and protection. A major challenge is to address the determinants of health through "upstream" policy and advocacy and "downstream" personal skills, development, community empowerment and action. These actions are achieved through strategic partnerships to create health opportunities for all.

REVIEW QUESTIONS

1. What are the strengths of a "settings" approach for health promotion?
2. Is there a role in health promotion for most health professionals?
3. How do the levels of prevention influence the choice of health promotion strategies in developing a health promotion program?
4. What is the difference between an individual and a population approach to prevention?
5. Why are some of the future challenges for prevention important to lay a foundation for the future of public health practice?

USEFUL WEBSITES

Australian Health Promotion Association: http://www.health-promotion.org.au

Public Health Association of Australia (PHAA): phaa.net.au

Hauora Health Promotion Forum of New Zealand: http://www.hauora.co.nz

International Union for Health Promotion and Education: http://www.iuhpe.org

Victoria Health Promotion Foundation: http://www.vichealth.vic.gov.au

REFERENCES

Australian Health Promotion Association (AHPA) and Public Health Association of Australia (PHAA) 2021 Health promotion and illness prevention policy position statement. Available: https://www.healthpromotion.org.au/images/AHPA_PHAA_Health_Promotion_and_Illness_Prevention_Policy_2021_.pdf

Barry MM 2021 Transformative health promotion: what is needed to advance progress? *Global Health Promotion* 28(4), 8–16. doi:10.1177/17579759211013766

Buck D, Bayliss A, Dougall D et al 2018 A vision for population health: towards a healthier future. The Kings Fund. Available: https://www.kingsfund.org.uk/sites/default/files/2018-11/A%20vision%20for%20population%20health%20online%20version.pdf

Department of Health (DoH) 2021 National preventive health strategy 2021-2030. Canberra: Commonwealth of Australia

Gugglberger L 2021 A brief overview of a wide framework—Health promoting schools: a curated collection. *Health Promotion International* 36(2), 297–302. https://doi.org/10.1093/heapro/daab037

International Union for Health Promotion and Education (IUHPE) 2018 Beating NCDs equitably – ten system requirements for health promotion and the primary prevention of NCDs. Paris: IUHPE

Jackson H, Shiel A 2017 Preventive Health: How Much Does Australia Spend and Is It Enough? Canberra: Foundation for Alcohol Research and Education

Public Health Association of Australia (PHAA) 2018 Top 10 public health successes over the last 20 years. PHAA Monograph Series No. 2. Canberra: Public Health Association of Australia

Pulimeno M, Piscitelli P, Colazzo S et al 2020 School as ideal setting to promote health and wellbeing among young people. *Health Promotion Perspectives* 10(4), 316–24. doi:10.34172/hpp.2020.50

United Nations 2022 Do you know all 17 SDGs? Available: https://sdgs.un.org/goals

Vos T, Carter R, Barendregt J et al 2010 Assessing cost-effectiveness in prevention (ACE–prevention): final report. Melbourne: University of Queensland, Brisbane and Deakin University

World Health Organization (WHO) 1978 Declaration of Alma-Ata. International conference on primary health care, Alma-Ata, USSR, 6–12 September 1978. Geneva: WHO. Available: https://www.who.int/teams/social-determinants-of-health/declaration-of-alma-ata

World Health Organization (WHO) 1986 The Ottawa Charter for Health Promotion. 1st International Conference on Health Promotion, Ottawa, 21 November 1986. Geneva: WHO. Available: http://www.who.int/healthpromotion/conferences/previous/ottawa/en/

World Health Organization (WHO) 1988 Adelaide recommendations on healthy public policy. Second International Conference on Health Promotion, Adelaide, South Australia, 5–9 April 1988. Geneva: WHO. Available: https://www.who.int/teams/health-promotion/enhanced-wellbeing/second-conference

World Health Organization (WHO) 1991 Sundsvall statement on supportive environments for health. 3rd International Conference on Health Promotion, Sundsvall, Sweden, 9–15 June 1991. Geneva: WHO. Available: https://www.who.int/teams/health-promotion/enhanced-wellbeing/third-conference

World Health Organization (WHO) 1997 Jakarta statement on healthy workplaces. Symposium on Healthy Workplaces at the 4th International Conference on Health Promotion, Jakarta, Indonesia, July 1997. Geneva: WHO. Available: https://www.who.int/teams/health-promotion/enhanced-wellbeing/fourth-conference/jakarta-declaration

World Health Organization (WHO) 2000 The Fifth Global Conference on Health Promotion Health Promotion: Bridging the Equity Gap 5–9 June 2000, Mexico City. Geneva: WHO. Available: https://www.who.int/teams/health-promotion/enhanced-wellbeing/fifth-global-conference

World Health Organization (WHO) 2005 The Bangkok charter for health promotion in a globalized world. Geneva: WHO. Available: http://www.who.int/healthpromotion/conferences/6gchp/bangkok_charter/en/

World Health Organization (WHO) 2009 The 7th Global Conference on Health Promotion Promoting Health and Development: Closing the Implementation Gap. 26–30 October 2009, Nairobi, Kenya. Geneva: WHO. Available: https://www.who.int/teams/health-promotion/enhanced-wellbeing/seventh-global-conference

World Health Organization (WHO) 2013 The 8th global conference on health promotion. Health in All Policies (HiAP). Geneva: WHO. Available: http://www.who.int/healthpromotion/conferences/8gchp/en/

World Health Organization (WHO) 2016 The 9th global conference on health promotion. Promoting Health, Promoting Sustainable

Development: Health for All, and All for Health. 21–24 November 2016, Shanghai, China. Geneva: WHO. Available: https://www.who.int/publications/i/item/WHO-NMH-PND-17.8

World Health Organization (WHO) 2020 Community engagement: a health promotion guide for universal health coverage in the hands of the people. Geneva: World Health Organization; Licence: CC BY-NC-SA 3.0 IGO

World Health Organization (WHO) 2021 New cost effective updates from WHO-CHOICE. Available: https://www.who.int/news-room/feature-stories/detail/new-cost-effectiveness-updates-from-who-choice

World Health Organization (WHO) 2021a The Geneva Charter for Well-being. Available: https://www.who.int/publications/m/item/the-geneva-charter-for-well-being

World Health Organization (WHO) 2021b 10th global conference on health promotion. Available: https://www.who.int/teams/health-promotion/10th-global-conference-on-health-promotion

World Health Organization (WHO) 2022 The 1st international conference on health promotion, Ottawa, 1986. Available: https://www.who.int/teams/health-promotion/enhanced-wellbeing/first-global-conference

13

Applying Contemporary Approaches to Planning, Implementation, Evaluation and Learning for Public Health

Louise Baldwin

LEARNING OBJECTIVES

After reading this chapter, you should be able to:
- Understand complex communities, systems and settings.
- Understand and apply co-design principles to guide public health approaches.
- Understand the multiple contributing factors to health of communities.
- Identify different sources of data and methods of data collection to identify community needs.

- Understand the need for evidence-based approaches combined with co-design approaches for local adaption.
- Explore the use of Theories of Change to guide planning of public health approaches.
- Understand and apply logic modelling to public health approaches and critically analyse the benefits and pitfalls of these planning tools.
- Design and apply evaluation and learning processes as an integrated part of planning and implementation.

UNDERSTANDING COMPLEX COMMUNITIES, SETTINGS AND SYSTEMS

Public health programs and policies are often referred to as complex, in recognition of the multiple number of factors that contribute towards the health of communities and individuals, and, accordingly, the number of factors that programs and policies need to address.

Prevention of public health issues at the population level takes far more than education alone. As a student or early career practitioner, it is important to understand what causes risks for public health. For example, engaging in alcohol binge drinking, tobacco consumption or illicit drugs may be based on a number of social, personal, community and other factors that are underlying the risky behaviours. Figure 13.1 provides a simple overview of the public health process. Before undertaking public health planning it is important to understand the factors that contribute to the public health issues among communities. Issues are complex and integrated; for example, Australia's success in tobacco control to address preventable tobacco-related diseases has been based on extensive multi-strategy sustainable

approaches. This has included policy, legislation, education, economic strategies, provision of quit services, and so on.

UNDERSTANDING COMPLEX FACTORS THAT CONTRIBUTE TO THE HEALTH OF COMMUNITIES

Tackling public health issues in practice takes a population perspective. To do this, practitioners often take a "settings" approach where people live, work, play and learn. This means working within the environments where communities interact to create the healthiest possible opportunities for communities. This may be enabled by a range of approaches and policies, the physical environment, access to services, opportunities for engagement—and, most importantly, underpinned by equity for all. Planning public health approaches in settings requires consideration of the way the setting and that system works. If this does not occur, projects and programs can end up finishing abruptly or become resource intensive and lack the ability to sustainably change long-term health outcomes.

THE NEED FOR CO-DESIGN

Approaches to reduce public health risks among communities must be multi-strategy. To do this, we can take a number of lenses. We can build on the tradition of the seminal framework, the Ottawa Charter (World Health Organization, 1986), which identifies five frames for action: (1) healthy public policy; (2) creating supportive environments; (3) strengthening community action; (4) develop personal skills; and (5) reorienting health services towards prevention. What we can add to this is a suite of contemporary learnings, which firstly includes a lens of health literacy (Nutbeam, 2021) and secondly includes enablers and system requirements for health promotion such as advocacy, policy structures across sectors, support for implementation, workforce capacity and investment (Barry, 2021). This big-picture thinking for public health may seem too broad for the community or service or focus of your work or study. However, keeping this big picture frame in mind as a structure for public health is important, so that any smaller programs and policy approaches can eventually join together for collective impact.

In consideration of the broader determinants of health and issues surrounding social equity, the need to co-design approaches to reduce risk for preventable health issues with the community is essential. This process provides relevance, ownership and participation among the community. In fact, Meyer and colleagues (2022) note that the absence of community voices in programs may decrease the likelihood of programs creating improved health outcomes for communities.

Vargas and colleagues (2022) provide a useful series of six steps to consider for planning with a co-design approach:

1. Identify: identification of the structures and stakeholders relevant to the issue of interest. The focus of this step is on the identification of opportunities for value creation and solutions for problems. It is important to recognise all the stakeholders that should be included in the process.
2. Analyse: analysis of the stakeholder network and identification of shared and conflicting values to systematically clarify the processes and options for decision making, nature of relationships and relevant obligations among these relationships. Part of this process involves understanding how stakeholders interact together and understanding relevant experiences and ideas for possible solutions.
3. Define: built on the rights, obligations and ideas identified in previous steps, participants prioritise problems, next steps and actions.
4. Design: design of initiatives by setting goals, actions to achieve those goals, evaluation processes and allocation of resources and assets. To get the right initiative, stakeholders need to collaborate and adapt their positions of value from learnings gained through interactions.
5. Realise: during the implementation, stakeholders test the designed strategies and gather information. This realisation stage can remain continuous or occur in stages where testing ideas are reevaluated. It is essential to build structures that enable continual dialogue between stakeholders to implement ideas and generate further ideas for improvement and future implementation.
6. Evaluate: during the evaluation step, the proposed outcomes are assessed, as well as the way previous steps were taken, the learnings from the diverse stakeholders, the changes in the environment and ways for sustainability (e.g. resources, new partnerships, capacity building).

In providing these opportunities for co-design and the most collaborative and relevant methods for identifying what changes can be made to help build communities in the most locally, culturally and socially relevant manner, there is a need for succinct steps. To help guide this practical application, the Australian Institute of Family Studies (Haynes, 2021) provides a set of simple steps:

- What are the most common needs in this community?
- What are the needs affecting a particular segment of the community?
- What can be done to address a particular need?
- Who is most affected by this need?
- How does this need affect people?
- What has been done in other communities to address this need?

Data to inform needs assessments can take many forms. Primary data are known as data that would be derived directly from community through co-design, or through other consultation such as surveys, community meetings, observational methods or interviews. Secondary data can be gathered from other routine surveys and other data collection that may occur at the national, state or local level. This may include national data sets such as that from the Australian Institute of Health and Welfare or State/Territory Health departments. It may also include research and evaluation reports as well as other social and demographic data. This interaction of data should be considered in a cyclical format to inform planning, implementation and evaluation of public health approaches (Haynes, 2021).

DESIGNING PUBLIC HEALTH PROJECTS AND PROGRAMS: A CASE FOR THE EVIDENCE BASE

The terms "evidence-based interventions" or "evidence-based public health" relate to population approaches to public health that have shown to be effective elsewhere—either in practice or through research. Evidence-based interventions have stemmed from clinical public health approaches to inform treatment and clinical actions and have in recent decades been extended to prevention with community-based approaches. The findings from these interventions can help "scale" the strategies with greater confidence of the likelihood that preventative public health action will help to build healthy communities (Hailemariam et al, 2019). One of the constant challenges for public health practitioners is accessing the evidence or research to learn of effective public health projects and programs. At the time of writing there is an absence of accessible databases in Australia; however, some of the globally accessible resources are useful for Australian practice:

- https://prevention.nih.gov/research-priorities/dissemination-implementation/evidence-based-practices-programs.
- https://www.healthevidence.org.
- https://www.campbellcollaboration.org/evidence-portals.html.

THEORIES OF CHANGE

Once the needs for communities have been collectively identified using co-design approaches, and evidence from similar approaches have been summarised to inform your work, it is common practice to develop a public health plan. These plans are useful for project management, seeking funding, communicating with stakeholders, guiding evaluation and documenting learnings to continually build further evidence to inform future practice.

The recognition of the complexity that underlies public health makes way for the use of "Theory of Change" (ToC)

models to assist with planning public health action. This has been a shift in recent years from traditional public health planning of goals, objectives, strategies with more "linear" timelines that saw "start" and "stop" projects.

ToC models enable identification of underlying "root causes" or determinants of public health, the influences between these determinants and how a public health approach may influence these factors to create the desired change at the setting, community or population level (United Nations Development Program, n.d.). The ToC diagram should visually represent the changes that could occur with a series of actions. It is often based around a series of prompt questions that relate to the stages in change—for example, if we do this, then this will occur and over time, the change will be … There are many different ways to pictorially show a ToC—a very simple option is demonstrated in Figure 13.2.

A *program logic model* helps you write goals, objectives and strategies, identify a target group and needed resources and write an evaluation. It is a diagrammatic representation of the logical connections in a program plan. It can be displayed in a flow chart, map or table, and portrays the sequence of steps leading to program results (see Fig. 13.3).

The terms ToC and program logic are often used in parallel—usually program logic helps to "tease out" your ToC and put it into action. There are multiple tools and resources that can be used to help build a program logic

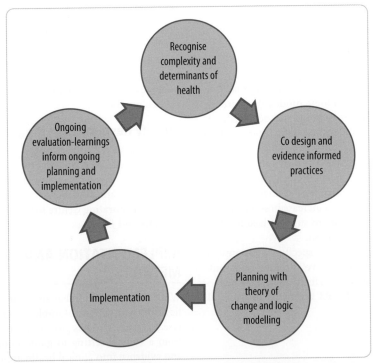

Fig. 13.1 An integrated approach to public health planning, implementation and ongoing evaluation and learning.

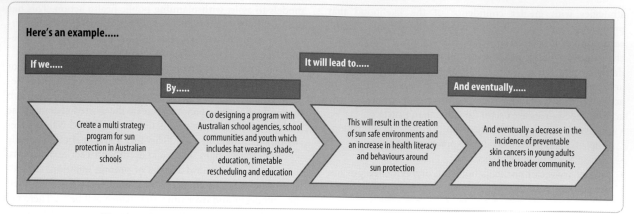

Fig 13.2 Basic Theory of Change Framework. From Theory of Change to program logic.

model. While the templates are often "linear" and look as if programs run from one step to another, it is important to have a "nimble" approach to a logic model, meaning that if some strategies are not working as planned, the team reviews the learnings and reconsiders with the community how the program is progressing.

When writing a program logic model and using the example in Figure 13.3, it can often be useful to write these "backwards", meaning starting with the desired outcomes and working backwards to identify what activities, outputs and inputs would be needed to achieve the desired outcomes and change for the community. Activity 13.1 enables you to think about why program logic models are useful in practice.

Outcomes (Objectives and Goals)

Outcomes identify what your public health approach or program is trying to achieve. In a logic model, these are the changes you have identified that could be achieved, informed through co-design and other data interpretation and sense-making.

Goals are the long-term outcomes the program desires and it is important to write this specifically so it can be measured. This may be a change in health outcomes; a change in social or economic conditions; or it may be an increase in service provision or the establishment of policies to support healthy environments such as smoke-free legislation.

Short-term outcomes or objectives specify the progressive changes that are considered to achieve the long-term outcomes—these need to be specific, realistic, logical, evidence-based and linked to goals. The SMART acronym can be useful:
- S—specific
- M—measurable
- A—achievable
- R—realistic
- T—time-limited.

A SMART objective could be: "Within 6 months, at least 80% of schools in our region will have been involved in co-design of a policy process to improve healthy eating for the whole school community".

Clear outcomes focus program goals and evaluation questions. This is important for many reasons in public health including continuing to build the evidence base of what works and does not work to improve health outcomes, for funding applications and for advocacy opportunities to change policy.

Write Strategies (Activities and Outputs)

Strategies are the activities chosen to reach your objectives or short-term results. A skin cancer prevention program may include sun-protective workplace policies (see Case Study 13.1), new sun-protective sporting uniforms, education on, and awareness of, correct use of sunscreens and integrated school curriculum tools.

Identify Resources: or Program "Inputs"

All programs require resources. How many staff/volunteers will be needed? Who will manage the program? Define the role of members of your planning group. Is the budget adequate? Useful tools are available—for example, the Canadian National Collaborating Centre for Methods and Tools (see Useful Websites and Books).

IMPLEMENTATION AND EVALUATION METHODS

While implementation has always been a strong focus of public health, a discipline of implementation science along with a research paradigm has grown over the past decade. Stemming from a clinical setting to guide implementation of research and evidence into clinical health approaches, implementation science has produced a number of useful frameworks to guide

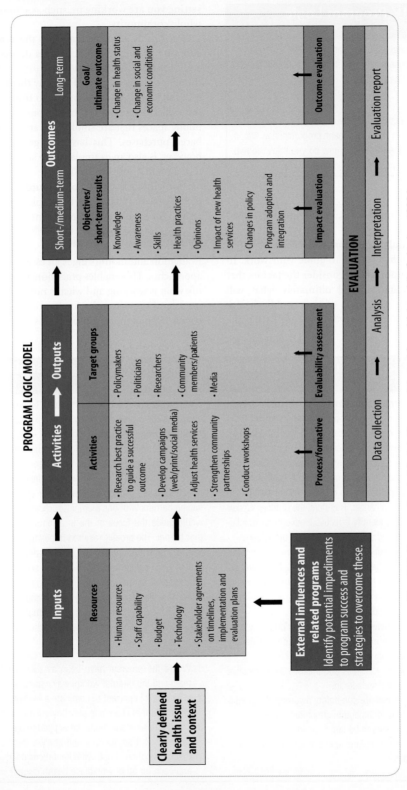

Fig. 13.3 Program Logic Model. (Source: Adapted from McLaughlin & Jordan, 1999.)

ACTIVITY 13.1 Program Logic Models

Why is a program logic model useful in planning public health initiatives? What are the components of a logic model and how does it compare with a Theory of Change?

Reflection

The chapter talks about the cyclical nature of planning, implementation and evaluation processes for public health programs; however, a logic model is generally a linear format—how do you think the two can be used in public health practice?

all levels of public health approaches, including primary and secondary prevention.

There are several implementation science frameworks, which can be freely searched online to guide your work. In using any of these it is important to consider the factors that will influence implementation and ultimately what will affect the ability for the outcomes of your public health approach to be integrated into everyday practice within the setting you are working in, such as schools, workplace or the whole community.

Put simply, implementation is the involvement, uptake or adoption of public health actions desired to improve health and social outcomes. This is not usually most effective when the actions become part of the way the setting or the community functions. A good example to think of is tobacco legislation, where in Australia it has become common law to provide public spaces that are smoke-free and limit availability for tobacco purchases. This has been great progress in Australia; however, is also an example where sustained action is required to maintain healthy outcomes.

In their work with schools, Jourdan and colleagues (2021) identify factors that affect the implementation of educational reform for health. These are outlined in Box 13.1.

Evaluation and Learning

Evaluation and monitoring is an essential part of public health approaches. This enables practitioners and researchers to identify what is working and what is not working, according to the needs and opportunities for improved health and social outcomes. Contemporary practice also incorporates a learnings

CASE STUDY 13.1 Outdoor Worker Sun Protection Project, Queensland University of Technology

Louise Baldwin and Monika Janda

Skin cancer places a huge burden on the health system, with Australia and New Zealand having the highest rates of this cancer in the world. Outdoor workers are at increased risk for developing skin cancer, due to the large amounts of time they spend outdoors and their consequent high exposure to ultraviolet radiation (UVR) from the sun. A combination of personal and environmental approaches to reducing UVR exposure can reduce the risk of developing skin cancer. Therefore, the Outdoor Worker Sun Protection project aimed to identify effective interventions to influence outdoor workers' sun-related attitudes, beliefs and behaviours.

A multi-strategy health promotion approach was taken and targeted a sample of small, medium and large-size workplaces. To ensure the project was low in cost and able to be replicated, a capacity-building approach was taken to reduce costly site visits and travel by staff. A six-stage approach was developed:

1. *Policy:* establish or review a workplace's sun-protection policy.
2. *Structural and environmental:* increase available shade and identify opportunities to reduce outdoor working times.
3. *Personal protective equipment:* assess and improve sun-protective clothing, hats, sunglasses and sunscreen.
4. *Education and awareness:* include sun-safety awareness and education around workplace locations and in structured sessions.
5. *Role modelling:* site supervisors to be sun-safe role models.
6. *Skin examinations:* encourage workers to check their own skin regularly and to visit their doctor.

A workplace champion was nominated by participating workplaces to help drive the project internally. A resource toolkit and online portal of resources were developed, along with each workplace's own action plan, blog, e-newsletter and Monday morning sun-safety alert email.

Staff maintained regular (at least weekly) contact with workplaces over the course of the project, which helped steer and guide strategies over the course of the intervention. For example, if workplaces were finding barriers with one element, such as sun-protective clothing, this would guide the focus of the intervention to assist with overcoming that barrier. The project resulted in positive changes for workers who received education or training in sun safety—for example, increased use of personal protective equipment such as broad-brimmed hats, long-sleeved shirts and long trousers. The project showed that sun-protection strategies could be implemented in workplaces with the support of a project team and an internal workplace champion, and that multi-strategies were effective (Rye et al, 2014).

Questions

1. Would the program have been as successful without the project team and the internal workplace champion?
2. Why was it important to nominate a workplace champion, and what role could that champion play beyond the initial project?
3. Could this six-stage model be applied to address mental health in a workplace? If so, identify and analyse each of the six stages and their application. If not, what limitations do you foresee in using this approach for other workplace health issues?

BOX 13.1 Factors Affecting Implementation of Educational Reforms for Health

Structural and Systems Factors
- School management
- School environment
- Services for vulnerable students
- School-family-community links

Policies
- Curriculum and assessment system
- Educational, health and intersectoral policies and plans
- Mobilisation of civil society

Practices
- Educational practices
- Public health intervention practices

Human Resources
- Professional development
- Staff support

Adapted from Jourdan D, Gray NJ, Barry MM, et al 2021 Supporting every school to become a foundation for healthy lives. The Lancet Child & Adolescent Health 5(4). 295-303, ISSN 2352-4642, https://doi.org/10.1016/S2352-4642(20)30316-3.

approach, meaning public health teams, along with stakeholders and community, interpret and reflect on the findings from progressive evaluations, and identify ways to put the learnings from these evaluations back into practice. Therefore, we represent evaluation as a cyclical approach—not just something that happens at a certain timepoint of a project or program.

Evaluation Purpose

Integrate short-, medium- and longer-term evaluation measures to guide your program, celebrate success along the way and modify elements that are not working as planned or intended.

In previous chapters we have discussed a systems approach, which recognises the complexity of factors that contribute to public health and, accordingly, the complexity of organisations, agencies, communities and factors that comprehensive approaches to public health should address. Evaluation of systems change approaches are also multi-faceted and may include systems mapping and modelling. There is a growing body of evidence on these approaches that can be accessed for further reference, such as McGill and colleagues (2021).

Program evaluation tools are more prolifically available to guide your study or practice. These may include tools such as the RE-AIM framework for evaluations and to formulate evaluation questions. Five factors are involved: reach, efficacy,

adoption, implementation and maintenance, as follows (adapted from Glasgow and colleagues [2019]):
- *Reach* captures the participation in a specific program (e.g, a patient counselling program at a clinic) or those in a community affected by a policy or program.
- *Efficacy* tests the effect of the design of a program. Would the design of a social media campaign be effective?
- *Adoption* measures the proportion of practices, or communities, that adopt the planned program.
- *Implementation* measures whether the program is being delivered as intended.
- *Maintenance* measures the extent to which the program is being sustained over time.

The US Centers for Disease Control and Prevention's (CDC) Evaluation tools provide a range of online tools and resources for practitioners and students (see: https://www.cdc.gov/evaluation/tools/index.htm). The CDC developed one of the seminal evaluation frameworks in 1999 and it continues to evolve today. The steps of the framework include:
1. Engage stakeholders (interested parties).
2. Describe the program and its context.
3. Focus the evaluation design.
4. Gather credible evidence.
5. Justify conclusions.
6. Ensure use of data and share the lessons.

These steps are underpinned by four key standards of utility, feasibility, propriety and accuracy (Kidder et al, 2018).

The Canadian program evaluation toolkit provides a series of steps for program evaluation. Prior to the evaluation, the toolkit provides a series of questions to consider:
- Who is the evaluation for?
- What do we need to find out from the evaluation?
- When will the findings be needed?
- Where will the findings be needed?
- Where should we gather information?
- How will the results be used? (Assoiants et al, n.d.)

Evaluation Designs

There are three commonly accepted levels of evaluation: process, impact and outcome. *Process evaluation* covers all aspects of program delivery, its quality and its target audience. *Impact evaluation* measures the immediate effect of the program (whether it met its objectives). *Outcome evaluation* measures the long-term effect of the program (whether it met its goals) (WHO, 2013). Bauman and Nutbeam (2014) present clearly detailed evaluation types and processes.

EVALUABILITY ASSESSMENTS

An evaluability assessment is a reflective process to identify if a program is ready for evaluation or what type of evaluation is relevant at that point in the evaluation. See Activity 13.2 to

---

ACTIVITY 13.2   Evaluability Assessments

Why is an evaluability assessment a significant part of the evaluation process? Why would program logic models be useful in an evaluability assessment?

Reflection

Evaluation should be part of public health practice; however, sometimes it is left to the end of projects or programs. Think about why evaluation should be integrated into usual practice and the values it would bring to project and program management.

ACTIVITY 13.3   Impact and Outcome Evaluations

What are some differences between impact and outcome evaluations? Research two of the evaluation designs suggested above, and compare their applications in measuring an impact and an outcome evaluation. You could do this by finding a journal article that contains both types of evaluation.

Reflection

Were you able to discern the differences between impact and outcome? One clue is that an impact evaluation measures the immediate impact of your program in making a difference to a population's awareness or knowledge, a change in attitude or change in practice in a service, whereas an outcome evaluation usually measures the long-term impact of a program on the population's health.

These long-term measures are also usually captured in broader reports, often produced by state health departments or the Australian Institute of Health and Welfare. Table 13.1 presents a checklist to guide your planning and evaluation.

---

think about how evaluation works as part of project and program management.

Process Evaluation to Measure Program Strategies and Activities

Process evaluation measures the activities of the program, program quality and target audience. It also can inform the measures for implementation, acceptance and population reach. Designing process evaluation reflects the activities in the logic model.

Impact Evaluation

Impact evaluation measures the short-term outcomes of the logic model. Learnings from process and impact evaluations are cycled back into reviews of program logic models to ensure public health approaches are responsive to the progressive evaluation and adapting as necessary based on findings.

Outcome Evaluation

Outcome evaluation measures the extent to which a program goal has been met and considers all aspects of the long-term outcomes. These are progressive learnings often informed by the findings from the process and impact evaluations. Is the health status changing? Are there changes in morbidity or mortality statistics in a population or short-term gains on a health problem? Your outcome measures, however, may be much smaller and relate to changes in the public's health in your local region. Activity 13.3 gives you an opportunity to research impact and outcome evaluations in practice.

Data Sources

When considering data sources for public health evaluation it is important to focus on relevant, useful data that are needed to communicate what is working and what is not working to relevant audiences. A mapping process is useful among the team to think about what data may already exist, what data need to be collected, how data could be collected in the most useful and efficient manner and who needs to know about the results.

Data sources for evaluation may include:
- Document review—where key themes from relevant documents are analysed and recorded to tell a story of findings.
- Surveys and questionnaire with key informant groups—it is important to test and validate survey tools to ensure these instruments will provide the data intended. Also give consideration to the relevance of surveying—ensure people are not overburdened with surveys already and that the pitch, language and style of the questionnaire is appropriate.
- Interviews—semi-structured interviews (meaning a discussion with guide questions) can provide rich insights from key informants on what is working and what is not working.
- Observation—depending on your public health approach, observations may be appropriate to consider.

Ethical requirements are essential to consider and all clearance and approvals should be considered prior to collecting or using any data.

A FINAL WORD

Robust planning, implementation and evaluation processes underpin public health practice. Some government departments have large data sets to analyse; non-government organisations' programs may be smaller in scale, but the principles of contemporary program planning and evaluation remain the same. This chapter has introduced the concepts of applying complexity-thinking to address public health needs and the importance of co-design with communities. Evidence continues to grow on effective public health approaches and

TABLE 13.1	**Planning and Evaluation Checklist: Evaluation and Dissemination**
Stage	**Action**
Problem analysis and needs assessment	Getting started—what issues do I need to consider in the planning and evaluation cycle?
	Engage stakeholders—who are they, and what are their values/expectations/concerns?
	Determine program objectives/mission—hierarchy of outcomes to guide action, and to link strategies and evaluation
	Pilot testing—how many participants?
Program planning and implementation	Select/describe strategies and methods—selection is linked to objectives
	Implementation process—needs to be managed in detail; suggested implementation and evaluation plan
	Evaluation procedures—qualitative, quantitative, or elements of both?
	Data collection—what, when and how to measure (pre-intervention testing; otherwise, there is no basis for doing a reasonable evaluation, and post-testing)
	Analysis of data—how much and what should be analysed?
	Costs, and what resources (human, financial, time) are available to meet the planned actions
	Using external evaluators—costs, expertise and independence of the evaluation
Evaluation and dissemination	Evaluation management
	Dealing with all of the players in the evaluation process and their individual expectations about program outcomes
	Participant burden—be aware of over-evaluating participants (the tyranny of evaluation)
	Process, impact, outcome levels—how do you make these judgments, and what are the implications for broader applications of the evaluation beyond the program?
	Investment in evaluation—money, time, personnel
	Evaluation outcomes—what did I learn, and how can I use that information for the future?
	Dissemination of the results—to whom and for what purpose?

Source: O'Connor-Fleming et al, 2006.

ensures the use of multi-strategy practice that is based on evidence while being adapted for community need and context. Theories of change are a contemporary and useful approach to guide public health planning underpinned by logic modelling to plan, review and guide project or program progress. Evaluation serves multiple purposes in public health project and program management and becomes integrated into planning and ongoing implementation, rather than at the "end" point of a project or program. These cyclical approaches enable ongoing monitoring and learning, guiding an understanding of what is working and not working across a range of factors related to intended outcomes and progress towards building healthy communities.

▌ R E V I E W   Q U E S T I O N S

1. What does complexity in public health refer to?
2. Thinking about complexity, why is co-design important in public health?
3. Why are planning and evaluation important practices in public health?
4. How are planning and evaluation linked, and why should these be integrated activities?
5. What is a Theory of Change and why is it useful in public health practice?
6. What data sources may be considered for integrated evaluation?
7. Why is evidence-based practice part of public health practice?

USEFUL WEBSITES AND BOOKS

Australian Health Promotion Association: https://www.healthpromotion.org.au/

Australian Institute of Health and Welfare: http://www.aihw.gov.au

Health*Info*Net: http://www.healthinfonet.ecu.edu.au/

International Union for Health Promotion and Education (IUHPE): http://www.iuhpe.org/index.php/en/

World Health Organization Western Pacific Region: http://www.wpro.who.int/southpacific/en/

REFERENCES

Assoiants A, Frampton N, Hickie C n.d. University of Calgary Program Evaluation Toolkit. Available: https://www.ucalgary.ca/live-uc-ucalgary-site/sites/default/files/teams/148/cmhs_program_evaluation_toolkit.pdf

Barry MM 2021 Transformative health promotion: what is needed to advance progress? *Global Health Promotion* 28(4), 8–16

Bauman A, Nutbeam D 2014 Planning and evaluating population interventions to reduce noncommunicable disease risk – reconciling complexity and scientific rigour? *Public Health Res Pract* 25(1), e2511402

Glasgow RE, Harden SM, Gaglio B et al 2019 RE-AIM Planning and Evaluation Framework: Adapting to New Science and Practice with a 20 Year Review Frontiers Public Health Sec. *Public Health Education and Promotion*. Available: https://doi.org/10.3389/fpubh.2019.00064

Hailemariam M, Bustos T, Montgomery B et al 2019 Evidence-based intervention sustainability strategies: a systematic review. *Implementation Science* 14, 57. https://doi.org/10.1186/s13012-019-0910-6

Haynes K 2021 Data sources in needs assessments Practice Guide. Available: https://aifs.gov.au/resources/practice-guides/data-sources-needs-assessments

Jourdan D, Gray NJ, Barry MM et al 2021 Supporting every school to become a foundation for healthy lives. *The Lancet Child & Adolescent Health* 5(4), 295–303. https://doi.org/10.1016/S2352-4642(20)30316-3

Kidder DP, Chapel TJ 2018 CDC's program evaluation journey: 1999 to present. *Public Health Reports* 133(4), 356–59. doi:10.1177/0033354918778034

McGill E, Er V, Penney T et al 2021 Evaluation of public health interventions from a complex systems perspective: a research methods review. *Social Science and Medicine* 272, 113697. https://doi.org/10.1016/j.socscimed.2021.113697

Meyer ML, Louder CN, Nicolas G 2022 Creating with, not for people: theory of change and logic models for culturally responsive community-based intervention. *American Journal of Evaluation* 43(3), 378–93. https://doi.org/10.1177/10982140211016059

Nutbeam D 2021 From health education to digital health literacy – building on the past to shape the future. *Global Health Promotion* 28(4), 51–5. doi:10.1177/17579759211044079.

Rye S, Janda M, Stoneham M et al 2014 Changes in outdoor workers' sun-related attitudes, beliefs, and behaviors: a pre-post workplace intervention. *Journal of Occupational and Environmental Medicine* 56(9), e62–72

United Nations Development Program (UNDP). Theory of Change UNDAF Companion Guidance. Available: https://unsdg.un.org/sites/default/files/UNDG-UNDAF-Companion-Pieces-7-Theory-of-Change.pdf

Vargas C, Whelan J, Brimblecombe J et al 2022 Co-creation, co-design and co-production for public health: a perspective on definitions and distinctions. *Public Health Research and Practice* 32(2), e3222211

World Health Organization (WHO) 1986 The Ottawa Charter for Health Promotion. Geneva: WHO. Available: https://www.who.int/teams/health-promotion/enhanced-wellbeing/first-global-conference

14

Global Health

Louise Baldwin and Ankur Singh

LEARNING OBJECTIVES

After reading this chapter, you should be able to:

- Understand the concept of global health and its key characteristics.
- Apply knowledge to think locally and act globally.
- Identify the key aspects of globalisation and how these are impacting on the health of populations worldwide.
- Identify and interpret key global collaborative action strategies for public health and understand how these affect country-level and local-level public health practice and research.

- Recognise the importance of the epidemiological studies such as the Global Health Observatory and the Global Burden of Disease Study in informing a global health approach.
- Understand the relationship between the Sustainable Development Goals and the broad determinants of health.
- Discuss some of the challenges of a human rights approach to the promotion of global health.

INTRODUCTION

Public health professionals need to have a robust understanding of health in a global context.

This chapter introduces the concept of global health and discusses the impact of globalisation on the health of populations. It also provides a brief overview of the global burden of diseases and highlights the key health issues for migrant populations. The chapter finishes with a brief discussion of the Sustainable Development Goals (SDGs) and the significance of a human rights approach when working in global health.

WHAT IS GLOBAL HEALTH?

How to define global public health remains a lively debate amongst researchers, practitioners and global health leaders, and as such, there is no commonly agreed definition of global health. However, several researchers have investigated what global health encompasses and how it relates to broader public health practice.

Recently, Salm and colleagues (2021) undertook a systematic review to identify common definitions and concepts of global health. The authors noted four theoretical aspects of global health:

1. "Global health is a multiplex approach to worldwide health improvement taught and pursued at research institutions

2. Global health is an ethically oriented initiative that is guided by justice principles

3. Global health is a mode of governance that yields influence through problem identification, political decision making as well as the allocation and exchange of resources across borders, and

4. Global health is a vague yet versatile concept with multiple meanings, historical antecedents and an emergent future" (Salm et al, 2021).

The Duke Global Health Institute (DGHI) define global health as a "field of study, research and practice that places a priority on achieving equity in health for all people" (DGHI, 2022). The Institute provides a useful comparison between global health and public health, as outlined in Table 14.1.

During your studies and early careers in public health, a range of competencies and skills are built. Whether public health work relates to local, state, national or global action, an awareness and understanding of global health, trends and strategies for wellbeing are important for public health research and practice. Sawleshwarkar and Negin (2017) reviewed global public health competencies for postgraduate students and identified some key themes that related to both study and practice. These include focus on the burden of disease and the determinants of

TABLE 14.1   Comparison Between Global Health and Public Health

	Global Health	Public Health
Area of impact	Issues that directly or indirectly impact health and can transcend national boundaries	Issues that impact the health of the population of a particular community or nation
Global cooperation	Development and implementation of solutions often require global cooperation	Development and implementation of solutions usually do not require global cooperation
Program focus	Embraces prevention in populations and clinical care of individuals	Mainly focused on prevention programs for populations
Health equity	Major objective is health equity among nations and for all people	Major objective is health equity within a nation
Disciplinary approaches	Interdisciplinary and multidisciplinary within and beyond health sciences	Encourages multidisciplinary approaches within the health and social sciences.

DGHI, 2022.

health, policy development, analysis and program management and, finally, action-related skills, including collaboration, partnering, communication, professionalism, capacity building and political awareness (Sawleshwarkar, 2017, p. 1).

The importance of global health is underlined by an increasingly globalised world and by major challenges in the 21st century that transcend national boundaries. These challenges include environmental degradation and climate change, antibiotic resistance, chronic health conditions due to unhealthy diets and tobacco smoking and increasing levels of migration and forced displacement due to economic inequality, violence and war. Undeniably the greatest and most notable impact on public health in recent times has been the COVID-19 pandemic. This unprecedented and rapid escalation of viral infection has been one of the most prominent public health emergencies in recent times. At the time of writing, the long-term public health impacts from this virus remain largely unknown; however, recent data, as at mid-2022, has shown that the pandemic infected more than 500 million people worldwide, led to 15 million deaths, disrupted health services in 92% of countries and halted progress on universal health coverage.

Furthermore, during the pandemic, global life expectancy has decreased, immunisation coverage of basic vaccines has decreased, the prevalence of anxiety and depression has increased and deaths from tuberculosis and malaria have increased (UN, 2022).

Activity 14.1 provides an opportunity to better understand the importance of global health in the public health context.

What are Global Health Challenges?

In 2020, the WHO released a summary of the pressing global health challenges for the next decades. It should be noted that this list was released in January 2020, prior to the escalation of the COVID-19 pandemic. However, it is pertinent to note that infectious diseases were noted as one of the pressing challenges. These are outlined in Box 14.1.

ACTIVITY 14.1   Global Health and Public Health

Thinking about global health, reflect on these questions to help apply your knowledge into practice:

- Why should public health students take an interest in global health?
- How do you think the student competencies listed above are relevant? List some examples of these competencies in action.
- Describe how global health reflects the interdependence of countries.
- Looking at the table from the Duke Global Health Institute, can you provide examples of global health action versus public health in your country or local area?
- Can you identify at least five international organisations that work in global health?

Reflection

Imagine you are working for one of the international organisations focusing on global health. Reflect on the values and skills required by public health professionals when working in global health. What values and skills do you already have? Which do you need to develop further?

Guiding Policies and Strategies for Global Health Action

When the World Health Organization was first formally recognised in 1948, the key priorities for worldwide action included malaria control, women's and children's health, tuberculosis, nutrition and environmental pollution (UN, 2022). Today, these issues still remain a priority for global action, thus demonstrating the long-term, sustained commitment required to adequately address global health issues.

1. Elevating health in the climate debate: the need to invest in clean air strategies and reducing health impacts of climate change.
2. Delivering health in conflict and crisis: protection of health workers in crisis situations and response to growing health needs in protracted conflict zones.
3. Making healthcare fairer: growing gaps in socioeconomic status contribute to growing gaps in health equity, meaning vulnerable groups fair worse in health and access to healthcare and services.
4. Expanding access to medicines: currently one-third of the world's population lacks accessibility to crucial medical and health supplies.
5. Stopping infectious diseases: investing in and implementing programs to support immunisation rates for vaccine-preventable diseases.
6. Preparing for epidemics, including infectious viruses and vector-borne diseases such as those spread by mosquitoes.
7. Protecting people from dangerous products: reducing the preventable disease burden including high fat, high salt and ultra-processed foods.
8. Investing in the people who defend our health: overcoming chronic underinvestment in the education and recruitment of health workers.
9. Keeping adolescents safe: overcoming the leading causes of adolescent death including injury, suicide, HIV, alcohol, tobacco and drug use.
10. Earning public trust: building evidence-based health education and scientific literacy for the public to get valid information circulated in a timely manner.
11. Harnessing new technologies, including artificial intelligence for healthcare and its challenges and opportunities.
12. Protecting the medicines that protect us, including overcoming microbial resistance.
13. Keeping healthcare clean, including basic water, sanitation and hygiene services (WASH).

WHO, 2020.

Leading global agencies such as the World Health Organization and the United Nations along with key government, community and professional associations, tend to set global targets and strategies for known diseases and risk factors that impact on public health and wellbeing. These strategies often set global and country targets or set a precedent for evidence-based ways of working to address burden of disease, determinants and related social and equity factors.

The Geneva Charter for Wellbeing 2021

Examples of these globally guiding strategies include The Geneva Charter for Wellbeing 2021. This landmark document is the next in a series of legacy documents that followed the development of the Ottawa Charter in 1986. In 2021, the Geneva Charter was launched after the 10th Global Conference on Health Promotion, held in Geneva, Switzerland. The Charter calls for a number of global public health actions, including healthy public policy for the common good, universal health coverage and planetary health (WHO, 2021).

The UNHCR Global Public Health Strategy 2021–2025

This strategy promotes health and human rights and focuses on the need for public health preparation for refugee emergencies. It calls on multi-stakeholder approaches to better respond to the refugee burden on communities and increases the self-reliance of refugees (UNHCR, 2021).

WHO Global Strategy on Health, Environment and Climate Change

Supported also by the World Health Assembly in 2019, this strategy aims to tackle environmental risks to health, underpinned by health in all policies approaches and upscaling health promotion and disease prevention (WHO, 2020a).

GLOBALISATION AND HEALTH

One aspect of global health to consider is globalisation, referring to a country's "openness to global collaboration and influence, through international economic activities and trade; exchange of culture, ideas and information; and collaboration between nations through international organisations" (Seferidi et al, 2022).

While globalisation can be beneficial for industry and trade, it can also have impacts on health. Seferidi and colleagues (2022) note that the impacts on food systems and diet-related outcomes can have enormous impacts on population health. While this can increase the availability and variety of foods for populations, it can also increase the quantity of and introduction of ultra-processed foods, having impacts on both undernutrition and overnutrition. This further reflects the social determinants of health, with the authors noting that associations differ across socioeconomic groups for diet-related outcomes due to globalisation.

To understand globalisation, Hanefeld and Lee (2015) have proposed to focus on three aspects of global change: spatial, temporal and cognitive. The term *spatial changes* refers to the way we understand and experience the physical (and virtual) space, and includes the increase in population mobility, which also involves animals and microbes, and the movement of information, wealth, goods and services. *Temporal changes* relates to the way we experience time. Technology has not only reduced the time required to travel between places, but has also made communication with others faster and easier. *Cognitive changes* refers to "how globalisation is changing what we think about ourselves and the world around us" (Hanefeld & Lee, 2015, p. 5). Our culture and beliefs are being substantially changed by mass and social media, religious and political groups, marketing and advertising agencies and research and educational institutions.

These three aspects of global change have had significant demographic, social, economic and environmental consequences that are impacting on the health of populations worldwide. Population growth and urbanisation have put considerable pressure on natural environments (e.g. soil and water depletion, loss of ecosystems) and are contributing to entrenched poverty and marginalisation. Social and cultural changes, along with increased population mobility and types of economic activity, have contributed to new and emerging infectious diseases, increasing rates of obesity and associated chronic health conditions, expansion of tobacco marketing and climate change (McMichael, 2013). Complete Activity 14.2 to reflect on the pros and cons of globalisation.

One example of the impact of globalisation on health is considering oral health in the Pacific Islands. The Pacific Islands have experienced increasing dental diseases between 1969 and 2018 (Pili et al, 2021). Globalisation has seen the introduction of sugary and processed foods to the Pacific Islands, along with tobacco. This has been associated with an increase in many oral health issues including oral cancers and periodontal disease. This has led to public health researchers calling for policy reform, increased access to health services and considering sugar taxes to reduce the burden of disease of high sugary foods on Pacific Island communities (Pili et al, 2021).

Global Health Data

With a focus on global action for public health through frameworks and priorities such as the Sustainable Development Goals (SDG), access to global data becomes more and more crucial for planning, implementation and monitoring of public health efforts. This is important not only for research and practice but also for funding and for advocacy.

The Global Health Observatory is one example of a publicly available data set for global health. It covers the 194 member countries of the World Health Organization (WHO) on more than 1000 indicators on priority health topics to monitor progress on the SDGs (Vardell, 2020). This includes the dedicated health SDGs but also those which relate to the determinants of health with 11 of the 17 goals having a health impact (Pang et al, 2021).

Developing indicators for global health data can be a complex process whereas, in fact, the ideal indicators are very simple measures that are useful and understandable to a range of different audiences. According to MacFarlane and colleagues (2019) the common types of indicators used in health include quantitative and qualitative indicators.

Quantitative

Proportion: this can include proportion of people with a disease or condition; proportion of population utilising a health service or other proportions such as health expenditure, population living in rural areas or use of substances such as tobacco.

Count: number of cases or events that relate to a population.

Ratio: one count divided by another such as ratio of males to females engaged in substance abuse.

Service density: number of service units e.g. hospital beds per population.

Qualitative

These can include assertions or opinions expressed as Satisfaction, or could include statements which people rank, e.g. wellbeing indicators include Life Satisfaction Scales (MacFarlane et al, 2019; Bagnall et al, 2017).

Using global health data to inform policy, advocacy and practice are important skills for public health practitioners. Activity 14.3 provides an opportunity to put these learnings into practice.

ACTIVITY 14.2   Pros and Cons of Globalisation

- How might globalisation impact on your life?
- How has globalisation impacted on your country of origin or the country you live in?
- Make a table, with one column for the positive aspects of globalisation and another for the negative aspects. List as many of these as you can think of.

Reflection

According to Professor John Rennie Short from the School of Public Policy, University of Maryland, in the United States:

> [G]lobalisation has now become the catchword to encompass the rapid and often disquieting and disruptive social and economic change of the past 25 years. No wonder there is significant backlash to the constant change—much of it destabilizing economically and socially disruptive. When traditional categories of identity evaporate quickly, there is a profound political and cultural unease. The globalisation project contains much that was desirable: improvements in living conditions through global trade, reducing conflict and threat of war through political globalisation and encouraging cultural diversity in a widening cultural globalisation. The question now, in my view, is not whether we should accept or reject globalisation but how to shape and guide it to these more progressive goals. We need to point the project toward creating more just and fair outcomes, open to difference but sensitive to cultural connections and social traditions. A globalisation project of creating a more connected, sustainable, just and peaceful world is too important to be left to the bankers and political elites.
>
> ***Short, 2016***

Reflect on current events around the world that suggest a backlash against globalisation. What can you do to create a more connected, sustainable, just and peaceful world?

MIGRATION AND HEALTH

Migration, or the movement of people living in a country other than where they were born is a global phenomenon. Migration can occur by choice for circumstances such as work, family or study. However sometimes migration can be forced, caused by factors such as conflict, war, natural disaster or politics (UN, 2022). In 2019, the United Nations estimated that approximately 272 million people were international migrants with nearly two-thirds of people classed as labour migrants, meaning they were moving countries for work and employment opportunities (UN, 2022). By the end of 2021, the UNHCR (2022) estimated that 89.3 million people worldwide were forcibly displaced. This was as a result of persecution, conflict, violence, human rights violations or events disturbing public order (UNHCR, 2022).

Mental health continues to be a major focus of migration and public health research, programs and policy. Healthy WA (2022) note that the process of resettlement can bear a huge burden on migrant mental health. This includes grief, loss, anxiety regarding family left in other countries, employment challenges, language barriers, isolation and trauma.

Health literacy, too, remains a constant challenge for migrants. While research remains very limited on health literacy, research on holistic mapping of migrant health literacy needs is much needed (Monani et al, 2021). As a student or early career public health practitioner, understanding health literacy needs spans all facets of the public health spectrum. Box 14.2 provides an excerpt from Monani and colleagues research (Monani et al, 2021), and the disparities in health literacy which became evident during the COVID-19 pandemic in 2020–2021. Activity 14.4 encourages you to apply upstream thinking and consider the social determinants of health and how they affect health literacy.

BOX 14.2 **Disparities in Health Literacy**

"Despite Australia's health and welfare policy commitment to health equity and social justice, the recent COVID-19 pandemic revealed – particularly in the Australian city of Melbourne – that residents in public housing were at a particularly high risk, with the majority of these being immigrants. Second, these were mostly immigrant men, or men who were welfare-dependent and had a drug and alcohol dependency. Studies both in the United Kingdom and United States have established that for Hispanic, Black and older men the ability to navigate the health care system, following that age-specific screening guidelines were far more challenging than any other category or group of persons. Additionally, low socioeconomic status and low education levels also meant that individual health literacy was significantly affected. As news unfolded on the COVID 19 pandemic in Melbourne, it became evident that immigrant men in Australia are frequently employed as front-line workers, in jobs such as security guards, cleaners and taxi drivers. They often work in underpaid, casual and precarious jobs, which adversely impacts their socioeconomic status and offers them little to no capacity to take time off from work and focus on activities to enhance their health and wellbeing. A comparative study on citizens from the European Union (EU) and non-EU migrants, revealed that health literacy is a complex "concept" and is even more complicated when measuring the equity outcomes for immigrants given the less favourable social position of migrants. That is, migration is a social determinant of health".

(Monani et al, 2021, p. 152.)

Excerpt from Monani and colleagues' research (Monani et al, 2021) on the disparities in health literacy, which became evident during the COVID-19 pandemic in 2020–2021.

SUSTAINABLE DEVELOPMENT GOALS AND GLOBAL HEALTH

As part of the 2030 Agenda for Sustainable Development, the Sustainable Development Goals (SDGs) are a global effort led by the United Nations Development Programme (UNDP) to "end poverty, protect the planet and ensure that all people enjoy peace and prosperity" (UNDP, 2017). The SDGs consist of 17 goals (see Figure 14.1), 169 targets and 230 indicators. As highlighted by Dr Margaret Chan, Director-General of the WHO from 2006 to 2017, the SDGs recognise in particular that:

> … health challenges can no longer be addressed by the health sector acting alone.… [H]ealth is an end-point that reflects the success of multiple other goals. Because the social, economic, and environmental determinants of health are so broad, progress in improving health is a

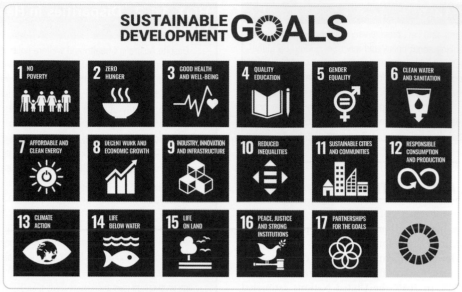

Fig. 14.1 Sustainable Development Goals. (Source: UNDP, 2017.)

---

reliable indicator of progress in implementing the overall agenda …[T]he ultimate objective of all development activities—whether aimed at improving food and water supplies or making cities safe—is to sustain human lives in good health [Chan 2016].

Activity 14.5 will help you to understand the relationship between the SDGs and the broad determinants of health.

The 2030 Agenda for Sustainable Development is both a local and a global agenda. At the core of the SDGs is the need for productive partnerships and global solidarity where wealthy countries are willing and able to support the most vulnerable countries. For instance, the Australian government has focused on advocating for strong "economic growth and development in the Indo-Pacific region, promoting gender equality, governance and strengthening tax systems" (Australian Government, Department of Foreign Affairs and Trade, 2017).

GLOBAL HEALTH AND HUMAN RIGHTS

The WHO's Constitution states that "the enjoyment of the highest attainable standard of health is one of the fundamental rights of every human being without distinction of race, religion, political belief, economic or social condition" (International Health Conference, 1946, p. 1). Although the right to health is codified in several international law and human rights instruments, such as the 1948 Universal Declaration of Human Rights (UN General Assembly, 1948) and the 1966 International Covenant on Economic, Social and Cultural Rights (ICESCR) (UN General Assembly, 1966), the highest attainable standard of physical and mental health remains an elusive goal for much of the world's population (OHCHR, 2022).

The United Nations has called for all of its organisations to apply a human rights approach across all of the work that they do. Such approaches reflect a systems-thinking approach to public health. To understand how human rights are implemented for the benefits of public health, Meier and colleagues (2019) explored four key areas:

1. The foundation of human rights as a framework for global governance: referring to the international norms to ensure global health and justice—including the need to define what the highest standard of health can be. These standards recognise that health-related disparities, including lack of

access to services and levels of care can be seen as rights violations for human health.

2. United Nations organisations mainstreaming health-related human rights: this not only recognised the work of the World Health Organization, but also international organisations that address the determinants of health. Combined with this, the work towards universal health coverage (UHC), which asserts human rights, specifically the rights to health, for vulnerable populations is a priority.

3. Funding agencies incorporating human rights in international health assistance: this includes the need and opportunity for international public health financing to enhance economic government for health-related human rights.

4. Human rights agencies advance the right to health: this recognises the impact that all agencies can have on health and the need for accountability to ensure efforts are being implemented to work towards the highest attainable health standards.

These joined-up efforts to mainstream human rights for global health demonstrate not only the interconnected nature of health across the determinants (e.g. the impact that the economy can have on health), but also lay the foundation to ensure sustainable approaches to health in all policies and universal public health benefits for populations.

A FINAL WORD

This chapter has introduced global health and the impact of globalisation, migration, displacement and human rights on the health of populations. It has also discussed the SDGs and their relationship with the broad determinants of health. With increasing levels of migration and forced displacement worldwide, a human rights approach to global health becomes an imperative for public health professionals.

REVIEW QUESTIONS

1. What are the key aspects that characterise global health?
2. What are some of the environmental changes associated with globalisation that impact on population health?
3. How do the Sustainable Development Goals relate to the broad determinants of health?
4. What are some of the public health-related obstacles that affect the health of migrants?

USEFUL WEBSITES

Global Burden of Disease—Institute of Health Metrics and Evaluation: http://www.healthdata.org/gbd
International Union for Health Promotion and Education: https://www.iuhpe.org/index.php/en/

Sustainable Development Goals: https://sustainabledevelopment.un.org/sdgs
United Nations High Commissioner for Refugees (UNHCR): http://www.unhcr.org/
WHO Global Health Observatory (GHO): http://www.who.int/gho/en/
WHO Human Rights and Health: http://www.who.int/mediacentre/factsheets/fs323/en/

REFERENCES

Bagnall AM, South J, Mitchell B et al 2017 Systematic scoping review of indicators of community wellbeing in the UK Version 1.2 August 2017. Available: https://whatworkswellbeing.org/wp-content/uploads/2020/02/community-wellbeing-indicators-scoping-review-v1-2-aug2017_0205746100.pdf
Chan M 2016 Health in the Sustainable Development Goals. Geneva: World Health Organization
Duke Global Health Institute (DGHI) 2002 Defining global health. Available: https://globalhealth.duke.edu/what-global-health
Hanefeld J, Lee K 2015 Introduction to globalization and health. In: Hanefeld J (ed), *Globalization and Health* (2nd ed., pp. 1–13) Maidenhead: McGraw-Hill Education.
Healthy WA 2022 Migrant and Refugee Mental Health. Available: https://www.healthywa.wa.gov.au/Articles/J_M/Migrant-and-refugee-mental-health
International Health Conference 1946 Constitution of the World Health Organization. New York: United Nations
International Union for Health Promotion and Education (IUHPE) 2021 Critical Actions for Mental Health Promotion. Paris: IUHPE
McMichael AJ 2013 Globalization, climate change, and human health. *The New England Journal of Medicine* 368, 1335–43
Monani D, Smith JA, O'Mara B et al 2021 Building equitable health and social policy in Australia to improve immigrant health literacy. *Health Promotion Journal of Australia* 32, 152–4. https://doi.org/10.1002/hpja.481
Pang T, Gayle G, Amul H 2021 Global health research changing the agenda. In: Benatar S, Brock G (eds). *Global Health Ethical Challenges*, 2nd ed. Cambridge: Cambridge University Press
Pili N, Nosa V, Tatui L 2021 Implementing policies and programmes to reduce the impact of globalisation on oral health in Pacific Island Countries and Territories. *Journal of Global Health Economics and Policy* 1, e2021012. doi:10.52872/001c.29655
Salm M, Ali M, Minihane M et al 2021 Defining global health: findings from a systematic review and thematic analysis of the literature. *BMJ Global Health* 6, e005292
Sawleshwarkar S, Negin J 2017 A Review of Global Health Competencies for Postgraduate Public Health Education. *Frontiers in Public Health*. doi:10.3389/fpubh.2017.00046
Seferidi P, Hone T, Duran AC et al 2022 Global inequalities in the double burden of malnutrition and associations with globalisation: a multilevel analysis of Demographic and Health Surveys from 55 low-income and middle-income countries, 1992–2018. Available: https://www.sciencedirect.com/journal/the-lancet-global-health/vol/10/issue/4
Short JR 2016 Globalization and its discontents: why there's a backlash and how it needs to change. The Conversation. Available:

https://theconversation.com/globalization-and-its-discontents-why-theres-a-backlash-and-how-it-needs-to-change-68800

United Nations Development Programme (UNDP) 2017 Sustainable Development Goals. New York: UNDP. Available: http://www.undp.org/content/undp/en/home/sustainable-development-goals.html

United Nations (UN) General Assembly 1966 International Covenant on Economic, Social and Cultural Rights. Geneva: UN

UNHCR 2021 UNHCR Global Public Health Strategy 2021-2025. Available: https://www.unhcr.org/en-au/publications/brochures/612643544/unhcr-global-public-health-strategy-2021-2025.html

United Nations Human Rights Office of the High Commissioner (OHCHR) 2022 International standards on the right to physical and mental health. Available: https://www.ohchr.org/en/special-procedures/sr-health/international-standards-right-physical-and-mental-health

Vardell E 2020 Global health observatory data repository. *Medical Reference Services Quarterly*, 39(1), 67–74. doi:10.1080/02763869.2019.1693231

World Health Organization (WHO) 2020 Urgent health challenges for the next decade. Available: https://www.who.int/news-room/photo-story/photo-story-detail/urgent-health-challenges-for-the-next-decade

World Health Organization (WHO) 2020a WHO global strategy on health, environment and climate change: the transformation needed to improve lives and wellbeing sustainably through healthy environments. Available: https://www.who.int/publications/i/item/9789240000377

World Health Organization 2021 Geneva Charter for Well-being. Available: https://www.who.int/publications/m/item/the-geneva-charter-for-well-being

15

Disasters, Emergencies and Terrorism

Gerry FitzGerald, Peter A. Leggat and Richard Franklin

LEARNING OBJECTIVES

After reading this chapter, you should be able to:
- Define "disasters" and discuss their causes and impacts.
- Identify trends in disasters and the factors influencing those trends.
- Identify and appraise the principles of disaster management in the modern context.
- Identify and defend the key public health implications of disasters.
- Identify and examine the role of public health practitioners in disaster management.

INTRODUCTION

Each year there are over 300 major disaster events worldwide resulting in an average of 61,212 deaths, 1903.4 million people affected and over US$150M in damages (Centre for Research on the Epidemiology of Disasters [CRED], 2022). Since 2020, the world has experienced the COVID-19 pandemic, which by the end of 2021 had resulted in an estimated 18.2 million excess deaths around the world (Lancet, 2022). Effective disaster management can reduce the health consequences of both natural and human-made disasters. As public health practitioners you will be often required to help plan and prepare for disasters, to respond to them and to aid community recovery. In particular, the community's response to outbreaks of disease is often led by public health practitioners.

WHAT ARE "DISASTERS"?

There are many definitions of "disasters", but little agreement on what does constitute a disaster. What is considered a disaster depends on your point of view and is influenced by a range of factors. Events including public health emergencies can range in scope and complexity from a small number of people affected, through to catastrophes that may destroy the fabric of society. While we may be clear about the ends of that continuum, there is no agreed point at which this transition to a disaster occurs. The core principle of most definitions is an event that requires us to do something different to "business as usual".

The United Nations defines disasters as:

*A **serious** disruption of the functioning of a community or a society involving widespread human, material, economic or environmental losses and impacts, which exceeds the ability of the affected community or society to cope using its own resources.*

(UNISDR, 2009)

The extent of the challenge to the health and wellbeing of the community is determined by the nature of the event, its location, spread and impact, and by the characteristics and size of the affected community. Similarly, the resources available to deal with the event are determined by the location, culture and socioeconomic status of the community. This imbalance between challenge and capability appears to capture the point at which an event is considered a disaster and requires effort outside of what the community can provide.

Thus, whether any single event or challenge to health and wellbeing is a disaster or not depends on the influence and interaction of many factors. Figure 15.1 seeks to demonstrate the variable nature of this relationship. The slide on the scale represents a particular event, but its position on the scale is determined by those factors that influence the mismatch of resources and challenges to health. It also depends on the perspectives and interest of those who seek to define the event.

We also use the term "disaster health" as a means of drawing focus to both the health consequences of disasters and the burden the event may impose on health services. Public health

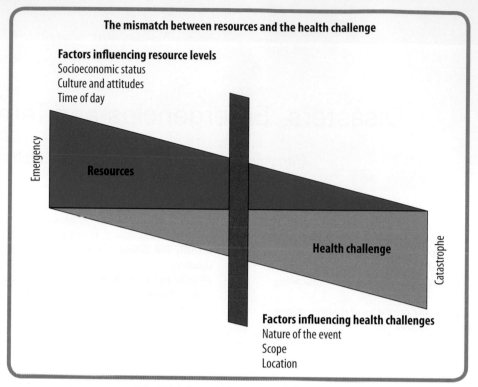

Fig. 15.1 The relative nature of disasters.

authorities must have in place scalable arrangements, whereby emergency responses may be escalated on the basis of standard principles and practices to such a level as to meet the particular challenge at that particular time. However, this approach can be overwhelmed when public health infrastructure is impacted.

Sundnes and Birnbaum (2003) described the context of disaster health as involving three essential domains: public health; emergency and risk management; and clinical and psychological care. Their conceptual map describes the interrelationship between these domains within a broader framework defined by community preparedness, response capability and resilience, political and social structures and the support resources available. The focus of this chapter is on the public health domain.

The other important consideration is the nature, structure and vulnerability of the community. Disasters are conceptualised as a *social phenomenon*. That is, hazards only become disasters when they affect a community. A cyclone is a hazard; however, unless is makes landfall in a populated area it will not become a disaster. Thus, the impact that the hazard can have depends on the resilience or vulnerability of the community, which in turn is determined by economic, social and cultural influences (think determinants of health). Any single event

may cause massive damage in a poor community and minimal damage in a rich well-structured community.

The ability of the community to withstand the impact of disasters is described in two conceptual notions: resilience and vulnerability.

Resilience is a concept that is also difficult to define, but incorporates elements of strength, flexibility, adaptability, responsiveness and recovery. Resilience can be applied at all levels from individuals and the communities they form, to the infrastructure that supports those communities. Socioeconomically advantaged communities have the resources and the capability to create resilience or buy it in when required.

Vulnerability implies that some individuals (or communities) are more susceptible to disasters than others. People may be more susceptible due to intrinsic factors such as disabilities restricting their mobility, while communities may be more vulnerable to extrinsic factors such as poor infrastructure. Disasters differentially affect poorer communities, women and children and those restrained because of disability (e.g. the elderly) or physical restraint (e.g. prisoners). However, vulnerability is not absolute. It depends on the nature of the event. For example, the elderly person may be more vulnerable if required to escape quickly from a hazard but less vulnerable to other hazards because of their prior experience and life knowledge.

However, the balance between risk and community values remains difficult to deliver. People living in rural areas wish to preserve their natural environment, even though it poses a significant bushfire risk. Consider the failure to obtain binding international agreement about dealing with climate change.

WHAT CAUSES DISASTERS?

Disasters occur when a "hazard" interacts with a community and causes harm to that community. As shown in Table 15.1, hazards have been categorised by the World Association for Disaster and Emergency Medicine (WADEM) into natural, man-made and mixed hazards (Sundnes & Birnbaum 2003).

Are disasters increasing? The number of recorded natural events and the number of people affected by those events continues to increase (CRED, 2018). Figure 15.2 incorporates two graphs from CRED, which demonstrate the number of events and the number of people killed in disasters over the past century. What these figures demonstrate is that, while the number of events has increased, the recorded number of people killed has declined because of the efforts of society to reduce disaster impacts.

Why are the number of events increasing? It is unclear whether the apparent increase is merely an increased level of recording or actual events. It is difficult to understand why the number of natural events such as earthquakes would be increasing, except where human activities may be contributing to an increase in the frequency or severity of events. In particular, global warming is contributing to an increased frequency and severity of heatwaves, forest fires, heavy precipitation and cyclones (Intergovernmental Panel on Climate Change [IPCC], 2022), and deforestation may be contributing to the frequency of mudslides.

However, at the same time, there have been significant improvements in the relative safety of transportation and occupational safety, and reductions in the level of major conflict. Conversely, population increases, greater urbanisation and the levels of human activity may increase the frequency of such adverse events.

The vulnerability of the community has changed. In developed countries resilient structures and sophisticated systems, including public health protections, have reduced the impact of disasters, whereas population growth and urbanisation has resulted in the growth of megacities on flood plains or in seismic areas. The social consequences of rapid urbanisation, including poverty and congestion, may lead to outbreaks of violence and diseases. Conflict over resources enhance risk. Either way, social change has increased the vulnerability of the community and the potential health consequences.

WHAT IMPACTS DO DISASTERS HAVE?

Disasters impact on the community in different ways, determined by the nature of the event and the vulnerability of the community. However, those impacts may be broadly categorised as health, economic, social and environmental (see Table 15.2)

The health consequences of any particular event can be mapped and strategies to reduce health consequences matched against particular risks. Thus, reduction in immediate direct effects may require immediate rescue or evacuation while strategies aimed at preventing long-term mental health consequences will include psychological first aid, follow-up and dealing with the economic and social uncertainties that often characterise a poorly managed recovery phase.

Health services are involved in disasters in two ways:
- Health services have a key role in the provision of healthcare or the protection of life.

TABLE 15.1 Types of Hazards

Type of Hazard	Definition	Examples
Natural hazards	Arising from the natural environment	- Biological: pandemics, etc. - Geophysical: volcanoes, landslides, earthquakes - Hydrological: floods and mudslides - Meteorological: storms and cyclones - Climatological: heatwaves and droughts
Human-caused hazards	Derived from the human environment	- Technological: including transport and industrial technology - Conflict: including armed and unarmed conflict (e.g. sanctions)
Mixed hazards	Resulting from the interaction of human development with the natural environment	- Desertification from land-clearing - Erosion and landslides from deforestation - Consequences of climate change on meteorological and climatological hazards

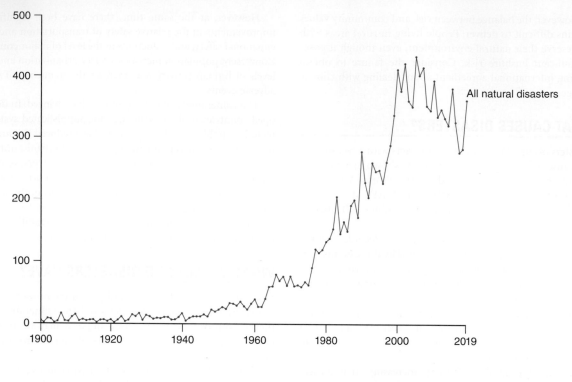

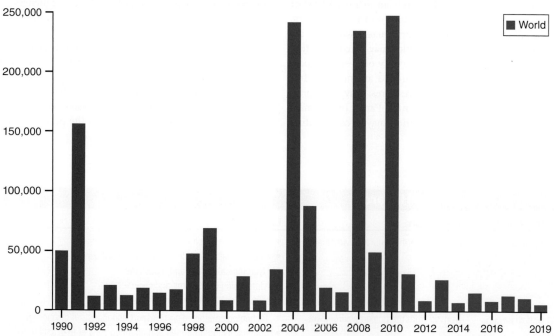

Fig. 15.2 Trends in incidents and deaths from natural disasters. (Source: Ritchie H, Roser M 2021 Natural disasters. Our World in Data. Available: https://ourworldindata.org/natural-disasters).

TABLE 15.2 Impacts of Disasters

Type of Impact	Description
Health impacts	May be conceptualised in three dimensions: (1) the timeliness of the consequences (immediate, medium-term and long-term); (2) the nature of the relationship (direct contact of humans with the hazard or indirect consequences as a result of damage to something else); (3) the health impacts on individuals (physical and mental) For example, the health impact of floods may be immediate, mid-term and long-term (Du et al, 2010). Direct effects are those related to exposure to the water or the debris contained within it. Thus, drowning and injury are direct, immediate consequences. On the other hand, floods may disrupt industry leading (indirectly) to longer-term economic constraints and the health consequences of poverty. The loss and grief that may accompany the flood, or the impact that the flood has on society, can have a long-term effect on an individual's mental health
Economic impacts	Include both actual costs (with a value) and intangible costs. Events can cause physical damage and the extent of that damage may not be immediately apparent. They can disrupt essential services, result in temporary or permanent evacuation of communities, damage commerce and community facilities. For example, consider the economic impact of a flood in a small rural town. The flood damages the social and economic fabric, particularly marginal industries, such as a corner store, which is vulnerable because of declining rural populations, reliance on tourists (which now find it hard to visit due to damaged roads) and competition from online shopping. The flood may damage the physical structure and (probably underinsured) stock making a marginal business unviable. The loss of the corner store reduces further the social attraction of the community, the opportunities for employment with flow-on impacts on the schools, health services and other element of social infrastructure. On the other hand, the economic standing of a community can directly affect its preparedness and vulnerability. Wealthier communities can afford more infrastructure and response resources and can meet the costs of evacuation and recovery
Social impacts	Disasters have a social impact on both the structure and the functioning of society, on its cohesion and effective functioning. The differential impacts of disasters can be quite disruptive to society and its smooth functioning. People's reactions vary. Mostly people do not panic; they generally respond in rational ways. People will act rapidly to protect their own life and safety, and at times this survival instinct is misinterpreted as panic. Disasters or subsequent evacuations may disrupt the normal social support arrangements, including the companionship of pets. Families may become stressed as competing demands of work and family are further complicated by the need to respond and recover. Children may not be able to access their friends and education, or they may be required to help with the recovery. Access to the workplace may be disrupted due to loss of the business or inability to reach the workplace due to disruptions to transportation and roads
Environmental impacts	Disasters impact on the environment just as the environmental management may contribute to, or mitigate, the impact of disaster. Cyclones will destroy vegetation, floods will change the course of rivers, toxic contaminants may be washed from storage locations into water courses, freshwater contamination of the Great Barrier Reef may challenge sustainability of corals and endangered species may be compromised by specific diseases. Land use planning and vegetation management can reduce water run-off. Alternatively, uncontrolled urban expansion can obstruct natural drainage and expose human populations to natural risk environments by building on flood plains. Fires can kill some species while allowing the rejuvenation of others. However, there are challenges in the active management of the environment to reduce risk. Communities object to fuel reduction burning on social, health or ecological grounds. People desire to live beside floodable waterways for the pleasing aspect it brings

• Health services are part of the community's critical infrastructure, which needs protection to maintain services. Health infrastructure may be subject to the same risks as the rest of the community (see Case Study 15.1 and Activity 15.1).

Perhaps the most common health impact of disasters is the loss of access to healthcare for patients who rely on that access to sustain their wellbeing. Disasters destroy health facilities and disruptions to transportation can prevent patients and staff accessing facilities, medication or other health-related material. Enhanced social distancing measures associated with attempts to reduce COVID-19 transmission have reduced healthcare access.

Mental health is a relatively silent but exceedingly important aspect of disaster health. Exposure to terrifying images or events, injury and permanent disability, loss and grief and the ongoing distress caused by the direct and indirect effects of disaster can have a long-lasting effect on individuals and

CASE STUDY 15.1   Evacuating Health Services

Health services are a critical component of any community's infrastructure, and during disasters health services are called upon to meet the increased demands associated with disasters. However, what happens when those facilities themselves are in danger, or are damaged, and patients have to be evacuated?

In February 2011, a category five tropical cyclone, Yasi, struck the north-east coast of Australia. As the cyclone approached the coast, a very real danger threatened the 330-bed Cairns Hospital, which is situated on the foreshore. The danger was posed by a combination of cyclonic conditions and storm surge. The decision was made to evacuate the patients to the state capital, Brisbane, an estimated 1700 km away. Thus, 356 patients, staff and family members were evacuated by ambulance from the hospital and taken to the airport, where they were loaded onto a number of military and civilian aircraft.

It is not common that health facilities require evacuation, but in this circumstance the physical threat from the cyclonic winds and the storm surge forced the decision. Because of the very broad nature of the physical threat, evacuation to a location well outside the danger zone was only sensible, and to one with sufficient resources to absorb the patients. No significant adverse events were observed in the patients' health.

ACTIVITY 15.1   Decision to Evacuate a Hospital

- What are some of the possible consequences of evacuating an acute-care hospital?
- What factors would influence your decision to evacuate?
- What are the factors that would influence where you would evacuate the patients to?

Reflection

Consider the impact on families of a decision to evacuate patients from one hospital to another hospital some considerable distance away. How could you provide support to those families? Consider how you would re-establish emergency health services once the immediate danger had passed.

therefore on the community. Effects can range from immediate distress and adjustment, through to chronic depression associated with posttraumatic stress disorder (PTSD). PTSD is the most significant long-term mental health consequence of disasters, which can impact on both those directly affected and those tasked with rendering aid.

Effective management of the mental health consequences of disaster can reduce their potential impacts. Effective psychological first aid will help individuals to adjust to often understandable reactions to traumatic events. The incidence of chronic issues is often associated with repeated exposure or the ineffective management of basic recovery issues, such as food, accommodation and protection. Monitoring of affected individuals will provide an opportunity for early recognition and intervention for those most at risk.

PRINCIPLES OF DISASTER MANAGEMENT

Effective disaster health management is complex and multifactorial, so there is potential for complexity to paralyse any action. However, a number of principles have been identified that should form the core of any management strategies.

An Engaged and Prepared Community

All disaster management is ultimately local. It is not possible for governments or external agencies to do everything without the direct involvement of the community in its own protection and recovery. In major events, particularly those associated with the destruction of major infrastructure, the community will be on its own until help can be organised. The initial response will be from local agencies, local resources and bystanders. The capacity of the community to provide assistance will be influenced not only by its resources but also its own needs, which in turn is determined by the health determinants and status of the community.

Critical to an engaged community is the concept of *community resilience*, which, while ill-defined, implies the capacity of the community to withstand challenges to its wellbeing and to "bounce back", taking control of its own destiny and restoring functionality.

Risk-Based Approach

Another concept important in disaster health is the concept of risk. Defining "risk" is difficult in this context. The terms "risk" and "hazard" are often used with little variation in meaning or understanding. A *hazard* is something that may cause damage. The *risk* to the community arising from that hazard is a combination of the nature of the hazard and the vulnerability of the community (risk = nature of hazard × vulnerability).

A risk-based approach involves the identification of hazards and their potential impact. The identified risks need to be evaluated and management strategies put in place to prevent, moderate or offset the risk. Risk is informed by a history of previous events such as floods, cyclones or earthquakes. But it may also be informed by research or by creative and analytical thought or mathematical modelling. An example of this is flood maps used by local councils to identify areas at risk.

All-Hazards Approach

Because of the diversity of risks, and because of the initial confusion that characterises major incidents, it is not possible, and potentially confusing, to separately prepare for individual hazards. The all-hazards approach seeks common approaches to preparation and response. Put simply, communities should respond in a standard way (at least initially), regardless of the challenge. This allows for standardised training and awareness, and for a relatively automated immediate response before the full extent or even the nature of the event may be known.

All-Agencies Approach

There is a risk that different agencies, or levels within individual agencies, may react to a major incident in different ways. The consequence could be confusion, gaps in response or overlap and wasted effort. A more effective approach is for all agencies to operate on the basis of similar and standard approaches.

Incident management systems seek a standardised approach to the response phase. There are several incident management systems used around the world, including the National Incident Management System (NIMS) in the USA and the Australian Inter-service Incident Management System (AIIMS). These outline the key elements of planning, operations, logistic and communications and help define roles and responsibilities which lead to action plans, teamwork and partnerships.

Familiarity

The principle of familiarity recognises that the most effective response to major incidents is achieved when those responding are familiar with their roles and responsibilities. This is best achieved if the response arrangements are based on those that people undertake on a daily basis.

An emergency is not the time to learn new tasks, but rather to utilise the expertise present within the community. Task allocation should, wherever possible, reinforce normal practice. Surgeons should do the surgery, and fire-fighters should rescue people and put out fires. Organised responses should reflect normal practice wherever possible. This not only reflects reality, but also ensures that the definitional issues discussed earlier become irrelevant. This minimises the aspects of disaster response that require unusual responses, and therefore specialised training. It is also recommended that these groups practise their response and review how well the response to the simulated disaster went in order to help strengthen the response and have people from multiple agencies become familiar with what others do.

Comprehensive Approach

The principle of a comprehensive approach seeks to ensure consistency throughout the continuum of *prevention*, *preparation*, *response* and *recovery* (PPRR).

Prevention and mitigation. Some hazards can be prevented, or at least reduced in likelihood. For example, road traffic management strategies reduce the frequency of major transportation incidents, and land use policies may reduce the impact of fires, desertification and flooding.

Other hazards are not preventable, but their impact can be mitigated by a combination of infrastructure investment and behavioural modification. Thus, while we cannot prevent cyclones, we can reduce their impact by imposing higher standards of building construction in cyclone-prone areas, having people clean up around their homes and evacuating people at risk into secure shelters. The use of early warning systems can help inform authorities and move people from high-risk areas.

Preparedness and planning. Preparing the community for major incidents is part of building community resilience. The most significant aspect of preparedness is planning.

Planning describes the process of identification, evaluation and management of risks, and the development of strategies to mitigate or respond to those risks. The process of planning may be more significant than the plan itself. The process engages the key agencies and leading individuals, ensures their interaction and helps identify the potential problems encountered during response and recovery. The planning process is educational and allows for the sharing of expertise. It also ensures that the key players know each other and are familiar with the capability of other individuals and agencies.

Plans are consistent with those of other agencies, and with international principles. For example, an agency's pandemic plan should be consistent not only with those of other agencies, but also with national and international pandemic preparedness plans. There will inevitably be a hierarchy of plans (international, national, provincial and local) that need to be consistent with each other. Figure 15.3 identifies a possible structure for a complex organisation, whereby the core plan is supported by operational plans for sub-units of the organisation, functional plans, which summarise the key functions, and special plans, which articulate the special requirements of particular hazards.

While planning is an essential component of preparedness, there is more to it than planning. Preparedness also includes surveillance and early warning, the provision of equipment and resources and the development of capability.

Surveillance is most obvious in pandemic surveillance, where close monitoring of infectious disease outbreaks is an essential component of preparedness for disasters. However, surveillance as a concept is equally appropriate for other hazards, such as the early warning system for tsunamis, flooding, tidal and wave activity, or the activities of security and protection agencies.

The physical resources, including capital infrastructure and consumables, needed for response and recovery need to be secured. For example, consumables may need to be identified or stockpiled. When considering the stockpiles required, it is important to take into consideration the "embedded" stockpiles. Many drugs and other consumables required in disasters are in everyday clinical use. For example, personal protective equipment such as masks and gloves will be required in a pandemic. During COVID-19, the supply of personal protective

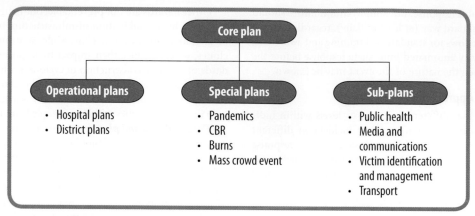

Fig. 15.3 Hierarchy of plans. (CBR = chemical, biological and radiological.)

equipment was seriously challenged at first. It is critical to identify where those existing supplies are, and also where they are manufactured and how they are supplied. Their production may be able to be scaled up within a relatively short timeframe. At the same time, drugs and other consumables are very costly to stockpile and often have use-by dates that need to be monitored.

People need to be prepared through *appropriate education and training*, and the testing of that familiarity through exercises.

Response and relief. The response and relief phase of disaster management concerns the period immediately following the event. This phase is the focus of much of disaster management, often led by key response agencies such as police, ambulance, fire or the state emergency management services. Health is not often the lead agency (sometimes referred to as "combat agency") except in the management of

major disease outbreaks. However, health is almost always involved as a partner agency in any event that is associated with significant injury to people.

The management of the response and relief phase is complex, but may distilled into the *eight Cs of response management* (see Table 15.3)

Look at the example of the eight Cs of response management in practice in Table 15.3, then consider Activity 15.2.

Recovery, Rehabilitation and Redevelopment. The aim of the recovery phase is to restore functionality. We may also use the opportunity posed by reconstruction to develop and improve. For example, after the destruction caused by cyclones it may be time to rebuild to more modern and resilient standards. The recovery phase is a critical aspect of disaster health management that is often relatively neglected or devalued by those interested in the emergency response aspects especially

TABLE 15.3 The Eight Cs of Response Management

Response Management	Description	Example (Queensland Floods 2010/2011)
Command, control and coordination	The means by which the resources are organised and applied to the task at hand. Command operates vertically within an organisation and refers to the direction of members to the delivery of its roles and responsibilities. Control operates horizontally across organisations and refers to the overall direction of emergency management activities. Coordination operates both vertically and horizontally and is mainly concerned with the systematic acquisition and application of resources from various agencies and locations	Command: the Premier took charge of the operation Control: the Disaster Management Group was established Coordination: the new Disaster Coordination Centre was activated
Communication	The provision of information, which facilitates an efficient and effective response. It includes the message as well as the means of communication. Communication is difficult to maintain and vulnerable to power failures affecting transmission towers, etc. Often redundant, non-technological means may need to be considered	Press conferences were conducted several times each day by the Premier

TABLE 15.3	**The Eight Cs of Response Management—cont'd**	
Response Management	**Description**	**Example (Queensland Floods 2010/2011)**
Clinical care	The management of the ill and injured. There are several key clinical concepts critical to effective care: • Triage: sorting of patients, according to their urgency and severity • Clinical standards directed at the particular challenge will be required • Clinical documentation is essential • Definitive diagnosis of the nature and extent of injuries or illness is required to define the healthcare requirements • Necessity to consider the family and contacts of those affected as well as their dependants including pets and livestock	Aerial retrieval of patients from vulnerable health facilities occurred
Capability and continuity	Strategies designed to maintain the functioning of health services. Attention must be given to: • Critical infrastructure protection, including workforce and public health infrastructure • Maintaining access to services through ensuring the stability of the infrastructure, the availability of key personnel and power, fuel and supplies • Creating additional capacity when required. In the first instance this may be achieved by concentration of expertise utilising existing infrastructure. However, as the demands increase, then the existing capability may need to be preserved functionally by early discharge of patients and limiting non-urgent activity. Further expansion of the health infrastructure may require system-wide management, growing capacity (using hotels) and importing capacity (e.g. field hospitals)	Capability: additional resources were sourced from unaffected areas and interstate Continuity: food and other supplies were flown into affected areas
Containment	Strategies required to limit the scope and spread of an event such as pandemics. Patients injured or exposed to a major toxin may independently seek medical aid and thus continue to spread the exposure. Likewise, people involved in a major traumatic incident often depart independently from the scene, making it difficult to determine the extent of the problem and ensure appropriate care. Containment in pandemic responses is achieved through isolation and quarantine, immunisation of family, contacts and neighbours, or through the prophylactic use of antiviral or antibacterial agents. Social distancing measures, such as school closure or the banning of mass gatherings, may reduce disease transmission opportunities	Evacuations occurred in vulnerable areas

after the first wave of health issues have been addressed. Poorly managed recovery can lead to the "secondary disaster", whereby the consequences of poor management create additional distress. Psychological effects may last a lifetime, and the cost of reconstruction leads to lost opportunities for development elsewhere. The need for financial and material assistance continues in the months and years after a disaster, when media scrutiny has stopped, and the world's compassion has shifted to the next issue.

The aim of recovery management is to restore both economic and social functioning. The key elements of the recovery phase are shown in Box 15.1.

Reporting is also a critical aspect of disaster management throughout the full cycle of disaster preparedness, response and recovery. It is important not only to contribute to the lessons learned and to research, but also as a means of reassuring the community and validating the experiences of people. Reporting is also important to improve the response to future events. Linked to reporting is the need for evaluation, which not only informs the community about what worked well and what did not, but it is also a means by which the community reaches some degree of closure, enabling it to move on to the new, and probably different, reality. It should be a means of informing and not serve as a medium for criticism. There is a

---

ACTIVITY 15.2   Managing Fukushima

- Imagine you were a public health official in the vicinity of the Fukushima nuclear power plant in northern Japan, which was disabled by an earthquake and subsequent tsunami, resulting in a loss of cooling to the reactor and the leakage of radioactive material into the seawater and atmosphere.
- What actions would you take to protect the health of the people in the surrounding community?

Reflection

Imagine the difficulty in responding to a tsunami warning at a five-storey hospital on the seafront in northern Japan. You have 20 minutes to respond. What would you do with the patients? You cannot move them outside as that would place them at added risk, and you have no idea how high the water might be or whether the building will withstand the waves.

BOX 15.1   Key Elements of the Recovery Phase

- *Restore essential services* to ensure that the basics of population health, water, food and security are restored
- *Rehabilitate the community* and its structures, including the functioning of community, systems of government and the societal structures, including community organisations
- *Provide for immediate needs*, including safe housing and financial support
- *Provide information*, including health and safety and public health information
- *Identify ongoing healthcare needs*, particularly mental health needs
- *Restore and develop the community infrastructure*
- *Develop the economy and restore economic activity*

---

real risk that the reporting and evaluation may be as destructive as the original event. Highly critical post-event inquiries may victimise and blame individuals rather than focus on system and structural issues. These may create a third wave of harm among the very people who sought to render aid.

SYSTEMS AND STRUCTURES

All nations have disaster management systems and structure in place to respond to major events. For example, in Australia the disaster management system is based on local authorities being the first responders, and the prime responsibility of district, state and national agencies is to assist the local authorities. Figure 15.4, from the Queensland Government Disaster Management website, outlines the coordination groups at each level. An essential component of disaster response is the establishment of central coordination and control centres (see Activity 15.3). Highly sophisticated centres are available in most jurisdictions.

The national government provides national standards and operational support and coordinates external assistance while each of the states and territories has in place arrangements to facilitate planning and to coordinate response and recovery arrangements. In addition, each of the states and territories also maintain a volunteer-based organisation. The State Emergency Service (SES) comprises volunteer units in each local authority.

Many agencies provide aid and assistance during disasters. These include government agencies, such as health, fire and police; non-government agencies, such as St John Ambulance, Médecins Sans Frontières and the Red Cross; and charitable and community organisations, such as Lions and Rotary. The Salvation Army, in particular, has a long tradition of providing immediate aid and support to emergency responders.

The military has traditionally played a significant role in disaster response, and generally has access to significant assets, such as aircraft and ships, which can facilitate responses, particularly for overseas disasters. In addition, the military has personnel who are rapidly deployable and are supported by appropriate resources to ensure that they are self-sustaining.

PUBLIC HEALTH IMPLICATIONS

Disasters can increase public health risks and at the same time damage public health protection. They can compromise clean food and water supplies and damage normal waste disposal. Displaced people may be separated from their normal public health protections and have to reconstruct health infrastructure in what may be austere environments.

Much of disaster health management is associated with the maintenance of public health systems. The key aspects include clean water, food, shelter and protection, waste disposal, immunisation for known risks, provisions of ongoing medication and support for those with chronic diseases and preventing the spread of vectors (e.g. mosquitoes breeding in flood waters). The risks of secondary complications in disasters are those associated with a breakdown in public health protection, or those associated with the collection of large numbers of people, which may facilitate person-to-person spread of illnesses.

COVID-19 demonstrated the particular impact that pandemics have on the public health workforce faced with managing surveillance, testing and tracing of contacts and reporting to inform public responses. There is insufficient space to consider the full range of public health implications of disaster health management. The following brief case studies include some common observations.

Floods

Flooding is the most common natural hazard, and causes almost half of all events, deaths and injuries. It has an extensive

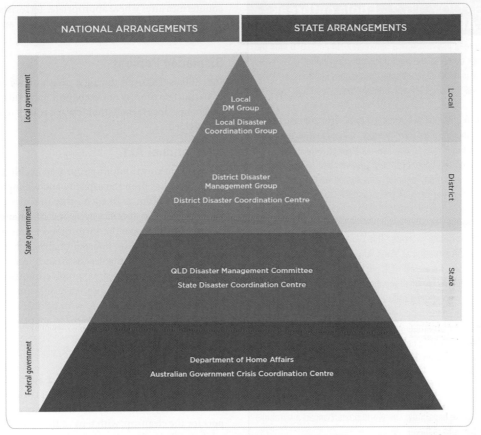

Fig. 15.4 Queensland Government disaster management arrangements. (Source: Queensland Government Disaster Management website 2014.)

ACTIVITY 15.3 **Local Disaster Health Committees**

Consider the structure of a local government disaster health committee. Who should be involved in the committee and what should their roles be?

impact on health, ranging from drowning through to the health consequences of poverty from destroyed livelihoods.

The key elements of flood management are mitigation strategies to divert or store water, construction standards to withstand the floods and evacuation strategies to remove people from the danger. In developed countries, most deaths occur due to the decision by individuals to enter floods, either in vehicles or on foot. In Australia, 90% of flood-related deaths occur in this way (FitzGerald et al., 2010). However, floods can also contaminate fresh water supplies and disrupt sewage disposal. Pooled water contributes to the growth of vectors of disease such as mosquitoes.

Pandemics

Pandemics are common. They may be relatively sudden, as exemplified by the outbreak of COVID-19, or slower in onset and relatively silent, such as the Human Immunodeficiency Virus (HIV) pandemic. The key aspects of pandemic management include:

- Early isolation and containment
- Enhanced infection-control procedures
- Rapid development and use of immunisation.

Consider Case Study 15.2 and place yourself in the decision-making position.

Mass Gatherings

Mass gatherings may be either spontaneous or planned. Mass gatherings are the accumulation of people to a level that exceeds the reasonable capacity of the area. The risks associated with mass gatherings are a combination of the risks of the event, determined by the nature and locality of the event, and the normal risks of so many people gathered together, aggravated by the often-confined nature of the location and the lack

CASE STUDY 15.2   Ebola outbreak in West Africa

The Ebola outbreak in West Africa between 2014 and 2016 was the worst and most complex outbreak in history (excluding COVID-19). The Ebola virus is resident in animals (particularly bats) and so there is a constant risk to human health and wellbeing resulting from exposure to native fauna.

The 2014/2016 outbreak overwhelmed local resources and the international community was slow to react. Initial identification was slow. Control was difficult to achieve because of local beliefs (the custom of washing the bodies of the deceased) and the lack of resources. As a result, many people were turned away from health services and left in the care of their families, thus continuing to spread the disease.

International responses were slow; compounded by concerns with the risk placed on health workers. The World Health Organization (WHO) declared the situation in West Africa a Public Health Emergency of International Concern (PHEIC), in recognition of the potential for international spread. A small number of cases occurred in other countries, mostly among expatriate health workers returning home, although there was some evidence of person-to-person spread.

Eventually massive international assistance was mobilised, and the epidemic brought under control. The epidemic lasted over 2 years and resulted in more than 28,600 cases and 11,325 deaths (CDC, 2018).

What would be different next time? There are experimental vaccines in production. The WHO recognised its failures and has increased its response capability. The world has enhanced awareness and a preparedness to respond.

Reflective Questions

1. Do you think health workers should be restrained from placing themselves at risk?
2. What would be the immediate public health implications of an Ebola outbreak?

of normal infrastructure. Risk mitigation can be achieved by careful planning, both for the ongoing health needs of the population as well as for the danger of major adverse events, including egress from stadiums and buildings due to fire.

Terrorism

Terrorism is not new as both government and non-government agencies throughout history have used terror to achieve political purposes. The aim of terrorists is to disrupt community functioning and therefore they will design and use methods that achieve that. Terrorist attacks result in injured people requiring healthcare. There are risks that terrorists may use agents targeting human health and wellbeing, such as chemical or biological agents, which require specific health responses. These may include specific immunisations and therapeutic countermeasures where appropriate. Terrorists have also demonstrated a preparedness to target health and humanitarian workers and health facilities.

Displaced Persons

Individuals displaced during a disaster have an increased risk of harm. The process of evacuation may endanger individuals in circumstances where their escape routes may be blocked or endangered.

International Aid

A significant contributor to improved health outcomes following disaster has been the capacity and willingness of countries to provide assistance to each other in times of need. This assistance may be specific in terms of finance or particular needs, or it may take the form of aid teams, including health teams. The nature of international health teams (often referred to as "disaster medical assistance teams") is determined by the event, but such teams should comprise individuals who are trained and aware of disaster health, are self-sufficient as to their own needs and operate with flexible management structures in place to enable the teams to adapt to the communities' needs.

Volunteers and Donations

Major incidents typically induce a significant outbreak of compassion and support. The 2011 floods in Brisbane, Australia were marked by an enormous outpouring of support for the clean-up, with tens of thousands of people volunteering to help clear the mud. However, the use of untrained volunteers has some risks. The volunteer teams may lack coordination and control, and at worst present an additional burden, such as when they require accommodation, food, water and sanitation.

Similarly, inappropriate donations can add to distress. Often, donors are generous in terms of things they do not need, but usually the recipients do not need them either. Culturally inappropriate donations (particularly food), or drugs that are past their use-by date, add to the confusion. Donations also have the potential, as mentioned earlier, to destroy the fragile attempts of local industry to return to full function.

Vulnerable Populations

There are a number of people who are particularly vulnerable in disasters. These include people who are unable to evacuate the area because they are isolated and unaware, physically incapable (disabled or ill) or contained (e.g. prisoners). The elderly are particularly vulnerable. Not only does their fragility make them vulnerable to injury, but they also often suffer from chronic illnesses and are dependent on medical care, which may become inaccessible. The evacuation of nursing homes is particularly troublesome, because of the combination of ill health and disability.

Management of Exercises

Exercises are an essential element of disaster preparedness, providing an opportunity not only to test plans and preparedness arrangements, but also to familiarise people with the concepts and practice of disaster health management, and with each other. The organisation of exercises requires reasonable experience and skills. Special tools are available—for example, the Emergo Train System (Emergo Train System, 2007)—to provide a structured approach to the management of exercises.

THE ROLE OF THE PUBLIC HEALTH PRACTITIONER

Public health practitioners have a critical role to play in disaster health management. Not only do they have a responsibility to be informed and be aware of disaster health requirements and principles, but they also need to be mindful that the restoration and maintenance of public health systems are critical to avoid the second wave of disaster health impacts.

Public health practitioners are responsible for planning and preparing for disasters, and for surveillance and early intervention. They are also responsible for monitoring the public health consequences of disasters, such as disease outbreaks, and for the provision of clean water, food and waste disposal (see Activity 15.3).

A FINAL WORD

Disaster health management is an important part of public health. However, effective management of disasters through preparation and response management can reduce the health consequences to the community. This chapter has provided you with an overview of the principles of disaster management to inform your understanding (see Activity 15.4).

ACTIVITY 15.4 Disaster Health Management

Draw up a table that outlines the principal issues that public health practitioners may face in the prevention, preparedness, response and recovery phases of disaster health management.

Reflection

Community resilience describes the ability of a community to withstand and recover from major incidents. The concept implies that the whole community has a role in minimising the impact of disasters. Community resilience includes strategies to design infrastructure to withstand the event (e.g. cyclone-resistant buildings), effective community-wide planning and preparedness and whole-of-community commitment to response and recovery. Identify other strategies that you consider would build resilience in your community.

REVIEW QUESTIONS

1. What do the letters "PPRR" stand for?
2. What are the eight Cs of response management?
3. What are some of the key issues to be addressed in "clinical" response management?
4. Who are most likely to be more vulnerable to the impact of disasters?
5. What are the seven key elements of the recovery phase?
6. What is the role of the public health practitioner in disaster health management?
7. Why are exercises essential elements of disaster preparedness?
8. What are some of the impacts of disasters on mental health, and how can these impacts be managed?
9. What do you understand by the principle of familiarity with respect to disaster management?

REFERENCES

Centre for Research on the Epidemiology of Disasters (CRED) 2021 Disasters in numbers. Available: https://www.cred.be/publications (Accessed 21 Jun 2022)

CDC 2014-2016 Ebola Outbreak in West Africa. Atlanta USA: Centers for Disease Control and Prevention. Available: https://www.cdc.gov/vhf/ebola/history/2014-2016-outbreak/index.html (Accessed 9 June 2018)

Du W, FitzGerald G, Clark M et al 2010 Health impacts of floods: a comprehensive review. *Prehospital and Disaster Medicine* 25(3), 265–72

Emergo Train System 2007 Available: http://www.emergotrain.com

FitzGerald G, Du W, Clark M et al 2010 Flood fatalities in contemporary Australia (1997–2008). *Emergency Medicine Australasia* 22, 183–9

Intergovernmental Panel on Climate Change (IPCC) 2022 Climate Change 2022: Impacts, Adaptation, and Vulnerability. Contribution of Working Group II to the Sixth Assessment Report of the Intergovernmental Panel on Climate Change [Pörtner H-O, Roberts DC, Tignor M, et al (eds)]. Cambridge University Press. Available: https://www.ipcc.ch/report/sixth-assessment-report-working-group-ii/ (Accessed 9 Nov 2022)

Lancet COVID-19 Excess Mortality Collaborators 2022 Estimating excess mortality due to the COVID-19 pandemic: a systematic analysis of COVID-19-related mortality, 2020–21. *Lancet* 399(10334), 1513–36

Queensland Government Disaster Management Plan 2018 Available: https://www.disaster.qld.gov.au/cdmp/Documents/Queensland-State-Disaster-Management-Plan.pdf

Ritchie H, Roser M 2021 Natural disasters. Our World in Data. Available: https://ourworldindata.org/natural-disasters

Sundnes KO, Birnbaum ML 2003 Health disaster management: guidelines for evaluation and research in the Utstein style. (Ch 1: Introduction.). *Prehospital and Disaster Medicine* 17(Suppl. 3), 1–24

UNISDR Terminology on Disaster Risk Reduction. United Nations Switzerland. Available: https://www.unisdr.org/files/7817_UNISDRTerminologyEnglish.pdf (Accessed 22 April 2018)

16

Concluding Remarks

Mary Louise Fleming and Louise Baldwin

After reading this chapter you will be able to:
- Consolidate your learning about the future of public health.
- Analyse the impact of globalisation on public health in Australia.

- Describe the socioecological model of public health, and its influence on public health practice.
- Identify the global and local megatrends that are impacting on public health.

INTRODUCTION

Public health is both an art and a science. As a science, it challenges the notion that health alone can make a difference to the health of the population. By doing so it clearly recognises the role of emotional, social, environmental, economic and political impacts on health and wellbeing. The art of public health has also changed. This is partly because social norms, values and beliefs are constantly evolving, and public health practitioners and others are using new and innovative ways of working across sectors with the population and subpopulations towards achieving health and wellbeing.

The socioecological approach to public health, used throughout this textbook, takes a multifactorial approach. It examines factors that impact on individual and interpersonal issues, communities, institutions and social and economic policies across the life-course. These factors are framed at each level by environmental influences. Figure 16.1 illustrates this approach graphically.

In this textbook, we have covered a wide range of issues under the banner of public health. In Section 1, we addressed important introductory concepts, definitions and challenges and the underpinning principles of epidemiology. We discussed Aboriginal and Torres Strait Islander health as one of the most important challenges for public health in Australia, now and in the future. Section 2 covers policy, ethics and evidence. We help you understand policy debates, the important ethical considerations that should always underpin policy and practice and the use of evidence to make informed decisions. In Section 3 we focused our

attention on strategies to promote, protect and restore the health of the population. The socioecological model is used to examine strategies at the "people", "place" and "enabling environmental" levels. Our final section covers important contemporary public health approaches, and how we might reimagine public health in the 21st century. We considered what contemporary practice looks like and reinforce the global nature and scope of public health. We examined disasters, emergencies and terrorism from a public health perspective, and why such issues are now a part of the global public health lexicon.

The textbook concludes with an examination of global megatrends and their impacts on health and wellbeing. There is a body of literature that discusses the global trends and health trends impacting on how public health develops and advances into the 21st century.

MEGATRENDS AND THEIR HEALTH IMPACTS

In 2022, the CSIRO released "Our Future World: Global megatrends impacting the way we live over coming decades" (Naughtin et al, 2022). A megatrend is described as a major trend or movement (Oxford English Dictionary, 2022). The authors preference their comments by suggesting that factors influencing such changes include the COVID-19 pandemic and the war in Ukraine. The impact of changes has consequently influenced global trade, businesses, communities and governments in Australia and exposed new risks and opportunities (Naughtin et al, 2022). The report concludes that technological change, the inability to access information and

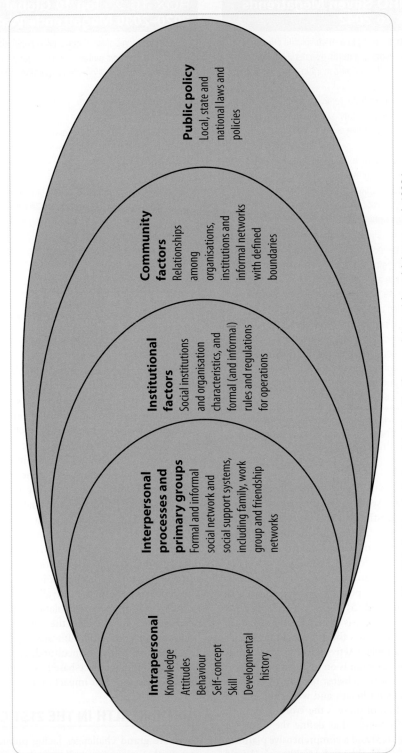

Fig. 16.1 Socioecological model of health. (Source: Adapted from McLeroy et al, 1988.)

Public policy
Local, state and national laws and policies

Community factors
Relationships among organisations, institutions and informal networks with defined boundaries

Institutional factors
Social institutions and organisation characteristics, and formal (and informal) rules and regulations for operations

Interpersonal processes and primary groups
Formal and informal social network and social support systems, including family, work group and friendship networks

Intrapersonal
Knowledge
Attitudes
Behaviour
Self-concept
Skill
Developmental history

BOX 16.1 CSIRO Seven Megatrends with an Outlook to 2042

1. Climate change adaptation: living in a more volatile climate with unprecedented weather events; natural disasters may cost the Australian economy almost three times more in 2050 when compared with 2017.
2. Leaner, cleaner and greener: in 2025, renewables are expected to surpass coal as the primary energy source; solution focused through synthetic biology, alternative proteins, advanced recycling and net-zero energy transition.
3. The escalating health imperative: existing health challenges posed by an ageing population, growing burden of chronic disease and the post-pandemic world; high or very high levels of psychological distress, heightened risk of infectious diseases and pathogens resistant to modern antibiotics.
4. Geopolitical shifts: an uncertain future, characterised by disrupted patterns of global trade, geopolitical tensions and growing investment in defence. Shrinking global economy, increased global military spending, and increase in cybercrime.
5. Diving into digital: increased digitisation, including teleworking, telehealth, online shopping and digital currencies.
6. Increasingly autonomous: increased artificial intelligence discoveries and applications across many industry sectors.
7. Unlocking the human dimension: consumer and citizen push for decision makers to consider trust, transparency, fairness and environmental and social governance; post the pandemic, societal trust in business and trust in government is declining.

Adapted from Naughtin C, Hajkowicz S, Schleiger E et al 2022 Our Future World: Global megatrends impacting the way we live over coming decades. Brisbane: CSIRO.

BOX 16.2 Top 10 Global Megatrends: 2020–2030 Megatrends Watch

1. *Demographic shift*: global ageing population to increase by 60%.
2. *Rising demand*: global energy demand to rise by almost a third.
3. *Economic expansion*: global economy to double in size to about $150 trillion.
4. *Hyperconnected Earth*: connected devices to surge eightfold reaching 125 billion.
5. *Ecological overshoot*: human ecological footprint will demand two planet Earths.
6. *Mega urbanisation*: another 15 cities with populations above 10 million.
7. *Resource scarcity*: half of the global population to face severe water shortage.
8. *Multipolar globalisation*: emerging economies (E7) will overtake developed economies (G7).
9. *Artificial intelligence*: computer power to match the intelligence of humans.
10. *Climate change*: global temperature to rise by about 1.5°C.

Data from Megatrends Watch Institute, Think Tank Institute for Future Research 2022. Available: http://www.megatrends2050.com/ (Accessed 10 August 2022).

data, and the requirement to use them, universally cause new socioeconomic inequalities (see Box 16.1).

The Megatrends Watch Institute (2022) identified 10 global megatrends between 2020 and 2030 and the Institute suggests that global megatrends can be traced back to five distinct, yet interrelated, pillars that include: (1) the rapidly changing demographics; (2) scarcity of natural resources; (3) the emergence of new global economic powers; (4) the exponential technological advancement; and (5) the ever-increasing environmental and climate-change crisis (The Megatrends Watch Institute, 2022). Box 16.2 describes the 10 global megatrends between 2020 and 2030. Complete Activity 16.1 to consider the impact of these and other megatrends on population health.

We have selected two more websites for you to consider that have a particular focus on health and wellbeing and the global health sector. The first of these is the World Economic Forum (2022) and the "6 trends that define the future of health and wellness" (Box 16.3) and a comprehensive platform for "Shaping the Future of Health and Healthcare" (World Economic Forum, 2022). They suggest that the "capital intensive,

hospital-centric model is unsustainable and ineffective". They argue that healthcare needs to be delivered in appropriate settings, through data-enabled delivery systems, virtual care and integrated across the continuum of care.

Finally, Deloitte imagines six global health sector issues (Box 16.4), caused by what they describe as a "seismic shift in health care". The catalysts for this shift in the clinical, financial and operational transformation of healthcare include: a global pandemic; rapidly advancing medical science; enhanced digital technologies, data access and analytics; consumer activism; and a shift from disease care to prevention and wellbeing (Deloitte, 2021).

While the authors and organisations have identified some different trends, or used other descriptions, it is perhaps not surprising that the megatrends have a similarity about them. Maybe this is because they are all based on research data, and its interpretation and extrapolation into the future. Complete Activity 16.2 to examine the relationship between global health megatrends and healthcare megatrends.

There are clearly sociocultural, economic, environmental and ethical and evidence-based extrapolations that influence future trends and their impact on health.

PUBLIC HEALTH IN THE 21ST CENTURY

There are grand challenges facing public health in the 21st century that, according to Freudenberg (2021), require incremental and transformative change committed to health justice

ACTIVITY 16.1 Megatrends Watch Institute and CSIRO Seven Megatrends

Go to the following Megatrends Watch Institute (MWI) websites. The website at http://www.megatrendswatch.com/megatrends-2050.html examines megatrends up until 2050. It is an ongoing research project that has identified 10 mega-challenges 2020–2030 that might give us an idea about the type of world we are likely to be living in over the coming decades. Now look at the CSIRO Seven Megatrends website (https://www.csiro.au/en/research/technology-space/data/our-future-world). You may want to compile a table with the two lists placed side-by-side in order to examine their similarities and differences.

How many of these trends do you believe are likely to impact on population health, and in what way might they have an impact? What are the likely major shifts shaping the world, and how will these shifts transform our landscape in the next 10 years and beyond?

The MWI website also identifies what it calls five distinct yet interrelated pillars. What are the five pillars? How might these interrelated pillars have an impact on population health?

What would you suggest could be done to reduce the impact of a potential megatrend, particularly if it is likely to have a negative impact on the public's health? You may want to work as a group to select a megatrend and use evidence to develop a case for and against it. Select another megatrend and follow it from global to local impacts on public health.

Reflection

It is quite realistic for us to assume that the current pace of change is rapid and never-ending. What is certain is that living with uncertainty has become the new norm. Do you think health professionals need to know about megatrends, and why that would be the case? Do you believe that integrating megatrends into your thinking might help you to consider population health trends, opportunities and risks? Why would this help your practice? (You may wish to consider some of the chapters in this text that examine global issues and their impact on health, such as Chapters 2, 6 and 14.)

BOX 16.3 World Economic Forum "6 Trends that Define the Future of Health and Wellness"

1. An ageing population: growing crises in care and advances in innovative products and services.
2. More virtual healthcare: use of telemedicine for consultations, use of apps and websites.
3. Customised personal diets: to meet individual health needs, 3D print their own food from ingredients stored in their smart fridges—appliances, smart devices will tell people what to buy and when to buy it.
4. Removing mental-health taboos: mental health is ranked third globally, younger generations more in tune with their mental health.
5. Environmental concerns: concerns about climate change, living environments.
6. Tech to the rescue?: advanced technology enables people to regulate their behaviour; devices connected to the Internet of Things could help safeguard people's health in the home and improve their wellness.

Data from World Economic Forum 2022 6 trends that define the future of health and wellness. Available: https://www.weforum.org/agenda/2022/02/megatrends-future-health-wellness-covid19/ (Accessed 10 August 2022).

BOX 16.4 Six Global Healthcare Sector Issues

1. Health equity.
2. Environmental, social and governance.
3. Mental health and wellbeing.
4. Digital transformation and healthcare delivery model convergence.
5. Future of medical science.
6. Public health reimagined.

Source: Data from Deloitte 2021 Global Health Care Outlook: are we finally seeing the long-promised transformation? Available: https://www..deloitte.com/content/dam/Deloitte/global/Documents/Life-Sciences-Health-Care/gx-health-care-outlook-Final.pdf (Accessed 10 August 2022)

that searches for common ground, shared agendas and collective strategies for the future. Zang and colleagues (2021) furthered this notion of a global challenge for health and health systems by suggesting the relationship between climate change and COVID-19. The primary step according to Monti and colleagues (2021) is the creation of a new and comprehensive model of the determinants of health for the 21st century and implementation of the concept of One Health at all levels of society. The authors argue that One Health sits at the interface between humans, animals and the natural environment. Consider Activity 16.3 in the context of how you might make a difference at the local level to support a planetary health vision.

The future of public health is also guided by the United Nations Sustainable Development Goals (SDGs). The interconnection of the 17 goals replicates the interconnected nature of health, climate, poverty and other determinants, and considers health in its broadest sense. Using the SDGs as a guide, national and state/territory public health will be important to ensure effective approaches that comprehensively address the social and other determinants of health for the greatest public

ACTIVITY 16.2   Global Health and Healthcare Megatrends

The World Economic Forum and Deloitte examine health and healthcare megatrends. How do you think they are similar, and how do they differ? Many of the issues discussed by both groups have a bearing on the provision of healthcare, and on changes in population health mortality and morbidity in the future. Working in a group, examine the global health megatrends and the health megatrends by making up a table with two columns, listing the similarities between the two organisations and the differences. In doing this activity, compare with your group how you have allocated similar trends and those that stand out as unique. Think about being an employee in a health department, and consider how such trends might have an impact on your planning for the future. Discuss these issues as a group. Now compare the megatrends with the health megatrends.

Reflection

Did you find many similarities between the two lists of health megatrends and between the general and the health megatrends? Having

been through this book we are hoping that you feel there are many megatrends that impact on health. How do you think you may be able to use the megatrend information to influence your own practice? For example, you might expect to see more technology in the workplace, such as the use of artificial intelligence or robots. The sequencing of the human genome has opened up many new and targeted interventions in healthcare, as well as some social and ethical issues. However, if you think back to the broad range of issues we have considered in this book, you will clearly get a sense that health is not just about genes and physiology. It is very much about the social determinants of health, and factors such as health literacy. It is also, importantly, about economic circumstances, environments and climate change, to name just a few influencers. More recently, COVID-19 has been very much in the forefront of healthcare thinking, technology and social and economic issues. This is why public health is so interesting but also so challenging!

---

health outcomes (UN, 2022). In economic and political terms, a failure to recognise the value of investment in the future needs to be changed to make it easier for governments to invest in health systems and public health. A global agenda is being advocated by the Pan-European Commission on Health and Sustainable Development, established by the WHO Regional Office for Europe, which is designed to achieve a healthy and secure future for all (Monti et al, 2021).

ACTIVITY 16.3   Planetary and One Health Vision for Global Health

Access the short article by Correia T, Daniel-Ribeiro CT, Ferrinho P 2021 "Calling for a planetary and one health vision for global health". One Health 13:100342, available at: https://www.ncbi.nlm.nih.gov/pmc/articles/PMC8555336/pdf/main.pdf

 Working in a group, define the terms "global health", "one health" and "planetary health". Then consider the editors' question about whether the concepts and related frameworks of global, one and planetary health are independent of one another, as suggested by the 2030 agenda for sustainable development. Alternatively, is there a commitment to inter- and transdisciplinary actions related to sustainable development goals? How do the editors answer this question? How do they suggest evidence should be utilised?

Reflection

There are many big questions here linked to our conversation about global and health megatrends. The important issue for you is not just to know about these trends, but to think about how they could be incorporated into your local practice. Collective action with a single vision would be a great start. How could this be achieved? Think about how the Editors suggest evidence should be used.

What political developments are happening in Australia? Recently, a new Federal Government suggested the development of an Australian Centre for Disease Control and Prevention. Many authors are calling for coordination at both the global and the national level. The journey travelled has traversed a socioecological model of health but also paid attention to economic and political dimensions of health.

Consider Case Study 16.1 "An Australian Centre for Disease Control". Read the following article by Wilson A, Rychetnik L 2022 "A centre for disease control and prevention – let's work together to be clear on the problems it must solve", available at: https://intouchpublichealth.net.au/a-centre-for-disease-prevention-and-control-lets-work-together-to-be-clear-on-the-problems-it-must-solve/. Answer the questions posed in Case Study 16.1.

A FINAL WORD

Public health faces many challenges in the 21st century, as we have demonstrated throughout this book. However, it has the will and the expertise to meet these challenges. In this chapter, we have presented you with what many authors believe are the global megatrends and health megatrends for the future. One of our main objectives in this book is to demonstrate that multiple strategies are required at multiple levels to make a real difference to the health of the Australian population. Importantly, single-focused solutions are unlikely to be cost-effective or efficient. We argue that health promotion and other prevention actions to reduce the burden of chronic and infectious diseases on our health system and improve health outcomes are cost-effective.

CASE STUDY 16.1 An Australian Centre for Disease Control

Read the article and then consider the benefits and the likely problems with an Australian centre for disease control (ACDC) that is designed to work to prevent both non-communicable (chronic) and communicable (infectious) diseases. It is noted that preventing chronic disease is still our greatest burden, killing eight out of 10 Australians. Over a third of Australia's total burden of death and disability is attributed to preventable risk factors (Wilson and Rychetnik, 2022). While there are advantages in a national system, Wilson and Rychetnik (2022) ask a series of questions about why a commonwealth agency would add value and if it can be sustained in our federation.

Questions

1. What are the benefits of an ACDC?
2. What are the likely negative aspects of a centralised ACDC?
3. Why would there be a renewed focus on chronic disease?
4. What is the relationship between the ACDC and the National Preventive Health Strategy (NPHS) 2021–2030?
5. Why should we continue to focus on chronic disease instead of infectious disease?
6. What could an ACDC offer to the debate about health inequities?
7. What are the three questions posed by the authors?
8. Draw up three columns to describe what the authors consider are the important aspects of each of these questions they pose to the reader.

We also strongly suggest that public health leadership should be focused on mobilising resources that use transdisciplinary strategies across multiple sectors to ensure that a broader range of determinants are addressed. Leadership should be at both the individual and the collective levels through supportive organisations and institutions, and be framed within SDGs. Changing public health requires "a social movement to support collective public health action at all levels of society—personal, community, national, regional, global, and planetary" (Horton et al, 2014, p. 847). As a practitioner, you may not initially have the ability to influence global public health issues; however, attention to building healthy, sustainable and equitable societies that has a focus on acting locally and thinking globally means that the focus shifts from advocacy for personal health alone to advocacy for sustainable health for the population.

REVIEW QUESTIONS

1. What are the elements of the socioecological model of health?
2. Why is it important to consider a model such as this to guide public health strategies?
3. What is a megatrend, and how is it defined?
4. Why is it important to consider large global trends if we are interested in public health in Australia?
5. Describe the global megatrends and health megatrends impacting on health into the future.
6. What are some of the key public health challenges for the future?
7. How might such global trends influence a health practitioner working in a rural or city area in Australia?

USEFUL WEBSITES

Australian Government Department of Health and Aged Care: https://www.health.gov.au/resources/publications/national-preventive-health-strategy-2021-2030

CSIRO: https://www.csiro.au/en/research/technology-space/data/our-future-world

Deloitte: https://www..deloitte.com/content/dam/Deloitte/global/Documents/Life-Sciences-Health-Care/gx-health-care-outlook-Final.pdf

McKinsey & Company: https://www.mckinsey.com/featured-insights/leadership/the-next-normal-arrives-trends-that-will-define-2021-and-beyond

Megatrends Watch Institute. Key megatrends for economic, social and environmental change: http://www.megatrends2050.com/

Planetary Health Alliance: https://planetaryhealthalliance.org/

Shaping the Future of Health and Healthcare 2022 Available: https://www.weforum.org/platforms/shaping-the-future-of-health-and-healthcare/articles

Rockefeller Foundation: https://www.rockefellerfoundation.org/initiative/precision-public-health/

United Nations (UN) 2022 Make the SDGs a reality: https://sdgs.un.org

World Economic Forum. 8 predictions for the world in 2030: https://www.weforum.org/agenda/2016/11/8-predictions-for-the-world-in-2030

REFERENCES

Correia T, Daniel-Ribeiro CT, Ferrinho P 2021 Calling for a planetary and one health vision for global health. *One Health* 13, 100342

Deloitte 2021 Global Health Care Outlook: Are we finally seeing the long-promised transformation? Available: https://www2.deloitte.

com/content/dam/Deloitte/global/Documents/Life-Sciences-Health-Care/gx-health-care-outlook-Final.pdf (Accessed 10 August 2022)

Freudenberg N 2021 At what cost: Modern capitalism and the future of health. New York: Oxford University Press

Horton R, Beaglehole R, Bonita R et al 2014 From public to planetary health: a manifesto. *The Lancet* 383(9920), 847. doi: 10.1016/S0140-6736(14)60409-8

Megatrends Watch Institute Think Tank Institute for Future Research 2022 Available: http://www.megatrends2050.com/ (Accessed 10 August 2022)

Monti M, Torbica A, Mossialos E et al 2021 A new strategy for health and sustainable development in the light of the COVID-19 pandemic. *The Lancet* 398(10305), 1029–31

Naughtin C, Hajkowicz S, Schleiger E et al 2022 Our Future World: Global megatrends impacting the way we live over coming decades. Brisbane: CSIRO

Oxford English Dictionary 2022 Definition of a megatrend. Available: https://www.collinsdictionary.com/dictionary/english/megatrend (Accessed 10 August 2022)

United Nations 2022 Sustainable Development Goals. Available: https://sdgs.un.org/goals#icons (Accessed 15 July 2022)

Wilson A, Rychetnik L 2022 A Centre for Disease Prevention and Control – let's work together to be clear on the problems it must solve. Available: https://intouchpublichealth.net.au/a-centre-for-disease-prevention-and-control-lets-work-together-to-be-clear-on-the-problems-it-must-solve/ (Accessed 15 July 2022)

World Economic Forum 2022 6 Trends that Define the Future of Health and Wellness. Available: https://www.weforum.org/agenda/2022/02/megatrends-future-health-wellness-covid19/ (Accessed 10 August 2022)

World Economic Forum 2022 Shaping the Future of Health and Healthcare. Available: https://www.weforum.org/platforms/shaping-the-future-of-health-and-healthcare (Accessed 10 August 2022)

Zang SM, Benjenk I, Breakey S et al 2021 The intersection of climate change with the era of COVID-19. *Public Health Nursing* 38(2), 321–35

INDEX

161